MW00453478

Mechanisms and Management of Pain for the Physical Therapist

Mission Statement of IASP Press®

IASP brings together scientists, clinicians, health care providers, and policy makers to stimulate and support the study of pain and to translate that knowledge into improved pain relief worldwide. IASP Press publishes timely, high-quality, and reasonably priced books relating to pain research and treatment.

Mechanisms and Management of Pain for the Physical Therapist

Editor

Kathleen A. Sluka, PT, PhD

Graduate Program in Physical Therapy and Rehabilitation Science,
The University of Iowa, Iowa City, Iowa, USA

Arcadia University
Department of Physical Therapy
450 S. Easton Road
Glenside, PA 19038-3295

IASP PRESS® ◈ SEATTLE

© 2009 IASP Press®
International Association for the Study of Pain®

All rights reserved. No part of this publication may be reproduced, stored in a retrieval system, or transmitted, in any form or by any means, electronic, mechanical, photocopying, recording, or otherwise, without the prior written permission of the publisher.

Timely topics in pain research and treatment have been selected for publication, but the information provided and opinions expressed have not involved any verification of the findings, conclusions, and opinions by IASP®. Thus, opinions expressed in *Mechanisms and Management of Pain for the Physical Therapist* do not necessarily reflect those of IASP or of the Officers and Councilors.

No responsibility is assumed by IASP for any injury and/or damage to persons or property as a matter of product liability, negligence, or from any use of any methods, products, instruction, or ideas contained in the material herein. Because of the rapid advances in the medical sciences, the publisher recommends that there should be independent verification of diagnoses and drug dosages.

Library of Congress Cataloging-in-Publication Data

Mechanisms and management of pain for the physical therapist / editor, Kathleen A. Sluka.
    p. ; cm.
Includes bibliographical references and index.
Summary: "This new volume covers the basics of pain neurobiology and reviews evidence on the mechanisms of action of physical therapy treatments as well as their clinical effectiveness in specific pain syndromes. It is a comprehensive textbook for the management of pain for the physical therapy student and the practicing physical therapist"--Provided by publisher.
ISBN 978-0-931092-77-0 (softcover : alk. paper)
1. Pain--Physical therapy. 2. Pain. 3. Analgesia. I. Sluka, Kathleen A. (Kathleen Anne), 1963- II. International Association for the Study of Pain.
[DNLM: 1. Pain--therapy. 2. Musculoskeletal Manipulations--methods. 3. Physical Therapy Modalities. WL 704 M486 2009]
RB127.M415 2009
616'.0472--dc22
                            2009023668

Published by:
IASP Press®
International Association for the Study of Pain
111 Queen Anne Ave N, Suite 501
Seattle, WA 98109-4955, USA
Fax: 206-283-9403
www.iasp-pain.org

Printed in the United States of America

Contents

List of Contributing Authors   *vii*

Foreword   *ix*

Preface   *xi*

Section I: Basic Concepts and Mechanisms

1. Definitions, Concepts, and Models of Pain   3
   Kathleen A. Sluka

2. Peripheral Mechanisms Involved in Pain Processing   19
   Kathleen A. Sluka

3. Central Mechanisms Involved in Pain Processing   41
   Kathleen A. Sluka

4. Individual Differences and Pain Variability   73
   Laura Frey Law and Steven Z. George

Section II: Physical Therapy Pain Management

5. Pain Assessment   95
   Josimari M. DeSantana and Kathleen A. Sluka

6. General Principles of Physical Therapy Practice
   in Pain Management   133
   Kathleen A. Sluka

7. Exercise-Induced Hypoalgesia: An Evidence-Based Review   143
   Marie Hoeger Bement

8. Transcutaneous Electrical Nerve Stimulation
   and Interferential Therapy   167
   Kathleen A. Sluka and Deirdre M. Walsh

9. Overview of Other Electrophysical and Thermal Agents   191
   G. David Baxter and Jeffery R. Basford

10. Manual Therapy   205
    Kathleen A. Sluka and Stephan Milosavljevic

Section III: Interdisciplinary Pain Management

11. Interdisciplinary Pain Management   217
    Harriët Wittink

12. Medical Management of Pain   231
    Eva Kosek

13. Psychological Approaches in Pain Management   257
    Dennis C. Turk and Hilary D. Wilson

Section IV: Pain Syndromes

14. Myofascial Pain and Fibromyalgia Syndrome   279
    Kathleen A. Sluka

15. Temporomandibular Disorders and Headache   299
    Kathleen A. Sluka

16. Spinal Pain   317
    Steven Z. George

17. Neuropathic Pain and Complex Regional Pain Syndrome   337
    Kathleen A. Sluka

18. Osteoarthritis and Rheumatoid Arthritis   349
    Kathleen A. Sluka

19. Case Studies   361
    Kathleen A. Sluka and Carol Vance

Index   397

Contributing Authors

Jeffrey R. Basford, MD, PhD *Department of Physical Medicine and Rehabilitation, Mayo Clinic, Rochester, Minnesota, USA*

G. David Baxter, TD, PT, MBA, DPhil *School of Physiotherapy, University of Otago, Dunedin, New Zealand*

Josimari M. DeSantana, PT, PhD *Department of Physical Therapy, Federal University of Sergipe, Aracaju, Sergipe, Brazil*

Laura Frey Law, PT, PhD *Graduate Program in Physical Therapy and Rehabilitation Science, The University of Iowa, Iowa City, Iowa, USA*

Steven Z. George, PT, PhD *Center for Pain Research and Behavioral Health and Brooks Center for Rehabilitation Studies, Department of Physical Therapy, University of Florida, Gainesville, Florida, USA*

Marie Hoeger Bement, PT, PhD *Department of Physical Therapy, Marquette University, Milwaukee, Wisconsin, USA*

Eva Kosek, MD *Department of Clinical Neuroscience, Karolinska Institute, and Stockholm Spine Center, Stockholm, Sweden*

Stephan Milosavljevic, PhD *Centre for Physiotherapy Research, School of Physiotherapy, University of Otago, Dunedin, New Zealand*

Kathleen A. Sluka, PT, PhD *Graduate Program in Physical Therapy and Rehabilitation Science, The University of Iowa, Iowa City, Iowa, USA*

Dennis C. Turk, PhD *Department of Anesthesiology, University of Washington, Seattle, Washington, USA*

Carol Vance, PT, MA *Graduate Program in Physical Therapy and Rehabilitation Science, The University of Iowa, Iowa City, Iowa, USA*

Deirdre M. Walsh, PT, PhD *Health and Rehabilitation Sciences Research Institute, University of Ulster, Northern Ireland, United Kingdom*

Hilary D. Wilson, PhD *Department of Anesthesiology, University of Washington, Seattle, Washington, USA*

Harriët Wittink, PT, PhD *Lifestyle and Health Research Group, Faculty of Health Care, University of Applied Sciences, Utrecht, The Netherlands*

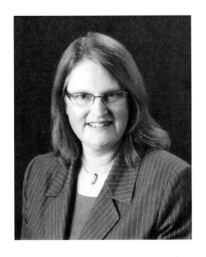

Kathleen A. Sluka, PT, PhD, is a professor in the Physical Therapy and Rehabilitation Science Graduate Program at the University of Iowa. She is also a member of the Pain Research Program and the Neuroscience Graduate Program. She received a physical therapy degree from Georgia State University and practiced physical therapy pain management in Houston, Texas, before obtaining a PhD in Anatomy from the University of Texas Medical Branch in Galveston. After a postdoctoral fellowship with Dr. William D. Willis, she joined the faculty at the University of Iowa. Dr. Sluka developed and currently teaches a course in the doctoral of physical therapy curriculum on Mechanisms and Management of Pain, which served as the basis for this text.

Dr. Sluka's research focuses on the neurobiology of musculoskeletal pain as well as the mechanisms and effectiveness of nonpharmacological pain treatments commonly used by physical therapists. She has published over 100 peer-reviewed manuscripts and numerous book chapters and reviews. Dr. Sluka has been awarded the Distinguished Service Award from the American Pain Society and received the prestigious Marian Williams Research Award from the American Physical Therapy Association.

Dr. Sluka is actively involved in the International Association for the Study of Pain (IASP) and its local chapter, the American Pain Society, as well as the American Physical Therapy Association. Currently, Dr. Sluka is a councilor of the IASP and serves on the board of the American Pain Society. Dr. Sluka reviews for more than 20 journals and holds editorships as follows: U.S. Section Head, *Pain and Analgesia, Rheumatology and Clinical Immunology,* and *Faculty of 1000 Medicine*; Editorial Board for *Journal of Pain*; and Associate Editorial Board for *PAIN*.

Foreword

Pain has an element of blank;
It cannot recollect
When it began, or if there were
A day when it was not.

It has no future but itself,
Its infinite realms contain
Its past, enlightened to perceive
New periods of pain.[1]

It has taken the biomedical community a very long time to begin to understand what Emily Dickinson meant when she wrote about pain. It is clear, however, that Kathleen Sluka and her outstanding assembly of international colleagues get it. I have been involved in teaching neuroscience and electrical modalities to physical therapy students for more than 25 years. The revolution in thinking about pain management during the 25 years parallels the development of more realistic animal models of pain, new techniques to explore the neural mechanisms associated with sustaining the perception of pain, a far greater understanding of personal and environmental factors that influence pain behavior, a broader array of intervention strategies based on a much more rational theoretical framework, and clinically relevant research findings. The breadth of topics in this textbook helps the reader to understand the scope of issues that fit under the umbrella of pain. After reading this text, the reader should be aware that pain, in many instances, is so much more than a single impairment in body structure and function. And, it should also be clear that the effective management of pain requires an interdisciplinary approach rather than just a pill or a TENS unit. The authors skillfully argue and justify that various modalities used alone will probably not lead to clinically meaningful change in a visual analog pain scale or a sustained increase in the patient's level of activity or participation. Sluka et al. have provided a rich, evidence-based framework to understand the mechanisms for and the management of this mysterious four-letter word—pain.

Section I contains four chapters that provide an excellent and clear infrastructure for the rest of the book: giving terms clear definitions, summarizing the vast literature on putative mechanisms to describe why pain remains when the tissue is healed, and introducing the reader to the concepts of how human individual differences lead to variability in response to pain. It is fascinating to watch the story

[1]Dickinson E. *The complete poems of Emily Dickinson.* Boston: Little, Brown, 1924. Available at: www.bartelby.com/113/. Accessed June 2, 2009.

of basic science research move from the study of tail-flick behavior in the rat to indicate thermal hyperalgesia to today's sophisticated animal models where pain is induced via a pharmacological agent or a special diet and where mediating factors such as gender, age, and diet are examined. The behavioral studies are coupled with mechanistic studies so that insight into the spinal mechanisms is not just hypothetical; recordings from neuronal and non-neuronal cell populations, the presence of synaptic plasticity, and specific types of neuroimmune reactions are being examined in the context of pain.

Some textbooks were published on physical therapy procedures without citing a single clinical research study reference as recently as the 1970s. These earlier "how to" books did not offer guidance in selecting an intervention to match the examination findings or to select a particular procedure over another. If we use the earlier books as a frame of reference, the shift in physical therapy practice is dramatic. The rest of this book illustrates the shift. Section II of this text focuses attention on pain regardless of medical diagnosis and provides guidance and evidence to support sound clinical decision making. The chapters in this section demonstrate the importance of the clinical examination, selecting the best tools to classify the pain behavior and providing help with the right tool to determine the effect of treatment outcome. Chapters on pain management in this section and Section III go beyond physical agents to provide evidence to support the use of exercise and manual therapy and to emphasize the need for interdisciplinary collaboration. Section IV provides a series of chapters that discuss a series of pain syndromes.

It is so exciting to see the exponential growth in research that can be used by the clinician. Mechanisms can be described that may account for the pain behavior, and evidence is available to aid in the selection of the most *effective* plan of care. We are finally making major strides in examining the effectiveness of particular interventions in relevant patient populations. No, we do not have the "final answers," but evidence is beginning to emerge that guides the rejection of certain approaches because studies in patients with pain do not indicate improvement with particular interventions. The interdisciplinary authors who wrote this book are conducting research at the bench or in the clinic around the world. They are passionate about providing knowledge and skills that will be translated into clinical practice for the benefit of patients who have suffered because of our ignorance for far too long. Thank you.

Rebecca L. Craik, PT, PhD, FAPTA
Professor and Chair, Department of Physical Therapy
Arcadia University, Glenside, Pennsylvania, USA

Preface

Since the formation of the International Association for the Study of Pain (IASP) more than 35 years ago, the practice of pain management, including the role of physical therapy, has changed dramatically. Further, knowledge about the role of the peripheral and central nervous systems in processing pain signals from uninjured and injured tissue has expanded exponentially. One important recent realization is the importance of altered processing in the central nervous system, with both enhanced excitability and reduced inhibition now seen as significant contributing factors to the pain of chronic diseases.

Pain severely affects function and is the main reason why people seek treatment in physical therapy. However, education about pain in physical therapy, as well as in medicine, has historically been minimal and is usually integrated into existing courses such as neuroscience, orthopedics, or physical agents. Given pain's importance in affecting an individual's function and quality of life, I believe it is important for all physical therapy students and practitioners to gain an up-to-date understanding of pain mechanisms and management. The IASP and its chapters have significantly enhanced the understanding and treatment of pain worldwide, emphasizing an interdisciplinary approach. I have developed and currently teach a stand-alone course to entry-level physical therapy students on pain mechanisms and management. This course emphasizes the latest knowledge on pain mechanisms and promotes an evidence-based and multidisciplinary approach to the management of both acute and chronic pain. This book parallels and continues to emphasize these concepts.

I believe it is important to understand the mechanisms underlying pain conditions in order to better understand appropriate treatment strategies. I propose that there are essentially three potential categories into which a pain condition can fall. One group has a strong peripheral component that drives central excitability and pain. In this group, when the peripheral generator of pain is removed, the pain is goes away. Acute pain syndromes commonly fall into this category. The second group has a strong central component that is independent of a peripheral pain generator. There may have been an initial peripheral pain generator, but it is no longer present, and the pain is maintained by enhanced central excitability. In this case, treatment must focus on techniques that enhance central inhibition and decrease central excitation. This category includes chronic pain conditions such as nonspecific low back pain, fibromyalgia, and temporomandibular joint disorder. The third group entails a combination of both peripheral and central sensitization so that both sites must be adequately treated in order to relieve the pain. This third group probably involves subacute as well as some chronic pain conditions.

This book has been organized into three sections. The first discusses important issues in pain terminology, epidemiology, and basic science mechanisms and emphasizes the heterogeneity of pain. Importantly, this section attempts to integrate pain assessment results with basic underlying mechanisms. It further emphasizes the importance of individual pain variability by discussing differences associated with sex, gender, and age, as well as genetic determinants of variability. The second section discusses the physical therapy management of pain. We include chapters on each treatment area—exercise, electrical stimulation, physical agents, and manual therapy—in the management of pain. Each chapter discusses the evidence for the basic science mechanisms underlying how the treatments reduce pain, as well as the clinical evidence to support their use in patients. We emphasize an interdisciplinary approach to pain, with chapters discussing the physical therapist's role in interdisciplinary pain management, which includes medical and psychological management of pain. The last section includes chapters on common syndromes including myofascial pain, fibromyalgia, spinal pain, migraine, temporomandibular disorder, osteoarthritis and rheumatoid arthritis, neuropathic pain, and complex regional pain syndrome. Each of these chapters describes the pathophysiology of the disease, as well as an evidence-based approach to medical management, psychological management, and physical therapy management. The last chapter gives 10 case studies with explanations of the physical therapy treatment and the evidence to support that treatment.

I felt it was important for this book to emphasize an evidence-based approach to the management of pain. The practice of physical therapy has changed dramatically over the last 10–15 years from one that based treatments on empirical evidence to one that bases treatments on high-quality evidence. The evidence base is incredibly important to making educated decisions in the treatment of pain. Evidence can come from strong basic science studies, experimental pain studies, and randomized controlled trials. Systematic reviews and meta-analysis combine the data from randomized controlled trials to come up with a recommendation for the use of a particular treatment in a specific condition. If there is strong evidence from systematic reviews and meta-analysis, the treatment should be used in these patients. If the primary evidence is weak or inconclusive, however, the conclusions of reviewers should be interpreted with caution because the evidence is only as good as the randomized controlled trials on which the review was based. In researching the literature for this book, I realized that a large amount of evidence has been generated over the last 5 to 10 years. This growth in evidence shows the escalation of research in physical therapy and rehabilitation over this time frame. This research is vitally important to the physical therapy community in terms of acceptance of techniques used in the profession, reimbursement for treatments, and the clinician's ability to make informed decisions in the management of pain.

This book was designed to fill a gap in the education of physical therapists by supporting a more comprehensive education in the management of pain. It is designed not only to be used by students, but to be a primer for practicing physical therapists actively involved in the treatment of pain. The book will also be useful in helping other professionals involved in rehabilitation to gain a better understanding of an evidence-based approach to the management of pain. I hope this book fills a need for physical therapy students, educators, and practitioners with an interest in an improved understanding of pain mechanisms and management.

I would like to thank the many people who made this book possible, particularly the chapter authors and coauthors who gave up their precious time to write a chapter in this book. I thank Carol Leigh at the University of Iowa for secretarial support in assisting with editing and formatting the book prior to submission, the IASP staff for their amazing dedication and assistance in the editing and designing this book, and the Editor-in-Chief of the IASP Press, Dr. M. Catherine Bushnell, for reading the chapters and supporting the publication of the book. I hope this book will lead to a better understanding and improved treatment of pain by physical therapists and rehabilitation professionals worldwide so that patients can get the pain relief they desperately seek.

Kathleen A. Sluka, PT, PhD

Section I

Basic Concepts and Mechanisms

Definitions, Concepts, and Models of Pain

Kathleen A. Sluka

Graduate Program in Physical Therapy and Rehabilitation Science,
The University of Iowa, Iowa City, Iowa, USA

Pain is a complex experience that is unique to each individual. As such, the experience of pain is difficult to define and difficult to treat. Pain can arise as a result of damage to any tissue that is innervated by nociceptors, or it can occur in the absence of tissue damage. For a clinician, the treatment of pain, particularly chronic pain, is difficult and unique to each patient. Everyone will experience pain at some point in his or her life. The impact of this pain may spread well beyond the perception of pain. For example, one may not be able to go to work, attend a significant family function, or participate in social activities because of pain. Pain is now considered the "fifth vital sign," along with the measurement of blood pressure, tempera-ture, heart rate, and respiratory rate. The Joint Commission on Accredita-tion of Healthcare Organizations mandates that effective pain manage-ment is appropriate for all patients.

The International Association for the Study of Pain (IASP) was founded in 1973, with the impetus of John Bonica, to bring together cli-nicians and researchers in an attempt to improve the treatment of pain. From its beginnings the IASP was multidisciplinary and international. In

Mechanisms and Management of Pain for the Physical Therapist
edited by Kathleen A. Sluka
IASP Press, Seattle, © 2009

2009, the association had 6,860 members in 117 countries and 77 national chapters. As such, it is the leading professional organization for science, practice, and education in the field of pain. Membership of IASP is open to all professionals involved in pain research or in the diagnosis and treatment of pain. The association holds a biennial World Congress on Pain, which is international and multidisciplinary, and publishes the leading journal in pain research, *PAIN*. The IASP and its chapters have made a huge impact on the understanding of pain, pain education, and pain management worldwide. IASP has published guidelines for education for almost all disciplines including medicine, nursing, psychology, and physical therapy. These guidelines will be the basis for the information presented in this book.

Pain Definitions

IASP defines pain as an unpleasant sensory and emotional experience associated with actual or potential tissue damage or described in such terms (www.iasp-pain.org). Inherent in this definition is the underlying premise that pain does not have to be associated with observable tissue damage or have a detectable underlying cause. Pain is multidimensional, involving not only the sensation of pain but also the emotional experience associated with it. Importantly, pain is subjective, and if it is described by the patient it is real.

Melzack and Casey propose three dimensions of pain: sensory-discriminative, motivational-affective, and cognitive-evaluative [9]. The sensory-discriminative dimension of pain refers to the sensation of pain and includes its location, quality (e.g., burning, dull, or sharp), intensity, and duration. The motivational-affective dimension refers to the unpleasantness of pain or how much the pain bothers the patient (e.g., nauseating, sickening). The cognitive-evaluative dimension puts pain in terms of past experiences and probability of outcome and can modify both the sensory-discriminative and the motivational-affective dimension. The cognitive dimension can thus negatively or positively affect the outcome. It is based on patients' beliefs, which may arise from their cultural background and from previous experiences of pain (their own or that of others). For example, if a person experiences low back pain for the second time, he may be more likely to do well if treatment during the first experience resolved the pain quickly. On the other hand, if a person with low back pain has had multiple episodes of pain that were not adequately treated or resolved in prior occurrences, the pain may be more difficult to treat. All three dimensions are linked, and they interact to affect the motor and behavioral consequences responsible for the complex pattern of responses to pain.

Several definitions provided by the IASP are useful for describing pain (Table I). *Hyperalgesia* is an increased sensitivity to noxious stimulus and can occur both at the site of injury (primary hyperalgesia) and outside the site of injury (secondary hyperalgesia). Hyperalgesia may include both a decrease in threshold and an increase in suprathreshold response. *Allodynia* is a term used to describe pain from a non-nociceptive stimulus. Thus, brushing the skin after a sunburn could be considered allodynia, whereas pressure applied to an inflamed joint could be considered hyperalgesia. Basic research suggests that the underlying neural mechanisms for primary hyperalgesia involve increased responsiveness of nociceptors (see Chapter 2). On the other hand, the underlying mechanisms of secondary hyperalgesia and allodynia appear to involve increased responsiveness of central neurons (see Chapter 3). *Referred pain,* common in both acute and chronic pain conditions, is spontaneous pain perceived outside the area of injury. It usually, but not always, follows a dermatome or spinal segmental area. However, it can be referred to areas quite distant from the site of injury. The most common example of referred pain is pain that radiates down the arm during a heart attack. Table I lists other terminology useful to the assessment and understanding of pain.

Acute and Chronic Pain

Pain can be referred to as either acute or chronic pain. There are distinct differences between these two pain conditions that should be recognized. Specifically, acute pain occurs as a direct result of tissue damage or potential tissue damage and is a symptom. It has a well-defined time of onset with clear pathology. Acute pain serves to protect from tissue damage and, if tissue damage has occurred, to allow time for healing. Acute pain that requires clinical treatment usually results from observable tissue damage, including injury, surgery, or procedures such as wound debridement. Acute

K.A. Sluka

Table I
Pain terminology

Term	Definition
Pain	An unpleasant sensory and emotional experience associated with actual or potential tissue damage, or described in terms of such damage
Hyperalgesia	An increased response to a stimulus that is normally painful
Allodynia	Pain due to a stimulus that does not normally provoke pain
Hypoalgesia	Diminished pain in response to a normally painful stimulus
Dysesthesia	An unpleasant abnormal sensation, whether spontaneous or evoked
Neurogenic pain	Pain initiated or caused by a primary lesion, dysfunction, or transitory perturbation in the peripheral or central nervous system
Neuropathic pain	Pain initiated or caused by a primary lesion or dysfunction in the nervous system
Pain threshold	The least experience of pain that a subject can recognize
Pain tolerance	The greatest level of pain that a subject is prepared to tolerate
Pain behavior	A pattern of audible or observable actions, posture, facial expressions, and verbalizations
Referred pain	Spontaneous pain outside the area injury
Noxious stimulus	An actually or potentially tissue-damaging stimulus
Nociceptor	A sensory receptor that is capable of transducing and encoding a noxious stimulus
Nociceptive neuron	A central or peripheral neuron that is capable of encoding noxious stimulation
Nociception	The neural process of encoding and processing noxious stimuli
Nociceptive pain	Pain arising from activation of nociceptors
Sensitization	Increased responsiveness of neurons to their normal input or recruitment of a response to normally subthreshold inputs
Peripheral sensitization	Increased responsiveness and reduced threshold of nociceptors to stimulation of their receptive fields
Central sensitization	Increased responsiveness of nociceptive neurons in the central nervous system to their normal or subthreshold afferent input

Source: Adapted from pain definitions of the International Association for the Study of Pain (www.iasp-pain.org).

pain can be adequately treated with pharmacological and nonpharmacological treatments aimed at the peripheral tissue damage. For example, nonsteroidal anti-inflammatory drugs or ice are commonly used to treat acute inflammation associated with ankle sprain. Thus, acute pain serves a useful and protective function.

Chronic pain, on the other hand, is not protective and does not serve a biological purpose. Pain can be considered chronic if (1) it outlasts normal tissue-healing time, (2) the impairment is greater than would be expected from the physical findings or injury, and/or (3) it occurs in the absence of identifiable tissue damage. In addition, many clinicians define chronic pain in terms of the number of months after the initial injury, usually 3–6 months. The use of a time frame to diagnose chronicity of pain is useful for some conditions such as osteoarthritis. It is not useful, however, for other conditions that may take a long time to heal, for conditions that were not adequately treated at the time of onset such that healing did not occur, or in the case of an athlete who constantly re-injures a joint because he will not wait an adequate amount of time for healing to occur. Although the majority of acute pain cases resolve within 3 months, the remaining cases that are now considered chronic cost billions of dollars per year in health care and lost wages. Thus, when pain becomes chronic, it is no longer a symptom but is considered the disease itself. Chronic pain is difficult to treat and responds best to an interdisciplinary approach.

Cutaneous Versus Deep-Tissue Pain

Pain from deep somatic tissues is different from cutaneous pain. Cutaneous pain is generally sharp and easy to locate, and it is not usually referred to other parts of the body. On the other hand, deep-tissue pain from the muscles, joints, or viscera can be diffuse and difficult to locate, and it is routinely referred to other structures, sometimes distant from the site of injury [6,8,14]. For example, visceral pain is often referred to muscles and cutaneous structures. In fact, people with visceral pain conditions such as irritable bowel syndrome show development of referred pain and muscle hyperalgesia [5]. Similarly, people with somatic deep-tissue pain, such as osteoarthritis or myofascial pain, also develop referred pain and muscle hyperalgesia outside the site of injury [5]. For muscle pain, the size of the area of referred pain correlates with the intensity and duration of the primary muscle pain [14]. In human subjects, painful intramuscular stimulation is rated as more unpleasant than painful cutaneous stimulation [15]; the pain from intramuscular stimulation lasts longer, and referred pain is more frequent than with cutaneous stimulation [17].

Thus, differentiation of primary and secondary hyperalgesia is critical for accurate treatment of patients with pain. This may prove difficult in some patients who show tenderness and increased muscle activity, as well as visceral or deep somatic pain.

Pain Theories and Models

Initial theorists attempted to describe all sensory experiences—touch, heat, cold, and pain—with a single theory. The proposed explanations included the specificity theory and the pattern theory. There was evidence to support the specificity theory for most sensations. However, both theories were inadequate to describe the sensation of pain.

Specificity Theory

The specificity theory suggests that there are separate nerve endings for each variety of sensation arising from cutaneous stimulation—touch, cold, warmth, and pain. For pain, the theory suggests that there are "pain receptors" that when stimulated always produces the sensation of pain and only pain. However, this theory cannot fully explain certain phenomena elicited by a painful stimulus or certain pain conditions. For example, phantom limb pain persists in the absence of the nociceptor, lesions of the central pain pathways do not completely abolish pain, and pain can return after the lesion. Further, touch can elicit pain (allodynia), and pain can continue after removal of the noxious stimulus (hyperpathia).

Pattern Theory

The pattern theory suggests that pain results from a patterned input from sense organs in the skin and consists of spatial and temporal impulses in the central nervous system (CNS). Sensation is thus a learning event that does not require a specific sensory channel. However, it is clear that there are specialized sensory endings that respond to noxious stimuli and that there are central pathways that transmit pain sensation (the spinothalamic tract).

Gate Control Theory

In 1965, Melzack and Wall proposed the gate control theory of pain, using concepts from both the specificity theory and the pattern theory [10]. This integrative model took into account both the physiological and psychological components of pain. The gate control theory profoundly influenced the study of pain and was the stimulus for development of new pain treatments. The theory suggests that there are specialized nerve endings, nociceptors, whose response is modulated in the dorsal horn of the spinal cord (Fig. 1). Input from large-diameter afferents (non-nociceptors) and small-diameter afferents (nociceptors) is "gated" in the spinal cord. These two inputs converge on a substantia gelatinosa (SG) neuron in the dorsal horn of the spinal cord, as well as a "T cell" (transmission cell). The SG neuron is inhibitory to the T cell, which initiates the consequences of pain—motor, sensory, and autonomic responses. The theory suggests that there is a balance between large- and small-diameter afferent input that under normal conditions favors an inhibition of the system, and thus no pain is experienced. Input from nociceptors inhibits the SG neuron, allowing the T cell to fire, "opening the gate," thus resulting in pain. The theory further suggests that increasing input from large-diameter afferents results in a "closing of the gate" by increasing firing of the SG neuron to inhibit nociceptor activity and subsequently decreasing firing of the T cell to result in a reduction in pain. In addition, the theory proposes that this system is

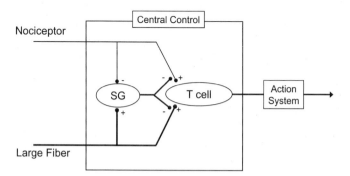

Fig. 1. The gate control theory of pain as initially described by Melzack and Wall in 1965. SG = substantia gelatinosa neuron in the spinal cord; T cell = transmission cell that activates the "action system" or the response to pain; "+" = excitatory synapse; "-" = inhibitory synapse. Redrawn from [12], with permission of the American Association for the Advancement of Science.

under the control of supraspinal sites that could further modulate pain. This theory was used to explain sensory phenomena unique to pain, such as the facts that stimulation of a single nociceptor does not always elicit pain, that repetitive noxious stimulation results in increasing pain, and that large-fiber input inhibits pain. It was also used to explain clinical pain conditions such as phantom limb pain and causalgia.

Many criticize the theory, however, calling it an oversimplification and stating that several of the tenets of the original theory have not held up over the past 40 years. For example, the theory suggests that nociceptors are tonically active. Subsequent neurophysiological studies have shown that nociceptors are not spontaneously active but rather fire in response to a noxious stimulus applied to uninjured tissue. The theory also suggests that nociceptors are directly inhibitory to the SG cell, but again this tenet has not held true: nociceptors are in fact excitatory. The theory further proposes that neurons respond to both noxious and innocuous stimuli. However, subsequent studies have shown that some neurons in the SG respond only to noxious stimuli and do not receive input from large-diameter afferent fibers. The theory also relied heavily on the concept of presynaptic inhibition, for which there is strong evidence. Since the time the theory was proposed, it has also become clear that there are postsynaptic mechanisms responsible for inhibition in the spinal cord as well. Further, substantial evidence has emerged to show that the central control system (supraspinal sites) both facilitates and inhibits pain at the level of the spinal cord (see Chapters 2, 3).

Regardless of these details, the idea of central control and modulation of pain remains valid, and it is used to explain a variety of pain conditions and treatments. Treatments such as transcutaneous electrical nerve stimulation (TENS) were initially designed based on the gate control theory to increase large-diameter input to the spinal cord to inhibit pain. Subsequent research has shown that that TENS additionally targets supraspinal control sites to inhibit activity of dorsal horn neurons in the spinal cord. Thus, the gate control theory of pain generated a substantial amount of research that has advanced the field tremendously in the last 40-plus years. It has resulted in the recognition that pain is a CNS phenomenon, that treatments for pain must be aimed not only at the peripheral nervous system but also at modulating the CNS, and that pain is multidimensional.

Biomedical Model

The biomedical model assumes that all pain has a distinct physiological cause and that clinicians should be able to find and treat that physiological problem. Indeed, for treatment of acute pain the biomedical model is appropriate and necessary. For example, if a person sprains his ankle, treatment of the sprain with adequate medical management—pharmacology, bracing, physical therapy, and techniques to promote healing—will resolve the pain. In this case, pain is considered a symptom of the initial injury, and the treatments are geared toward treating the injury. However, for the treatment of chronic pain, the biomedical model is inadequate.

Biopsychosocial Model

The biopsychosocial model is an alternative approach to the biomedical model that is particularly useful for the treatment of chronic pain. It views pain as an interaction among biological, psychological, and sociocultural variables. This model has been described in a variety of ways by a number of investigators. A schematic diagram is often drawn to represent the different aspects of the pain experience (see Fig. 2). In all variants of the model, nociception is the first component and represents the detection of tissue damage and the activation of nociceptors and the nociceptive pathway in the CNS. The second component is pain and involves recognition of pain at the cortical level as a consequence

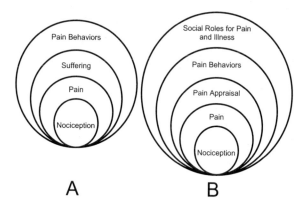

Fig. 2. Schematic diagram showing the biopsychosocial model of pain as conceived (A) by Loeser [7] (reprinted with permission of Lippincott, Williams & Wilkins) and (B) by Turk et al. [16] (reprinted with permission of the American College of Physicians).

of nociception. It is important to recognize that pain does not occur until the signal reaches the cortex and the patient recognizes the perception of pain. The psychosocial aspects of pain come into play at that time. Loeser's model [7] suggests the next component to be suffering, a state of emotional distress associated with events that threaten the biological and psychosocial integrity of the individual. Suffering is the negative affective response brought about by pain, such as depression, anxiety, or fear. Suffering often accompanies severe pain, but it can occur with pain that is less severe, or in conditions that do not give rise to pain. It should be clear that pain and suffering are distinct phenomena. The fourth component is pain behavior or the outward manifestation of the pain event. Pain behaviors are influenced by cultural background and environmental factors and include both verbal and nonverbal behaviors. Examples of pain behaviors include simple facial expressions, but they may also include complex behavior such as not returning to work or avoiding physical activity (i.e., fear avoidance). The avoidance of activity stems from a fear of re-injury or harm and makes it particularly problematic for physical therapists to engage patients in an active treatment program. Turk has added (or used to replace "suffering") a component called "pain appraisal," which refers to the meaning that is attributed to the pain experience [16]. As an example, a person with pain may choose either to continue working and socializing or to avoid all activity and work. Social roles or environmental factors, which take into account how the pain affects the person's role in society, have also been added [16].

All of these factors together represent the biopsychosocial model that must be addressed to adequately resolve issues associated with chronic pain. All factors will not be present in all individuals with chronic pain, but multiple factors are likely to be responsible for the chronic pain experience. Further, these factors vary across time within a patient's life. In addition, many of these factors will also pertain to acute pain conditions, and if not addressed at that time they can play a significant role in the development of chronic pain. For example, an anterior cruciate ligament tear and surgery will probably result in significantly more suffering and illness behavior for the professional basketball player than for the computer programmer, who may not experience suffering.

Disablement Model

The American Physical Therapy Association in 2001 released its *Guide to Physical Therapy Practice* [2]. In this guide it describes and adopts a disablement model initially proposed by Nagi in 1969. Although other models exist and are described in the guide, we will describe the domain of physical therapy practice for pain within Nagi's model. *Pathology* refers to the ongoing pathological state. For acute pain this condition is usually the physician's diagnosis and is related to the site of tissue injury. For chronic pain, the pain is typically the disease itself, and in many cases it is not directly associated with observable or measurable physiological changes or tissue damage. *Impairments* are usually the consequence of the disease or pathology. The guide defines an impairment as an "abnormality of structure or function." The impairment may be an alteration in anatomical, physiological, or psychological functions. Physical therapists typically quantify the signs and symptoms of the impairment that are associated with movement, such as changes in range of motion or decreases in strength. Further, they attempt to quantify pain as an impairment. A *functional limitation* occurs when impairments result in a reduced ability to perform functional tasks or activities that are "usual" for the patient. A functional limitation includes activities of daily living such as walking, grooming, or housekeeping. Physical therapists are generally concerned with physical function, but they should be aware of the impact that other

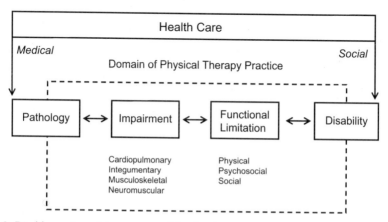

Fig. 3. Disablement model as proposed by the American Physical Therapy Association. Modified from Nagi [2], with permission of the American Physical Therapy Association.

domains such as cognition might have on physical function. For example, a person with shoulder pain may not be able to brush or wash her hair because of the pain. *Disability* is broadly defined by the guide to physical therapy practice as "an inability or restricted ability to perform actions, tasks, and activities related to required self-care, home management, work, community and leisure roles." Disability is an extension of functional limitations that become so severe that they cannot be overcome to allow those affected to maintain their normal role in society. Disability would occur when the patient with shoulder pain not only cannot perform normal grooming (brushing her hair) but now cannot go to work or socialize with friends and family due to the pain and other functional limitations. Rehabilitation and physical therapy must work to reduce disability and functional limitations to improve quality of life.

The role of the physical therapist is to determine which impairments are related to the patient's functional limitations and determine which impairments can be reduced or eliminated. If they cannot be reduced or eliminated, then the physical therapist's role is to educate the patient on how to compensate to perform a given task. The biopsychosocial model, together with the disablement model, suggests that the treatment of functional limitations and disability will require an interdisciplinary approach. It is imperative that physical therapists and other rehabilitation specialists be aware of psychological and social factors and how they can affect quality of life.

International Classification of Functioning, Disability and Health Model

The World Health Organization in 2001 published the International Classification of Functioning, Disability and Health (ICF) [18]. The ICF is a classification of human functioning and disability. Its goal is to provide a unified and standard language for the description of health and health-related components of well-being. There are two basic lists: (1) body function and structures and (2) activities and participation. Functioning encompasses body functions, activities, and participation, whereas disability encompasses impairments, activity limitations, and participation restrictions (see Table II). Health conditions are classified with the ICD-10 (*International Classification of Diseases*, 10th revision) [19], and functioning and disability are classified in the ICF. The ICD-10 provides a diagnosis of disease or health condition and should be combined with the ICF to classify the impact of the disease on functioning and disability. Therefore, the ICF, when combined with the ICD-10, provides a means to diagnose a pain condition, to evaluate the impact of the condition on the individual's function, and to recognize the disability that may result from the condition.

Table II
Classification of functioning and disability and contextual factors

	Part 1: Functioning and Disability		Part 2: Contextual Factors	
Components	Body functions and structures	Activities and participation	Environmental factors	Personal factors
Domains	Body functions and structures	Life areas (tasks, actions)	External influences	Internal influences
Constructs	Change in body functions (physiological), change in body structures (anatomical)	*Capacity:* executing tasks in a standard environment; *Performance:* executing tasks in the current environment	Facilitating or hindering the impact of the physical, social, and attitudinal world	Impact of attributes of the person
Positive aspects	Functional and structural integrity, functioning	Activities, participation	Facilitators	N/A
Negative aspects	Impairment, disability	Activity limitation, participation restriction	Barriers/ hindrances	N/A

Source: Adapted from the *International Classification of Functioning, Disability and Health* [18], with permission from the World Health Organization.

Epidemiology of Pain

Pain, whether acute or chronic, is the number one reason for people to seek medical attention. All pain should be addressed, and everyone has a right to pain relief. Acute pain associated with frank injury can be severe enough that it needs to be adequately treated with pharmacological and nonpharmacological treatments to allow the patient to engage in the healing process. Pain in children, in older adults, and in those with cognitive impairments is frequently undertreated [3,4]. For example, cognitively impaired older adults with hip fractures are less likely to receive adequate pain medication than those who can verbally express their pain [11].

A survey of the United States population (1,004 adults) by Research America in 2003 showed that 57% of those surveyed experienced chronic or recurrent pain in the last 12 months [13]. A survey of persons with chronic pain in the United States by the American Pain Foundation in 2006 showed that pain has a significant effect on everyday activities, interfering with recreational activities, household chores, and work in 40–60% of those surveyed [1]. For those with chronic pain, participation in recreational activities was limited in 85% of those surveyed, which is a much greater percentage than for acute pain, in which 59% of those surveyed had limitations [1]. Similarly, for the activities of daily living surveyed (running errands, household chores, taking care of oneself and others, traveling, and attending a public event), individuals with chronic pain had greater limitations than those with acute pain [1]. It should be emphasized, however, that 30–60% of respondents with acute pain have significant limitations in their activities of daily living as a result of the pain [1]. Interestingly, only 25% of respondents saw a physical therapist or performed exercises (45% of those with chronic pain and 14% of those with acute pain) [1]. The Centers for Disease Control and Prevention's National Center for Health Statistics reports that pain is evenly distributed between genders, across the lifespan, across ethnic groups, geographically, and across socioeconomic boundaries. The incidence of pain is highest for low back pain (28%), but there is also a significant percentage of the population with neck pain (15%), migraine (15%), and peripheral joint pain (30%, with knee pain in 18% and shoulder pain in 9%) [12]. Thus, both acute and chronic pain are common problems that can significantly affect quality of life by interfering with social and work activities.

Physical Therapy Practice

The practice of physical therapy is typically aimed at finding and eliminating the physical cause of the pain using a variety of techniques, including exercises as well as manual therapies and modalities. For acute pain conditions associated with tissue damage and nociceptive pain, this biomedical approach to pain management is adequate and likely to be successful. However, once pain becomes chronic, this model of practice needs modification and should include an interdisciplinary approach to treatment. At this stage, physical therapy practice should shift to enhance the active involvement of the patient with education on activity modification and exercise while minimizing passive treatments such as manual therapy and physical modalities. Manual therapy and physical modalities should only be used in patients with chronic pain as an adjunct to the active, exercise-oriented approach. Further, in some patients with the acute pain, the pain is not proportional to the amount of tissue damage and thus is likely to involve significant CNS changes and psychosocial variables that need to be addressed. Upcoming chapters will discuss in more detail a general approach to physical therapy treatment of pain and explore the underlying mechanisms and clinical evidence for such treatments. In addition, chapters will address the basic science mechanisms of pain transmission, the interdisciplinary management of pain, including medical and psychological approaches, and common pain syndromes.

References

[1] American Pain Foundation. Voices of chronic pain patient survey. May 2006.,Available at: http://www.painfoundation.org.
[2] American Physical Therapy Association. Guide to physical therapy practice, 2nd ed. Phys Ther 2001;81:9–744.
[3] Bernabei R, Gambassi G, Lapane K, Landi F, Gatsonis C, Dunlop R, Lipsitz L, Steel K, Mor V. Management of pain in elderly patients with cancer. SAGE Study Group. Systematic assessment of geriatric drug use via epidemiology. JAMA 1998;279:1877–82.
[4] Feldt KS, Ryden MB, Miles S. Treatment of pain in cognitively impaired compared with cognitively intact older patients with hip-fracture. J Am Geriatr Soc 1998;46:1079–85.
[5] Giamberardino MA. Referred muscle pain/hyperalgesia and central sensitisation. J Rehabil Med 2003;85–8.
[6] Kellgren JH. Observations on referred pain arising from muscle. Clin Sci 1938;3:175–90.
[7] Loeser J. Concepts of pain. In: Stanton-Hicks J, Boaz R, editors. Chronic low back pain. New York: Raven Press; 1982. p. 109–42.
[8] Marchettini P, Cline M, Ochoa J. Innervation territories for touch and pain afferents of single fascicles of the human ulnar nerve. Brain 1990;113:1491–500.
[9] Melzack R, Casey KL. Sensory, motivational, and central control determinants of pain: a new conceptual model. In: Kenshalo D, editor. The skin senses. Springfield: Thomas; 1968. p. 423–43.
[10] Melzack R, Wall PD. Pain mechanisms: a new theory. Science 1965;150:971–8.
[11] Morrison RS, Siu AL. A comparison of pain and its treatment in advanced dementia and cognitively intact patients with hip fracture. J Pain Symptom Manage 2000;19:240–8.
[12] National Center for Health Statistics. Health, United States. With chartbook on trends in the health of Americans. Hyattsville, MD: National Center for Health Statistics; 2007.

[13]   Peter D. Hart Research Associates. Americans talk about pain. Washington, DC: Peter D. Hart
       Research Associates; 2003.
[14]   Simone DA, Marchettini P, Caputi G, Ochoa JL. Identification of muscle afferents subserving
       sensation of deep pain in humans. J Neurophysiol 1994;72:883–9.
[15]   Svensson P, Beydoun A, Morrow TJ, Casey KL. Human intramuscular and cutaneous pain: psy-
       chophysical comparisons. Exp Brain Res 1997;114:390–2.
[16]   Turk DC, Okifuji A, Sherman J. Behavioral aspects of low back pain. In: Taylor J, Twome L, edi-
       tors. Physical therapy of the low back. New York: W.B. Saunders; 2000. p. 351–68.
[17]   Witting N, Svensson P, Gottrup H, Arendt-Nielsen L, Jensen TS. Intramuscular and intradermal
       injection of capsaicin: a comparison of local and referred pain. Pain 2000;84:407–12.
[18]   World Health Organization. International classification of functioning, disability and health. Ge-
       neva: World Health Organization; 2001.
[19]   World Health Organization. International statistical classification of diseases and related health
       problems, 10th revision. Geneva: World Health Organization, 1992.

Correspondence to: Prof. Kathleen A. Sluka, PT, PhD, Graduate Program in Physical Therapy and Rehabilitation Science, The University of Iowa, 1-252 Medical Education Building, Iowa City, IA 52242-1190, USA. Tel: 1-319-335-9791; fax 1-319-335-9707; email: kathleen-sluka@uiowa.edu.

Peripheral Mechanisms Involved in Pain Processing

Kathleen A. Sluka

*Graduate Program in Physical Therapy and Rehabilitation Science,
The University of Iowa, Iowa City, Iowa, USA*

Sensory Receptors and Pathways

Cutaneous sensory receptors convey electrical signals from encapsulated touch receptors to the central nervous system (CNS) via Aβ fibers. Muscle spindles are mechanoreceptors that are specialized to respond either to the rate of change in muscle length or to muscle length, and their signals are carried to the CNS through Group Ia and Group II fibers, respectively. Group II primary afferents that innervate joints are large myelinated afferents that transmit information about proprioception of the joint. Other specialized nerve endings carried by large-diameter afferents from the skin, muscles, and joints are listed in Table I. On the other hand, nociceptors are unencapsulated receptors, termed free nerve endings, which respond to noxious stimuli; they include Aδ fibers (Group III; thinly myelinated axons) and C fibers (Group IV; unmyelinated axons).

Primary afferent neurons are unipolar neurons with a cell body located in the dorsal root ganglia (DRG), a peripheral process innervating peripheral structures, and a central process terminating in the spinal cord

Table I

Peripheral afferent fiber classification

Axon Class	Myelinated	Conduction Velocity (m/s)	Specialized Ending	Receptor Location	Sensation
Group Ia	Yes	70–120	Muscle spindle	Muscle	Proprioception
Group Ib	Yes	70–120	Golgi tendon organ	Tendon	Muscle stretch or contraction
Aβ (Group II)	Yes	25–70	Meissner corpuscle, Merkel's cell, Pacinian corpuscle, Ruffini ending, hair follicle, Paciniform endings, muscle spindle	Skin, joint, muscle	Touch, pressure, vibration, position sense, stretch of muscle
Aδ (Group III)	Yes (thinly)	2–25	Free nerve ending	Skin, muscle, joint, tendon, intervertebral disk, bone, periosteum, fascia	Noxious stimuli
C (Group IV)	No	<2	Free nerve ending	Skin, muscle, joint, tendon, intervertebral disk, bone, periosteum, fascia	Noxious stimuli

dorsal horn or medulla. For the limbs and trunk, the cell bodies of the sensory neurons are located in the DRG. For the head and face, the sensory neuron cell bodies are located in the trigeminal ganglia (Fig. 1A). Primary afferent fibers vary in size and conduction velocity from thickly myelinated (Ia) to unmyelinated (C) fibers (Table II).

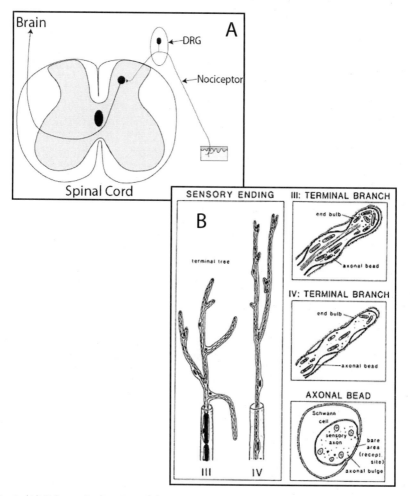

Fig. 1. (A) Schematic drawing of the nociceptor innervation of the skin, the cell body in the dorsal root ganglion (DRG), and the peripheral and central terminals of the nociceptor. The nociceptor synapses in the spinal cord with a spinothalamic tract neuron that transmits nociceptive information to the brain for perception of pain. (B) Serial reconstructions of the free nerve endings of nociceptors innervating the knee joint. Terminal branches of Groups III and IV show axonal beads, where they probably release neurotransmitters; they contain receptors capable of transducing mechanical, thermal and chemical stimuli. Reproduced from [112] with permission of IASP Press.

Table II
Definitions relevant to nociception

Noxious stimulus	An actually or potentially tissue-damaging stimulus
Nociceptor	A sensory receptor that is capable of transducing and encoding a noxious stimulus
Nociceptive neuron	A central or peripheral neuron that is capable of encoding noxious stimulation
Nociception	The neural process of encoding and processing noxious stimuli
Nociceptive pain	Pain arising from activation of nociceptors
Sensitization	Increased responsiveness of neurons to their normal input or recruitment of a response to normally subthreshold inputs
Peripheral sensitization	Increased responsiveness and reduced threshold of nociceptors to stimulation of their receptive fields
Central sensitization	Increased responsiveness of nociceptive neurons in the central nervous system to their normal or subthreshold afferent input

Source: Adapted from pain definitions of the International Association for the Study of Pain (www.iasp-pain.org).

All sensory neurons are activated by adequate stimuli. For nociceptors, these stimuli reflect tissue-damaging stimuli unique to the innervated tissue, while for non-nociceptors these stimuli are typically involved in sensation unique to the structure of the innervated tissue. For example, the adequate stimulus to activate a Pacinian corpuscle is vibration, whereas that for a muscle spindle is muscle length or the rate of change in muscle length.

Nociceptors

A *nociceptor* is a sensory receptor that is capable of transducing and encoding actually or potentially tissue-damaging stimulus (*noxious stimulus*) (Table II). Nociceptors convert mechanical, thermal, and chemical energy into electrical signals and carry this information to the CNS. The peripheral terminals of nociceptors, free nerve endings, are found in and around most tissues including the skin, muscles, tendons, joint structures, periosteum, intervertebral disks, and even within peripheral nerves (nervi nervorum) [145]. For nociceptors from different tissues, the adequate stimulus is distinctly different. For example, one of the adequate stimuli to activate a cutaneous nociceptor is cutting the skin; however, cutting the viscera does not activate visceral nociceptors.

Cutaneous Nociceptors

The free nerve endings of cutaneous $A\delta$ and C nociceptors respond to noxious mechanical and/or thermal stimuli. Many cutaneous nociceptors respond to multiple noxious stimuli, including mechanical, thermal, and chemical stimuli, and hence are called *polymodal* nociceptors [113,145]. A third group of nociceptors has been identified as silent or mechanically insensitive and may be activated by inflammatory mediators such as prostaglandins. The adequate stimulus to activate a cutaneous nociceptor is a noxious mechanical, heat, or cold stimulus.

Muscle and Joint Nociceptors

The primary afferent fibers innervating muscle and joint nerves are classified as Groups II, III, and IV [55,79,107,108,111,145]. Group III primary afferent fibers are thinly myelinated, and Group IV fibers are unmyelinated. Both Group III and Group IV fibers transmit nociceptive information from free nerve endings in the periphery to the spinal cord dorsal horn. The adequate stimulus to activate a joint nociceptor is mechanical and usually involves stretching of the capsular tissue at the end of its range, or pressure applied directly over the capsule. Adequate stimuli to activate a muscle nociceptor are pressure and ischemia [32,79,81].

Visceral Nociceptors

Primary afferent fibers innervating the viscera consist entirely of $A\delta$ and C fibers [47]. Nociceptors of the viscera are considered polymodal, responding not only to mechanical stimuli, but also to heat and chemical stimuli [47]. For hollow visceral organs, the adequate stimulus to activate visceral nociceptors is distension [47]. However, 68% of visceral mechanonociceptors are activated by low-intensity distension, while the remaining 32% are activated by high-intensity distension.

Silent Nociceptors

Some nociceptors are normally silent, but after tissue injury, they become activated and respond to noxious stimuli. For example, Schaible and colleagues showed that prior to experimental knee joint inflammation, some Group III and IV nociceptors do not spontaneously fire or respond to

noxious knee joint movement [111]. After inflammation, however, these nociceptors fire spontaneously, and now respond to noxious joint movement.
Substances released as a result of the injury may sensitize the nociceptors,
allowing them to fire in response to lower intensity stimuli (see below under
"Peripheral Sensitization"). Silent nociceptors were initially located in joint
tissue but have since been located in the skin and viscera as well [47,109,113].
Approximately one-third of nociceptors innervating the joint, skin, or viscera are silent [47,109,113] and become activated after tissue damage.

Peripheral Sensitization

The sensitivity of nociceptors to painful stimuli is modifiable, increasing
or decreasing in response to peripherally applied mechanical, thermal, or
chemical stimuli. "Sensitization" is a term used to describe changes in nociceptive neurons after tissue injury. It is defined as an increased responsiveness of neurons to their normal input or recruitment of a response to
normally subthreshold inputs (Table II). Peripheral sensitization refers to an
increased responsiveness and reduced threshold of nociceptors to stimulation of their receptive fields. A number of neuronal and non-neuronal substances are capable of sensitizing primary afferent fibers, as described below.
        Sensitization of a neuron is characterized by an increase in spon-
taneous activity, a decrease in response threshold to noxious stimuli, an
increase in responsiveness to the same noxious stimuli, and/or an increase
in receptive field size. Recording the activity of the peripheral nerves before and after induction of acute inflammation, Schaible and Schmidt
[108,111] showed increased spontaneous activity and responsiveness
to noxious and innocuous joint movement in primary afferent fibers of
Groups II, III, and IV. Similar changes occur after inflammation of the
muscle with carrageenan [7,31] or after ischemia of the muscle [81]. Following peripheral inflammation, silent nociceptors begin to respond to
both innocuous and noxious stimuli, such as pressure and joint movement
(Fig. 2). Brennan and colleagues [53,95], using a model of postoperative
pain, found a decrease in threshold and an increased responsiveness to
cutaneous mechanical stimuli, as well as a small increase in receptive field
size of the neuron (Fig. 2), indicating sensitization of the cutaneous nociceptors in response to injury. Taken together, these data indicate a general

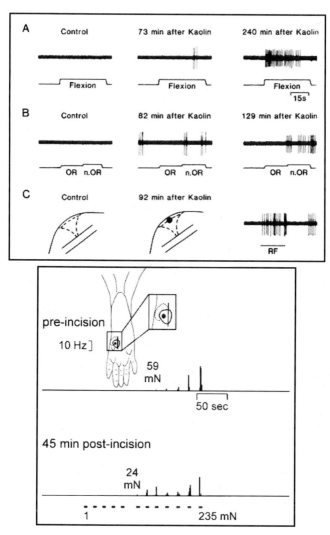

Fig. 2. Sensitization of primary afferent fibers is observed by recording from isolated afferents before and after tissue injury. The top figure shows the recordings from a silent nociceptor (A) prior to induction of knee joint inflammation and (B) for up to 4 hours after inflammation. (C) Development of a mechanical receptive field after inflammation. Notice that the neuron did not respond prior to inflammation (induced by kaolin/carrageenan). After inflammation the neuron responded to noxious and innocuous movement of the knee joint. Reproduced from [110], with permission of the American Physiological Society. The bottom figure shows recordings from a primary afferent nociceptor prior to hindpaw incision, and 45 minutes after incision. Responses to different forces of mechanical stimuli applied with a von Frey filament are shown. Notice that there was a decrease in threshold after injury, as well as an increase in responsiveness of the neuron to repeated stimulation. Also notice that there was a small increase in the receptive field after incision. Reproduced from [53], with permission of the American Physiological Society.

increase in the activity of nociceptors after tissue injury, which would increase the number of afferents firing after a peripheral insult and increase input to the CNS. This sensitization increases the responsiveness of primary pain afferent nociceptors to noxious stimuli and hence constitutes an explanation for hyperalgesia at the site of injury (i.e., primary hyperalgesia).

Neurotransmitters of Primary Afferent Fibers

A number of neurotransmitters, receptors, and ion channels located within or on the peripheral terminals of primary afferent fibers are capable of producing pain and inflammation. Neurotransmitters in primary afferent fibers have been identified, predominantly in neurons located in the DRG, that send axons to the periphery. In some cases neurotransmitters and receptors have been located within the peripheral terminals. Mediators of the inflammatory process can also activate primary afferent nociceptors to initiate the nociceptive or painful response to injury. This field has expanded tremendously in the last decade, with continued advances occurring exponentially. Therefore, we will only touch the surface of the pharmacology of peripheral nociceptors, highlighting a few well-established mechanisms (for a more extensive review, see references [99,145]).

Neuropeptides

Although blood-borne factors are considered to be the major initiator of inflammation, a substantial literature beginning in the late 1800s is devoted to the involvement of the peripheral and sympathetic nervous systems in this process (see references in [127,144]). *Neurogenic inflammation* is a term used to describe the role of the nervous system in the development and maintenance of peripheral inflammation. Neuropeptides such as substance P and calcitonin gene-related peptide (CGRP) are contained in small-diameter afferents (Groups III and IV). When released from primary afferent fibers in the periphery, they produce an inflammatory response [8,10,69,72,143,148], indicating that primary afferent neurons are involved in plasma extravasation during arthritis. In fact, substance P and CGRP are increased in the inflamed knee joint [2,69,69]. Further, peripherally, there are changes in the content of fibers labeled for substance P and CGRP, both in human inflammatory conditions and in animal models of inflammation

[75,76,93]. Elimination of primary afferent fibers by peripheral neurectomy or capsaicin (which destroys Group IV afferents) reduces the inflammatory response [25,66,67,120]. This neurogenic component of inflammation also involves the CNS through the generation of an action potential in the spinal cord that is transmitted to the periphery, termed the dorsal root reflex. The dorsal root reflex releases neuropeptides from the peripheral terminal to enhance the inflammatory response [102,103,124,126].

Opioids

Interestingly, after peripheral inflammation, in animals and human subjects, there is an upregulation of opioid receptors on the peripheral terminals of primary afferent fibers [131–133]. Additionally, macrophages, monocytes, and lymphocytes all contain opioids [97], and the amount of endogenous opioid peptides in these cells increases in inflamed tissues [132]. Thus, there appears to be a peripheral endogenous mechanism to reduce pain in inflamed tissues. Further, the effects of opioid agonists, such as morphine, could produce their actions through activation of peripheral opioid receptors.

Glutamate

Glutamate is an important excitatory neurotransmitter in the nervous system. It is found in primary afferent fibers [141], and its receptors are found on primary afferent terminals of nociceptors [14,16]. Injection of glutamate peripherally produces hyperalgesia in human subjects and animals and sensitizes primary afferent fibers [3,14,38,60,71,134]. Glutamate is upregulated in joint afferents after inflammation [142], and there is an increase in glutamate in inflamed tissues from humans and animals [70,78]. Further, there is an increase in the proportion of nociceptors expressing glutamate receptors after inflammation [15], and blockade of glutamate receptors reduces pain and hyperalgesia in human subjects and animals [13,17].

Ion Channels

Several ion channels, found on peripheral terminals of primary afferent fibers, may also be important in the response to noxious stimuli. Low pH is found in inflamed tissues and produces pain in humans and animals [54,101,119]. Acid-sensing ion channels are located in DRG neurons, are activated by low pH, and are importantly involved in pain arising from muscles and joints [59,83,96,121,122]. The vanilloid receptor, TRPV1, located in the DRG, is activated by the exogenous ligand capsaicin; it responds to low pH and mediates hyperalgesia to heat stimuli [18,19].

Sodium channels are involved in fast synaptic transmission and action potential propagation. The DRG neurons express six different sodium channels, including sensory-neuron-specific sodium channels not present within other parts of the nervous system. The involvement of sodium channels in the peripheral nervous system is complex but clearly important for both inflammatory and neuropathic pain (see [4,29,139]). The $Na_V1.7$ and $Na_V1.8$ channels play critical roles in nociception [9,29,37]. A change in sodium channel composition occurs after peripheral neuropathy, resulting in physiological changes that contribute to hyperexcitability of DRG neurons [48]. Recent evidence shows that mutations in the genes encoding for $Na_V1.7$ result in the painful syndrome erythromelalgia (also called erythermalgia) and in paroxysmal extreme pain disorder. In contrast, people with a complete loss of functional $Na_V1.7$ have been reported to be insensitive to pain [9,29,30,37,48]. Local anesthetics, such as lidocaine, mediate their effects by blocking sodium channels, and future pharmaceutical agents may be aimed at specific channels such as $Na_V1.7$ or $Na_V1.8$.

Non-Neuronal Activators and Inflammatory Mediators

A number of substances are released from inflammatory cells that can directly activate or sensitize primary afferent fibers (Fig. 3). These include serotonin, bradykinin, prostaglandins, and cytokines. Serotonin,

Fig. 3. Schematic drawing of the peripheral mediators of sensitization after inflammation. ⟶ Release of a variety of neurochemicals from non-neuronal cells may act directly or indirectly to sensitize nociceptors. Release of substance P, CGRP, or glutamate can further enhance the inflammatory response by acting on non-neuronal cells and capillaries to cause plasma extravasation and vasodilatation. ASIC = acid-sensing ion channel; AMPA/Ka = non-NMDA glutamate receptors; B2 = bradykinin 2 receptor; CGRP = calcitonin gene-related peptide; δ = delta-opioid receptor; Enk/Endo = enkephalins and endomorphins; EP1 = prostaglandin receptor; H1 = histamine 1 receptor; 5-HT = serotonin; IL = interleukin; μ = mu-opioid receptor; NK1 = neurokinin 1 receptor; NMDA = N-methyl-D-aspartate receptor; TNF = tumor necrosis factor; PGE_2 = prostaglandin E_2; PKA = protein kinase A; PKC = protein kinase C.

Inflammation

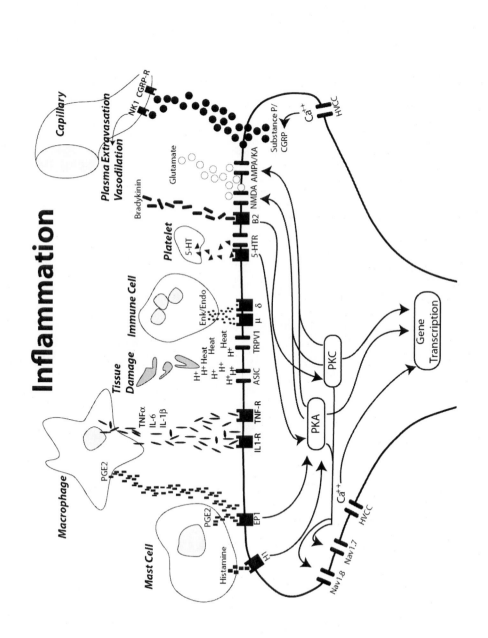

released from platelets, activates muscle nociceptors and causes pain in humans [45,106]. Bradykinin, which is released from plasma after tissue injury and is present in inflammatory exudates, sensitizes nociceptors and produces pain and heat hyperalgesia in humans [20,33,64,65,74,90,94]. Prostaglandins are metabolites of the arachidonic acid cascade and are produced in response to tissue injury. Prostaglandins directly excite and sensitize nociceptors through receptors located on primary afferent fibers [21,22,110]. The nonsteroidal anti-inflammatory drugs (NSAIDs) produce their effects by reducing prostaglandin production through inhibition of the enzyme cyclooxygenase, which is involved in the breakdown of arachidonic acid.

During inflammation, cytokines are released by macrophages. The proinflammatory cytokines, including interleukins (IL-1β, IL-6) and tumor necrosis factor alpha (TNF-α), are increased in the synovial fluid from patients with arthritis; they sensitize primary afferent nociceptors and produce mechanical and thermal hyperalgesia [27,43,44,61,62,77,91,137,138]. Blocking TNF-α receptors or reducing available TNF-α reduces hyperalgesia in animal models of inflammation and neuropathic pain [128–130]. Antibodies to TNF-α, which reduce TNF-α availability, are now considered an important disease-modifying drug in rheumatoid arthritis [43,56,100]. While the actions of each of these inflammatory mediators have been described individually, many mediators act together to enhance inflammation and hyperalgesia, producing a potentiated response.

Animal Models of Pain

Several animal models of pain have been designed to mimic clinical pain conditions (for review, see [39]). Animal models of pain can serve to probe the mechanisms behind the development and maintenance of different pain conditions. They also allow investigators to assess the initial efficacy and safety of pharmaceutical and nonpharmaceutical treatments, as well as the mechanisms of action of these treatments. Models exist for studying cutaneous pain, neuropathic pain, musculoskeletal pain, visceral pain, and postoperative pain. These models can broadly be classified as acute pain models, inflammatory pain models, and neuropathic pain models. Much of our knowledge on pain pathways, peripheral sensitization, and central sensitization has arisen from studies using these animal models of pain.

Acute Pain Models

Acute pain models generally involve testing responses to noxious mechanical or thermal stimuli in an uninjured animal. Such models have served for decades as screening tools to test the efficacy of pharmacological agents [42]. They do not typically result in tissue injury and thus do not cause hyperalgesia or neuron sensitization.

Cutaneous Pain Models

Generally, cutaneous pain models involve inflammation induced by injection of an irritant either into the skin or subcutaneously. Hyperalgesia is routinely assessed at the site of inflammation. These models of tissue injury were initially developed to more directly measure pain that might be similar to clinical syndromes. The most common inflammatory models involve injection of carrageenan or complete Freund's adjuvant into the paw to produce an acute or chronic inflammatory event, respectively, resulting in primary hyperalgesia [105]. Animals show increased responses and decreased thresholds to mechanical and thermal stimuli after the induction of inflammation [39,39,104]. In addition, the animals guard their limbs, decreasing the amount of weight on the inflamed extremity. Capsaicin, the substance found in hot chili peppers, activates TRPV1 channels and produces local inflammation, as well as hyperalgesia. This substance has been used in both animals and human subjects as an experimental model of pain [36,68,115,118,146]. All cutaneous pain models result in peripheral and central sensitization of neurons in the nociceptive pathway, which includes nociceptors, dorsal horn neurons, and thalamic, cortical, and descending pathways [49,51,52,58,73,116]. Formalin is an inflammatory irritant that produces spontaneous pain behaviors that last for up to 1 hour [1]. This test produces two phases of behaviors, phase I and II, which are thought to represent changes in the peripheral and central nervous system, respectively [1]. The formalin test has proven useful for screening pharmaceutical agents as well as for discriminating peripheral and central mechanisms.

Joint Pain Models

The most common model of joint pain involves injection of a mixture of kaolin and carrageenan into the knee joint [24,125]. This model mimics arthritic conditions and produces an acute, as well as a chronic, inflammatory phase [98]. As inflammation becomes more chronic, hyperalgesia spreads to include the contralateral hindlimb [98]. Intra-articular injection of complete Freund's adjuvant and capsaicin has also been used to model inflammatory joint pain [34,118]. These models are associated with primary hyperalgesia to mechanical pressure applied to the knee joint, and with secondary heat and mechanical hyperalgesia of the paw [98,117,136]. Inflammation of the joint results in peripheral as well as central sensitization of dorsal horn, thalamic, amygdalar, and cortical neurons [35,49,50,88,89,107].

A model of repetitive strain injury has been developed in which rats are trained to pull on a bar with or without force 4 times per minute for 2 hours per day, 3 days per week, for up to 12 weeks [23]. This model results in increases in inflammatory cytokines around the median nerve, as well as changes in substance P and neurokinin-1 in the dorsal horn [5,40]. However, at present we do not know if this repetitive strain injury produces pain behaviors.

Muscle Pain Models

The most common model of muscle pain is induced by injection of carrageenan into a muscle belly to mimic myositis [80,98]. Similar to the results observed with joint injection of carrageenan, there is an initial acute inflammation that converts to chronic inflammation [98]. The acute inflammation is associated with a unilateral primary and secondary hyperalgesia, whereas the chronic inflammation phase results in more widespread hyperalgesia that includes the contralateral hindlimb [98]. Inflammatory muscle pain also results in peripheral sensitization of Group III and IV afferents, as well as central sensitization of neurons in the spinal cord dorsal horn [57,79].

A non-inflammatory model of musculoskeletal pain was developed to mimic the chronic widespread pain observed clinically in people with low back pain or fibromyalgia. Repeated intramuscular acid injections are non-inflammatory but produce long-lasting mechanical hyperalgesia. Importantly, in this model there is no damage within the muscle tissue, and the hyperalgesia is maintained by changes in the CNS [119]. There is bilateral hyperalgesia of the muscle, as well as visceral hyperalgesia [82,119,135,149]. This model is unique in that it does not result in peripheral sensitization but is maintained by changes in the CNS, including sensitization of dorsal horn neurons and supraspinal pathways [119,123,135].

Neuropathic Pain Models

Several models of neuropathic pain have been developed and are used extensively in animal studies. The most common models are sciatic nerve ligation, induced by making loose ligations around the sciatic nerve [6]; spinal nerve ligation, induced by making tight ligations around the spinal nerves [63]; and spared nerve injury, induced by tight ligation of the tibial and peroneal nerve in the hindlimb [28]. Each of these neuropathic pain models produces a measurable, long-lasting hyperalgesia and changes in the CNS [6,28,63]. Further models of neuropathic pain induced by chemotherapy drugs or by diabetes also result in long-term hyperalgesia [140,147]. Neuropathic models result in sensitization of nociceptors and of central pathways, including the dorsal horn and supraspinal sites [12,92,114].

Visceral Pain Models

Visceral pain models include hollow organ distension and urinary bladder inflammation as models for generic visceral pain and cystitis, respectively [41,85]. Colorectal distension in awake, unanesthetized, unrestrained rats produces a quantifiable aversive behavior and cardiovascular and visceromotor responses indicative of acute visceral nociception [86]. After visceral inflammation or injury there is sensitization of visceral nociceptors, dorsal horn neurons, and supraspinal modulation sites [26,46,47,84,87].

Postoperative Pain

To study postoperative pain, Brennan and colleagues developed an animal model in which a longitudinal incision is made through the skin, fascia, and muscle of the plantar aspect of the hindpaw [11]. This model reflects both superficial and deep-tissue injury seen with surgical treatments and results in spontaneous pain and mechanical hyperalgesia around the site of injury. Sensitization of nociceptors and dorsal horn neurons occurs in response to incisional pain [53,95,150].

Summary

This chapter has described the peripheral nociceptors innervating a variety of tissue types and the adequate stimuli that are necessary to activate them. Tissue injury may cause changes in these nociceptors that include increases in spontaneous activity, increased responsiveness to noxious stimuli, and a decreased threshold to noxious stimuli. This process of peripheral sensitization involves the neurotransmitters and receptors located in nociceptors, as well as inflammatory mediators. A variety of animal models are used to study clinical pain conditions and the underlying mechanisms for these conditions. The use of these animal models has greatly enhanced the understanding of a variety of painful conditions, spurred the development of new pharmaceutical and nonpharmaceutical treatments, and increased our understanding of the efficacy and mechanisms of current treatments. The next chapter will discuss the nociceptive pathways and neurotransmitters in the CNS and explore the changes that occur in animal models of pain.

References

[1] Abbot FV, Franklin KBJ, Westbrook RF. The formalin test: scoring properties of the first and second phases of the pain responses in rats. Pain 1995;60:91–102.
[2] Appelgren A, Applegren B, Eriksson S, Kopp S, Lundeberg T, Nylander M, Theodorsson E. Neuropeptides in temporomandibular joints with rheumatoid arthritis: a clinical study. Scand J Dent Res 1991;99:519–21.
[3] Arendt-Nielsen L, Svensson P, Sessle BJ, Cairns BE, Wang K. Interactions between glutamate and capsaicin in inducing muscle pain and sensitization in humans. Eur J Pain 2008;12:661–70.
[4] Baker MD, Wood JN. Involvement of Na$^+$ channels in pain pathways. Trends Pharmacol Sci 2001;22:27–31.
[5] Barbe MF, Elliott MB, Abdelmagid SM, Amin M, Popoff SN, Safadi FF, Barr AE. Serum and tissue cytokines and chemokines increase with repetitive upper extremity tasks. J Orthop Res 2008;26:1320–6.
[6] Bennett GJ, Xie YK. A peripheral mononeuropathy in rat that produces disorders of pain sensation like those seen in man. Pain 1988;33:87–107.
[7] Berberich P, Hoheisel U, Mense S. Effects of a carrageenan induced myositis on the discharge properties of group III and IV muscle receptors in the cat. J Neurophysiol 1988;59:1395–409.

[8]   Bethel RA, Brokaw JJ, Evans TW, Nadel JA, McDonald DM. Substance P-induced increase in vascular permeability in the rat trachea does not depend on neutrophils or other components of circulating blood. Exp Lung Res 1988;14:769–79.

[9]   Black JA, Liu S, Tanaka M, Cummins TR, Waxman SG. Changes in the expression of tetrodo-toxin-sensitive sodium channels within dorsal root ganglia neurons in inflammatory pain. Pain 2004;108:237–47.

[10]   Brain SD, Williams TJ. Inflammatory oedema induced by synergism between calcitonin gene-related peptide (CGRP) and mediators of increased vascular permeability. Br J Pharmacol 1985;86:855–60.

[11]   Brennan TJ, Vandermeulen EP, Gebhart GF. Characterization of a rat model of incisional pain. Pain 1996;64:493–501.

[12]   Burgess SE, Gardell LR, Ossipov MH, Malan TP, Vanderah TW, Lai J, Porreca F. Time-dependent descending facilitation from the rostral ventromedial medulla maintains, but does not initiate, neuropathic pain. J Neurosci 2002;22:5129–36.

[13]   Cairns BE, Svensson P, Wang K, Castrillon E, Hupfeld S, Sessle BJ, Arendt-Nielsen L. Ketamine attenuates glutamate-induced mechanical sensitization of the masseter muscle in human males. Exp Brain Res 2006;169:467–72.

[14]   Cairns BE, Svensson P, Wang K, Hupfeld S, Graven-Nielsen T, Sessle BJ, Berde CB, Arendt-Nielsen L. Activation of peripheral NMDA receptors contributes to human pain and rat afferent discharges evoked by injection of glutamate into the masseter muscle. J Neurophysiol 2003;90:2098–105.

[15]   Carlton SM, Coggeshall RE. Inflammation-induced changes in peripheral glutamate receptor populations. Brain Res 1999;820:63–70.

[16]   Carlton SM, Hargett GL, Coggeshall RE. Localization and activation of glutamate receptors in unmyelinated axons of rat glabrous skin. Neurosci Lett 1995;197:25–8.

[17]   Castrillon EE, Cairns BE, Ernberg M, Wang K, Sessle BJ, Arendt-Nielsen L, Svensson P. Effect of a peripheral NMDA receptor antagonist on glutamate-evoked masseter muscle pain and mechanical sensitization in women. J Orofac Pain 2007;21:216–24.

[18]   Caterina MJ, Leffler A, Malmberg AB, Martin WJ, Trafton J, Petersen-Zeitz KR, Koltzenburg M, Basbaum AI, Julius D. Impaired nociception and pain sensation in mice lacking the capsaicin receptor. Science 2000;288:306–13.

[19]   Caterina MJ, Rosen TA, Tominaga M, Brake AJ, Julius D. A capsaicin-receptor homologue with a high threshold for noxious heat. Nature 1999;398:436–41.

[20]   Cesare P, McNaughton P. A novel heat-activated current in nociceptive neurons and its sensitization by bradykinin. Proc Natl Acad Sci USA 1996;93:15435–9.

[21]   Chen X, Levine JD. NOS inhibitor antagonism of PGE_2-induced mechanical sensitization of cutaneous C-fiber nociceptors in the rat. J Neurophysiol 1999;81:963–6.

[22]   Chen X, Tanner K, Levine JD. Mechanical sensitization of cutaneous C-fiber nociceptors by prostaglandin E2 in the rat. Neurosci Lett 1999;267:105–8.

[23]   Clark BD, Al-Shatti TA, Barr AE, Amin M, Barbe MF. Performance of a high-repetition, high-force task induces carpal tunnel syndrome in rats. J Orthop Sports Phys Ther 2004;34:244–53.

[24]   Coggeshall RE, Hong KAH, Langford LA, Schaible H-G, Schmidt RF. Discharge of fine medial articular afferents at rest and during passive movements of inflamed knee joints. Brain Res 1983;272:185–8.

[25]   Colpaert FC, Donnerer J, Lembeck F. Effects of capsaicin on inflammation and on substance P content of nervous tissues in rats with adjuvant arthritis. Life Sci 1983;32:1827–34.

[26]   Coutinho SV, Urban MO, Gebhart GF. Role of glutamate receptors and nitric oxide in the rostral ventromedial medulla in visceral hyperalgesia. Pain 1998;78:59–69.

[27]   Cunha FQ, Poole S, Lorenzetti BB, Ferreira SH. The pivotal role of tumour necrosis factor alpha in the development of inflammatory hyperalgesia. Br J Pharmacol 1992;107:660–4.

[28]   Decosterd I, Woolf CJ. Spared nerve injury: an animal model of persistent peripheral neuropathic pain. Pain 2000;87:149–58.

[29]   Dib-Hajj SD, Cummins TR, Black JA, Waxman SG. From genes to pain: Na$_v$1.7 and human pain disorders. Trends Neurosci 2007;30:555–63.

[30]   Dib-Hajj SD, Rush AM, Cummins TR, Hisama FM, Novella S, Tyrrell L, Marshall L, Waxman SG. Gain-of-function mutation in Nav1.7 in familial erythromelalgia induces bursting of sensory neurons. Brain 2005;128:1847–54.

[31] Diehl B, Hoheisel U, Mense S. Histological and neurophysiological changes induced by carra-geenan in skeletal muscle of cat and rat. Agents Actions 1988;25:210–3.

[32] Diehl B, Hoheisel U, Mense S. The influence of mechanical stimuli and of acetylsalicylic acid on the discharges of slowly conducting afferent units from normal and inflamed muscle. Exp Brain Res 1993;92:431–40.

[33] Di Rosa M, Giroud JP, Willoughby DA. Studies of the mediators of the acute inflammatory re-sponse induced in rats in different sites by carrageenan and turpentine. J Pathol 1971;104:15–29.

[34] Donaldson LF, Seckl JR, McQueen DS. A discrete adjuvant-induced monoarthritis in the rat: effects of adjuvant dose. J Neurosci Meth 1993;49:5–10.

[35] Dougherty PM, Sluka KA, Sorkin LS, Westlund KN, Willis WD. Neural changes in acute arthritis in monkeys. I. Parallel enhancement of responses of spinothalamic tract neurons to mechanical stimulation and excitatory amino acids. Brain Res Rev 1992;17:1–13.

[36] Dougherty PM, Willis WD. Enhanced responses of spinothalamic tract neurons to excit-atory amino-acids accompany capsaicin-induced sensitization in the monkey. J Neurosci 1992;12:883–94.

[37] Drenth JP, Waxman SG. Mutations in sodium-channel gene SCN9A cause a spectrum of human genetic pain disorders. J Clin Invest 2007;117:3603–9.

[38] Du J, Koltzenburg M, Carlton SM. Glutamate-induced excitation and sensitization of nocicep-tors in rat glabrous skin. Pain 2001;89:187–98.

[39] Dubner R, Ren K. Assessing transient and persistent pain in animals. In: Wall PD, Melzack R, editors. Textbook of pain. New York: Churchill Livingstone; 1999. p. 359–69.

[40] Elliott MB, Barr AE, Kietrys DM, Al-Shatti T, Amin M, Barbe MF. Peripheral neuritis and in-creased spinal cord neurochemicals are induced in a model of repetitive motion injury with low force and repetition exposure. Brain Res 2008;1218:103–13.

[41] Farquhar-Smith WP, Rice AS. Administration of endocannabinoids prevents a referred hyperal-gesia associated with inflammation of the urinary bladder. Anesthesiology 2001;94:507–13.

[42] Feldman RS, Meyer JS, Quenzer LF. Principles of neuropsychopharmacology. Sunderland: Sinauer; 1997.

[43] Feldmann M, Brennan FM, Elliott MJ, Williams RO, Maini RN. TNF-alpha is an effective thera-peutic target for rheumatoid arthritis. Ann NY Acad Sci 1995;766:272–8.

[44] Ferreira SH, Lorenzetti BB, Bristow AF, Poole S. Interleukin-1 beta as a potent hyperalgesic agent antagonized by a tripeptide analogue. Nature 1988;334:698–700.

[45] Fock S, Mense S. Excitatory effects of 5-hydroxytryptamine, histamine and potassium ions on muscular group IV afferent units: a comparison with bradykinin. Brain Res 1976;105:459–69.

[46] Friedrich AE, Gebhart GF. Effects of spinal cholecystokinin receptor antagonists on morphine antinociception in a model of visceral pain in the rat. J Pharmacol Exp Ther 2000;292:538–44.

[47] Gebhart GF. Visceral polymodal receptors. Prog Brain Res 1996;113:101–12.

[48] Gold MS, Weinreich D, Kim CS, Wang R, Treanor J, Porreca F, Lai J. Redistribution of $Na_v1.8$ in uninjured axons enables neuropathic pain. J Neurosci 2003;23:158–66.

[49] Guilbaud G. 15 years of explorations in some supraspinal structures in rat inflammatory pain models, some information, but further questions. Am Pain Soc J 1994;3:168–79.

[50] Guilbaud G, Benoist JM, Condes-Lara M, Gautron M. Further evidence for the involvement of SmI cortical neurons in nociception: their responsiveness at 24 hours after carrageenin-induced hyperalgesic inflammation in the rat. Somatosens Motor Res 1993;10:229–44.

[51] Guilbaud G, Benoist JM, Levante A, Gautron M, Willer JC. Primary somatosensory cortex in rats with pain-related behaviors due to a peripheral mononeuropathy after moderate ligation of one sciatic-nerve: neuronal responsivity to somatic stimulation. Exp Brain Res 1992;92:227–45.

[52] Guilbaud G, Kayser V, Benoist JM, Gautron M. Modifications in the responsiveness of rat ven-trobasal thalamic neurons at different stages of carrageenin-produced inflammation. Brain Res 1986;385:86–98.

[53] Hamalainen MM, Gebhart GF, Brennan TJ. Acute effect of an incision on mechanosensitive af-ferents in the plantar rat hindpaw. J Neurophysiol 2002;87:712–20.

[54] Hamamoto DT, Ortiz-Gonzalez XR, Honda JM, Kajander KC. Intraplantar injection of hy-aluronic acid at low pH into the rat hindpaw produces tissue acidosis and enhances withdrawal responses to mechanical stimuli. Pain 1998;74:225–34.

[55] Hepplemann B, Heuss C, Schmidt RF. Fiber size distribution of myelinated and unmyelinat-ed axons in the medial and posterior articular nerves of the cat's knee joint. Somatosens Res 1988;5:273–81.

[56] Hochberg MC, Tracy JK, Hawkins-Holt M, Flores RH. Comparison of the efficacy of the tumour necrosis factor alpha blocking agents adalimumab, etanercept, and infliximab when added to methotrexate in patients with active rheumatoid arthritis. Ann Rheum Dis 2003;62:ii:13–6.

[57] Hoheisel U, Koch K, Mense S. Functional reorganization in the rat dorsal horn during an experimental myositis. Pain 1994;59:111–8.

[58] Hylden JLK, Nahin RL, Traub RJ, Dubner R. Expansion of receptive fields of spinal lamina I projection neurons in rats with unilateral adjuvant-induced inflammation: the contribution of dorsal horn mechanisms. Pain 1989;37:229–43.

[59] Ikeuchi M, Kolker S, Burnes LA, Walder RY, Sluka KA. Role of ASIC3 in the primary and secondary hyperalgesia produced by joint inflammation in mice. Pain 2008;137:662–9.

[60] Jackson DL, Graff CB, Richardson JD, Hargreaves KM. Glutamate participates in the peripheral modulation of thermal hyperalgesia in rats. Eur J Pharmacol 1995;284:321–5.

[61] Kaneko S, Satoh T, Chiba J, Ju C, Inoue K, Kagawa J. Interleukin-6 and interleukin-8 levels in serum and synovial fluid of patients with osteoarthritis. Cytokines Cell Mol Ther 2000;6:71–9.

[62] Kaneyama K, Segami N, Nishimura M, Suzuki T, Sato J. Importance of proinflammatory cytokines in synovial fluid from 121 joints with temporomandibular disorders. Br J Oral Maxillofac Surg 2002;40:418–23.

[63] Kim SH, Chung JM. An experimental-model for peripheral neuropathy produced by segmental spinal nerve ligation in the rat. Pain 1992;50:355–63.

[64] Kirchhoff C, Jung S, Reeh PW, Handwerker HO. Carrageenan inflammation increases bradykinin sensitivity of rat cutaneous nociceptors. Neurosci Lett 1990;111:206–10.

[65] Koltzenburg M, Kress M, Reeh PW. The nociceptor sensitization by bradykinin does not depend on sympathetic neurons. Neuroscience 1992;46:465–73.

[66] Lam FY, Ferrell WR. Capsaicin suppresses substance P-induced joint inflammation in the rat. Neurosci Lett 1989;105:155–8.

[67] Lam FY, Ferrell WR. Specific neurokinin receptors mediate plasma extravasation in the rat knee joint. Br J Pharmacol 1991;103:1263–7.

[68] Lamotte RH, Lundberg LER, Torebjork HE. Pain, hyperalgesia and activity in nociceptive-C units in humans after intradermal injection of capsaicin. J Physiol 1992;448:749–64.

[69] Larsson J, Ekblom A, Henriksson K, Lundeberg T, Theodorsson E. Immunoreactive tachykinins, calcitonin gene-related peptide and neuropeptide Y in human synovial fluid from inflamed knee joints. Neurosci Lett 1989;100:326–30.

[70] Lawand NB, McNearney T, Westlund KN. Amino acid release into the knee joint: key role in nociception and inflammation. Pain 2000;86:69–74.

[71] Lawand NB, Willis WD, Westlund KN. Excitatory amino acid receptor involvement in peripheral nociceptive transmission in rats. Eur J Pharmacol 1997;324:169–77.

[72] Levine JD, Moskowitz MA, Basbaum AI. The contribution of neurogenic inflammation in experimental arthritis. J Immunol 1985;135:843–7S.

[73] Ma YT, Sluka KA. Reduction in inflammation-induced sensitization of dorsal horn neurons by transcutaneous electrical nerve stimulation in anesthetized rats. Exp Brain Res 2001;137:94–102.

[74] Manning DC, Raja SN, Meyer RA, Campbell JN. Pain and hyperalgesia after intradermal injection of bradykinin in humans. Clin Pharmacol Ther 1991;50:721–9.

[75] Mapp PI, Kidd BL, Gibson SJ, Terry JM, Revell PA, Ibrahim NBN, Blake DR, Polak JM. Substance P-, calcitonin gene-related peptide- and C-flanking peptide of neuropeptide Y-immunoreactive fibres are present in normal synovium but depleted in patients with rheumatoid arthritis. Neuroscience 1990;37:143–53.

[76] Mapp PI, Walsh DA, Garrett NE, Kidd BL, Cruwys SC, Polak JM, Blake DR. Effect of 3 animal models of inflammation on nerve fibers in the synovium. Ann Rheum Dis 1994;53:240–6.

[77] McNearney T, Baethge BA, Cao S, Alam R, Lisse JR, Westlund KN. Excitatory amino acids, TNF-alpha, and chemokine levels in synovial fluids of patients with active arthropathies. Clin Exp Immunol 2004;137:621–7.

[78] McNearney T, Speegle D, Lawand N, Lisse J, Westlund KN. Excitatory amino acid profiles of synovial fluid from patients with arthritis. J Rheumatol 2000;27:739–45.

[79] Mense S. Nociception from skeletal muscle in relation to clinical muscle pain. Pain 1993;54:241–89.

[80] Mense S, Skeppar P. Discharge behaviour of feline gamma-motoneurones following induction of an artificial myositis. Pain 1991;46:201–10.

[81] Mense S, Stahnke M. Responses in muscle afferent fibres of slow conduction velocity to contraction and ischaemia in the cat. J Physiol 1983;342:383–7.

[82] Miranda A, Peles S, Rudolph C, Shaker R, Sengupta JN. Altered visceral sensation in response to somatic pain in the rat. Gastroenterology 2004;126:1082–9.

[83] Molliver DC, Immke DC, Fierro L, Pare M, Rice FL, McCleskey EW. ASIC3, an acid-sensing ion channel, is expressed in metaboreceptive sensory neurons. Mol Pain 2005;1:35.

[84] Ness TJ, Gebhart GF. Characterization of neurons responsive to noxious colorectal distension in the T13–L2 spinal cord of the rat. J Neurophysiol 1988;60:1419–38.

[85] Ness TJ, Gebhart GF. Colorectal distension as a noxious visceral stimulus: physiologic and pharmacologic characterization of pseudaffective reflexes in the rat. Brain Res 1988;450:153–69.

[86] Ness TJ, Gebhart GF. Visceral pain: a review of experimental studies. Pain 1990;41:167–234.

[87] Ness TJ, Gebhart GF. Acute inflammation differentially alters the activity of two classes of rat spinal visceral nociceptive neurons. Neurosci Lett 2000;281:131–4.

[88] Neugebauer V, Li W. Differential sensitization of amygdala neurons to afferent inputs in a model of arthritic pain. J Neurophysiol 2003;89:716–27.

[89] Neugebauer V, Li W, Bird GC, Han JS. The amygdala and persistent pain. Neuroscientist 2004;10:221–34.

[90] Neugebauer V, Schaible HG, Schmidt RF. Sensitization of articular afferents to mechanical stimuli by bradykinin. Pflugers Arch 1989;415:330–5.

[91] Ozaktay AC, Cavanaugh JM, Asik I, DeLeo JA, Weinstein JN. Dorsal root sensitivity to interleukin-1 beta, interleukin-6 and tumor necrosis factor in rats. Eur Spine J 2002;11:467–75.

[92] Palecek J, Paleckova V, Dougherty PM, Carlton SM, Willis WD. Responses of spinothalamic tract cells to mechanical and thermal stimulation of skin in rats with experimental peripheral neuropathy. J Neurophysiol 1992;67:1562–73.

[93] Pereira da Silva JA, Carmo-Fonesca M. Peptide containing nerves in human synovium: immunohistochemical evidence for decreased innervation in rheumatoid arthritis. J Rheumatol 1990;17:1592–9.

[94] Petho G, Derow A, Reeh PW. Bradykinin-induced nociceptor sensitization to heat is mediated by cyclooxygenase products in isolated rat skin. Eur J Neurosci 2001;14:210–8.

[95] Pogatzki EM, Gebhart GF, Brennan TJ. Characterization of A-delta- and C-fibers innervating the plantar rat hindpaw one day after an incision. J Neurophysiol 2002;87:721–31.

[96] Price MP, McIlwrath SL, Xie J, Cheng C, Qiao J, Tarr DE, Sluka KA, Brennan TJ, Lewin GR, Welsh MJ. The DRASIC cation channel contributes to the detection of cutaneous touch and acid stimuli in mice. Neuron 2001;32:1071–83.

[97] Przewlocki R, Hassan AH, Lason W, Epplen C, Herz A, Stein C. Gene expression and localization of opioid peptides in immune cells of inflamed tissue: functional role in antinociception. Neuroscience 1992;48:491–500.

[98] Radhakrishnan R, Moore SA, Sluka KA. Unilateral carrageenan injection into muscle or joint induces chronic bilateral hyperalgesia in rats. Pain 2003;104:567–77.

[99] Raja SN, Meyer RA, Ringkamp M, Campbell JN. Peripheral neural mechanisms of nociception. In: Melzack R, Wall PD, editors. Textbook of pain. New York: Churchill Livingstone; 1999. p. 11–57.

[100] Ravindran V, Scott DL, Choy EH. A systematic review and meta-analysis of efficacy and toxicity of disease modifying anti-rheumatic drugs and biologic agents for psoriatic arthritis. Ann Rheum Dis 2008;67:855–9.

[101] Reeh PW, Steen KH. Tissue acidosis in nociception and pain. Prog Brain Res 1996;113:143–51.

[102] Rees H, Sluka KA, Westlund KN, Willis WD. Do dorsal root reflexes augment peripheral inflammation? Neuroreport 1994;5:821–4.

[103] Rees H, Sluka KA, Westlund KN, Willis WD. The role of glutamate and GABA receptors in the generation of dorsal root reflexes by acute arthritis in the anaesthetized rat. J Physiol 1995;484:437–45.

[104] Ren K, Hylden JLK, Williams GM, Ruda MA, Dubner R. The effects of a non-competitive NMDA receptor antagonist, MK-801, on behavioral hyperalgesia and dorsal horn neuronal activity in rats with unilateral inflammation. Pain 1992;50:331–44.

[105] Ren K, Williams GM, Hylden JL, Ruda MA, Dubner R. The intrathecal administration of excitatory amino acid receptor antagonists selectively attenuated carrageenan-induced behavioral hyperalgesia in rats. Eur J Pharmacol 1992;219:235–43.

[106] Richardson BP, Engel G. The pharmacology and function of 5-HT3 receptors. Trends Neurosci 1986;9:424–8.

[107] Schaible HG, Grubb BD. Afferent and spinal mechanisms of joint pain. Pain 1993;55:5–54.

[108] Schaible H-G, Schmidt RF. Effects of an experimental arthritis on the sensory properties of fine articular afferent units. J Neurophysiol 1985;54:1109–22.

[109] Schaible HG, Schmidt RF. Direct observation of the sensitization of articular afferents during an experimental arthritis. In: Dubner R, Gebhart GF, Bond MR, editors. Proceedings of the 5th World Congress on Pain. Amsterdam: Elsevier; 1988. p. 44–50.

[110] Schaible HG, Schmidt RF. Excitation and sensitization of fine articular afferents from cat's knee joint by prostaglandin E2. J Physiol 1988;403:91–104.

[111] Schaible HG, Schmidt RF. Time course of mechanosensitivity changes in articular afferents during a developing experimental arthritis. J Neurophysiol 1988;60:2180–94.

[112] Schmidt RF, Schaible HG, Meslinger K, Hepplemann B, Hanesch U, Pawlak M. Silent and active nociceptors: structure, functions, and clinical implications. In: Gebhart GF, Hammond DL, Jensen TS, editors. Proceedings of the 7th World Congress on Pain; Progress in pain research and management, Vol. 2. Seattle: IASP Press; 1994. p. 213–250.

[113] Schmidt R, Schmelz M, Forster C, Ringkamp M, Torebjork E, Handwerker H. Novel classes of responsive and unresponsive C nociceptors in human skin. J Neurosci 1995;15:333–41.

[114] Shim B, Kim DW, Kim BH, Nam TS, Leem JW, Chung JM. Mechanical and heat sensitization of cutaneous nociceptors in rats with experimental peripheral neuropathy. Neuroscience 2005;132:193–201.

[115] Simone DA, Baumann TK, Lamotte RH. Dose dependent pain and mechanical hyperalgesia in humans after intradermal injection of capsaicin. Pain 1989;38:99–107.

[116] Simone DA, Sorkin LS, Oh U, Chung JM, Owens C, Lamotte RH, Willis WD. Neurogenic hyperalgesia: central neural correlates in responses of spinothalamic tract neurons. J Neurophysiol 1991;66:228–46.

[117] Skyba DA, Radhakrishnan R, Sluka KA. Characterization of a method for measuring primary hyperalgesia of deep somatic tissue. J Pain 2005;6:41–7.

[118] Sluka KA. Stimulation of deep somatic tissue with capsaicin produces long-lasting mechanical allodynia and heat hypoalgesia that depends on early activation of the cAMP pathway. J Neurosci 2002;22:5687–93.

[119] Sluka KA, Kalra A, Moore SA. Unilateral intramuscular injections of acidic saline produce a bilateral, long-lasting hyperalgesia. Muscle Nerve 2001;24:37–46.

[120] Sluka KA, Lawand NB, Westlund KN. Joint inflammation is reduced by dorsal rhizotomy and not by sympathectomy or spinal cord transection. Ann Rheum Dis 1994;53:309–14.

[121] Sluka KA, Price MP, Breese NM, Stucky CL, Wemmie JA, Welsh MJ. Chronic hyperalgesia induced by repeated acid injections in muscle is abolished by the loss of ASIC3, but not ASIC1. Pain 2003;106:229–39.

[122] Sluka KA, Radhakrishnan R, Benson CJ, Eshcol JO, Price MP, Babinski K, Audette KM, Yeomans DC, Wilson SP. ASIC3 in muscle mediates mechanical, but not heat, hyperalgesia associated with muscle inflammation. Pain 2007;129:102–12.

[123] Sluka KA, Radhakrishnan R, Price, MP, Welsh MJ. ASIC3 mediates mechanical hyperalgesia-induced by muscle injury. In: Brune K, Handwerker HO, editors. Hyperalgesia: molecular mechanisms and clinical implications; Progress in pain research and management, Vol. 30. Seattle: IASP Press; 2004. p. 105–11.

[124] Sluka KA, Rees H, Westlund KN, Willis WD. Fiber types contributing to dorsal root reflexes induced by joint inflammation in cats and monkeys. J Neurophysiol 1995;74:981–9.

[125] Sluka KA, Westlund KN. An experimental arthritis model in rats: the effects of NMDA and non-NMDA antagonists on aspartate and glutamate release in the dorsal horn. Neurosci Lett 1993;149:99–102.

[126] Sluka KA, Westlund KN. Centrally administered non-NMDA but not NMDA receptor antagonists block peripheral knee joint inflammation. Pain 1993;55:217–25.

[127] Sluka KA, Willis WD, Westlund KN. The role of dorsal root reflexes in neurogenic inflammation. Pain Forum 1995;4:141–9.

[128] Sommer C, Schmidt C, George A. Hyperalgesia in experimental neuropathy is dependent on the TNF receptor 1. Exp Neurol 1998;151:138–142.

[129] Sommer C, Schmidt C, George A, Toyka KV. A metalloprotease-inhibitor reduces pain associated behavior in mice with experimental neuropathy. Neurosci Lett 1997;237:45–8.

[130] Sorkin LS, Xiao WH, Wagner R, Myers RR. Tumour necrosis factor-alpha induces ectopic activity in nociceptive primary afferent fibres. Neuroscience 1997;81:255–62.

[131] Stein C. The control of pain in peripheral tissue by opioids. N Engl J Med 1995;332:1685–90.

[132] Stein C, Hassan AH, Przewlocki R, Gramsch C, Peter K, Herz A. Opioids from immunocytes interact with receptors on sensory nerves to inhibit nociception in inflammation. Proc Natl Acad Sci USA 1990;87:5935–9.

[133] Stein C, Millan MJ, Shippenberg TS, Peter K, Herz A. Peripheral opioid receptors mediating antinociception in inflammation. Evidence for involvement of mu, delta and kappa receptors. J Pharmacol Exp Ther 1989;248:1269–75.

[134] Svensson P, Cairns BE, Wang K, Hu JW, Graven-Nielsen T, Arendt-Nielsen L, Sessle BJ. Glutamate-evoked pain and mechanical allodynia in the human masseter muscle. Pain 2003;101:221–7.

[135] Tillu DV, Gebhart GF, Sluka KA. Descending facilitatory pathways from the RVM initiate and maintain bilateral hyperalgesia after muscle insult. Pain 2008;136:331–9.

[136] Vance CG, Radhakrishnan R, Skyba DA, Sluka KA. Transcutaneous electrical nerve stimulation at both high and low frequencies reduces primary hyperalgesia in rats with joint inflammation in a time-dependent manner. Phys Ther 2007;87:44–51.

[137] Watkins LR, Maier SF, Goehler LE. Immune activation: the role of pro-inflammatory cytokines in inflammation, illness responses and pathological pain states. Pain 1995;63:289–302.

[138] Watkins LR, Wiertelak EP, Goehler LE, Smith KP, Martin D, Maier SF. Characterization of cytokine-induced hyperalgesia. Brain Res 1994;654:15–26.

[139] Waxman SG, Dib-Hajj S, Cummins TR, Black JA. Sodium channels and their genes: dynamic expression in the normal nervous system, dysregulation in disease states. Brain Res 2000;886:5–14.

[140] Weng HR, Cordella JV, Dougherty PM. Changes in sensory processing in the spinal dorsal horn accompany vincristine-induced hyperalgesia and allodynia. Pain 2003;103:131–8.

[141] Westlund KN, Lu Y, Coggeshall RE, Willis WD. Serotonin is found in myelinated axons of the dorsolateral funiculus in monkeys. Neurosci Lett 1992;141:35–8.

[142] Westlund KN, Sun YC, Sluka KA, Dougherty PM, Sorkin LS, Willis WD. Neural changes in acute arthritis in monkeys .II. Increased glutamate immunoreactivity in the medial articular nerve. Brain Res Rev 1992;17:15–27.

[143] White DM, Helme RD. Release of substance P from peripheral nerve terminals following electrical stimulation of the sciatic nerve. Brain Res 1985;336:27–31.

[144] Willis WD Jr. Dorsal root potentials and dorsal root reflexes: a double-edged sword. Exp Brain Res 1999;124:395–421.

[145] Willis WD, Coggeshall RE. Sensory mechanisms of the spinal cord. New York: Springer, 2004.

[146] Witting N, Svensson P, Gottrup H, Arendt-Nielsen L, Jensen TS. Intramuscular and intradermal injection of capsaicin: a comparison of local and referred pain. Pain 2000;84:407–12.

[147] Wuarin-Bierman L, Zahnd GR, Kaufmann F, Burcklen L, Adler J. Hyperalgesia in spontaneous and experimental animal models of diabetic neuropathy. Diabetologia 1987;30:653–8.

[148] Yaksh TL, Bailey J, Roddy DR, Harty GJ. Peripheral release of substance P from primary afferents. In: Gebhardt GF, Bond MR, editors. Proceedings of the 5th World Congress on Pain. Amsterdam: Elsevier; 1988. p. 51–4.

[149] Yokoyama T, Audette KM, Sluka KA. Pregabalin reduces muscle and cutaneous hyperalgesia in two models of chronic muscle pain in rats. J Pain 2007;8:422–9.

[150] Zahn PK, Brennan TJ. Incision-induced changes in receptive field properties of rat dorsal horn neurons. Anesthesiol 1999;91:772–85.

Correspondence to: Kathleen A. Sluka, PT, PhD, Graduate Program in Physical Therapy and Rehabilitation Science, The University of Iowa, 1-252 Medical Education Building, Iowa City, IA 52242-1190, USA. Tel: 1-319-335-9791; fax 1-319-335-9707; email: kathleen-sluka@uiowa.edu.

Central Mechanisms Involved in Pain Processing

3

Kathleen A. Sluka

Graduate Program in Physical Therapy and Rehabilitation Science,
The University of Iowa, Iowa City, Iowa, USA

The processing of nociceptive information and pain in the central nervous system (CNS) is complex, involving multiple anatomical pathways and brain sites. These pathways include reflexive responses that are coordinated within the spinal cord, ascending nociceptive pathways, descending facilitatory pathways, and descending inhibitory pathways. All of these are interrelated and control the level of pain at a given time. Thus, pain processing is plastic and modifiable.

According to the classical "three-neuron system" described in neuroscience textbooks, the transmission of nociceptive and temperature information involves the primary afferent fiber (first neuron), the spinothalamic tract (STT) neuron (second neuron), and the thalamocortical neuron (third neuron) (Fig. 1). Regarding large-afferent sensation, this system involves the primary afferent fiber relaying information to the ipsilateral nucleus cuneatus and gracilis in the medulla (first neuron). Neurons in the nucleus cuneatus and gracilis transmit information to the contralateral ventroposterior lateral nucleus of the thalamus (second neuron) and then from the thalamus to the somatosensory cortex (third neuron). As

Mechanisms and Management of Pain for the Physical Therapist
edited by Kathleen A. Sluka
IASP Press, Seattle, © 2009

will become apparent, this three-neuron system is overly simplified for transmission of nociceptive information. This chapter will describe spinal, supraspinal, and cortical processing of nociceptive information.

Spinal Cord

The spinal cord is the first site of termination of nociceptors in the CNS and integrates incoming information from primary afferent fibers, local spinal neurons, and supraspinal sites. The spinal cord is anatomically divided into 10 laminae [117] that correlate with function. Laminae I to VI comprise the dorsal horn, where the majority of sensory afferents terminate. In general, the fine sensory fibers conveying noxious information

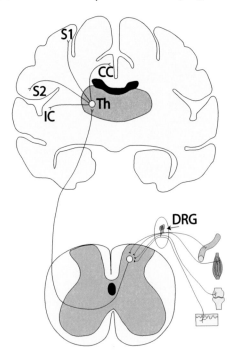

Fig. 1. Illustration of the convergence of nociceptive input from different tissue types in the periphery on dorsal horn neurons. Multiple tissue types (skin, muscles, joints, or viscera) can send input to the same dorsal horn neuron in the spinal cord. The nociceptive input is conveyed to a spinothalamic tract neuron in the dorsal horn that then conveys nociceptive information to the thalamus. From the thalamus, nociceptive information is conveyed to the cortex. CC = cingulate cortex; DRG = dorsal root ganglia; IC = insular cortex; Th = thalamus; S1 = primary somatosensory cortex; S2 = secondary somatosensory cortex.

from the skin terminate in the most superficial layers—laminae I, II, as well as laminae V. The terminals of larger fibers conveying tactile information are dispersed among laminae III and IV. Many of these fibers terminate on spinal interneurons that then relay information to cells deeper in the spinal cord. Primary afferent fibers from several peripheral structures (the skin, joints, muscles, and viscera) may converge on one neuron (Fig. 1). This convergence is thought to be the basis for referred pain.

The central projections from neurons innervating muscles and joints are distinctly different from those innervating the skin. Muscles and joints send nociceptive information predominantly to lamina I and the deeper dorsal horn, in contrast to those from cutaneous tissue, which have dense projections to lamina II [32,94,95,126].

Neurons in the dorsal horn of the spinal cord are classified as high-threshold, wide-dynamic-range (WDR), and low-threshold neurons. High-threshold neurons respond only to noxious stimulation, and low-threshold neurons respond only to innocuous stimuli, whereas WDR neurons respond to both noxious and innocuous stimuli. Thus, transmission of nociceptive information through the dorsal horn activates high-threshold and WDR neurons. Following tissue injury, sensitization of both high-threshold and WDR neurons occurs, termed *central sensitization.* This condition is manifested as an increase in receptive field size, increased responsiveness to innocuous or noxious stimuli, and/or decreased threshold to innocuous or noxious stimuli [68,71,105,128]. Unique to central neurons is an increased responsiveness to innocuous stimuli after tissue injury, which is probably the underlying basis for *allodynia,* a painful response to normally innocuous stimuli.

Enlargement of receptive fields occurs after tissue injury and can include the entire limb or even the contralateral hindlimb. For example, Schaible and colleagues showed that within hours after induction of joint inflammation by injection of kaolin and carrageenan, the receptive fields of spinal dorsal horn neurons enlarge to include the entire hindlimb [101,128] (Fig. 2). In a non-inflammatory model of muscle pain, the receptive fields enlarged to include the contralateral hindlimb (Fig. 2), which parallels the bilateral hyperalgesia observed in this model [144]. Interestingly, Mense and colleagues showed that within minutes, injection of the inflammatory irritant bradykinin outside a neuron's receptive field resulted in new receptive fields that included the site of injection, as well as additional sites [68] (Fig. 2). Thus, the expansion of receptive fields of central neurons is common and widespread, and it may explain the underlying referred and distant pain associated with deep-tissue injury.

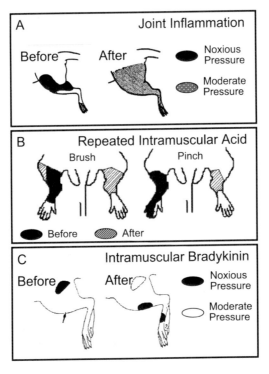

Fig. 2. Extracellular recordings from dorsal horn neurons before and after injury to deep tissue are increased. The receptive fields were assessed by application of stimuli to the periphery. (A) Receptive field changes in response to inflammation of the joint with kaolin and carrageenan. Prior to inflammation, noxious pressure applied to an area around the knee joint evoked activity in the dorsal horn neuron. After joint inflammation, moderate pressure evoked activity in the dorsal horn neuron across the entire hindlimb. Reproduced from [101] with permission of the American Physiological Society. (B) Responses of a wide-dynamic-range neuron to innocuous brushing of the skin and noxious pinching of the skin before (black) and after (diagonal hatching) the second injection of acidic saline into the gastrocnemius muscle. The receptive field increased ipsilaterally and spread to the contralateral limb after the second injection for the responses to both innocuous (brush) and noxious (pinch) stimuli applied to the skin. Reprinted from [144] with permission of IASP. (C) The receptive field of a dorsal horn neuron after intramuscular injection of bradykinin expanded to include the area of injection, as well as another area on the paw. In addition, the original receptive field showed a decreased threshold to activation, with moderate pressure now producing activity in the dorsal horn neuron. Reprinted from [68] with permission of Elsevier.

Sensitization of dorsal horn neurons, including STT neurons, to peripherally applied noxious and innocuous stimuli also occurs after tissue injury. Sensitization occurs not only in response to stimuli applied to the site of injury, but also after stimulation of uninjured tissue [40,101,128,178]. For example, recording from WDR neurons in the spinal cord, Schaible and colleagues reported a progressive increase in firing rate in response to compression of the knee joint or ankle after knee joint inflammation [101] (Fig. 3). Similarly, recordings from STT neurons show enhanced responsiveness to cutaneous noxious and innocuous stimuli after joint inflammation [40]. It should also be pointed out that changes occur not only in the dorsal horn neurons but also in motor neurons, as was shown in the original reports of central sensitization [178,179]. Further, electrical stimulation of muscle nociceptors produces a longer-lasting and more robust response of central neurons than does stimulation of cutaneous nociceptors [165].

Sensitization of dorsal horn neurons can be maintained by input from sensitized nociceptors. In this case, the goal of therapy is to reduce the input from peripherally sensitized nociceptors, which will decrease the sensitization of dorsal horn neurons and the consequent pain. However, central sensitization can be initiated by input from sensitized nociceptors and can persist in the absence of nociceptive input. For example, early studies showed that central sensitization and contralateral hyperalgesia induced by cutaneous insult continues after application of local anesthetics to the site of injury or deafferentation of the limb [26,27,181]. Similarly, the hyperalgesia associated with repeated intramuscular acid injections is independent of nociceptive input (which was abolished by dorsal rhizotomy or by local anesthetic injection into the muscle where the acid was injected) [142]. If the central sensitization predominates and remains after peripheral injury, treatments should focus on central mechanisms to reduce central sensitization.

Glial Cells and Pain

Glial cells in the CNS, particularly the spinal cord, play a critical role in the processing of nociceptive information (for review see [166,168]). Glia express receptors for many neurotransmitters, including glutamate receptors, and are involved in the clearance of neurotransmitters

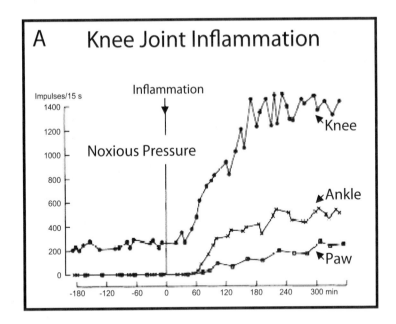

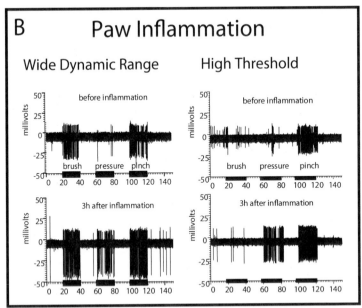

Fig. 3. (A) Extracellular recordings from dorsal horn neurons in response to noxious pressure of the knee, ankle, or paw before and after knee joint inflammation. After induction of knee joint inflammation (arrow), the dorsal horn neuron developed an increased response to noxious pressure applied to the knee and a new response to noxious pressure applied to the ankle and paw. Reproduced from [101] with permission of the

from the synaptic cleft. Activation of astrocytes and microglia occurs in a number of pain models, including neuropathic and inflammatory models [50,51,157]. Interestingly, glia release a variety of neuroactive substances known to sensitize neurons, such as glutamate, nitric oxide, and proinflammatory cytokines. Proinflammatory cytokines administered spinally produce nocifensive behaviors and sensitize dorsal horn neurons [35,115], and spinal blockade of proinflammatory cytokines reverses hyperalgesia [167] (Fig. 4).

Neurotransmitters of the Spinal Cord

For an extensive review of the neurotransmitters and receptors involved in nociceptive transmission in the spinal cord, see Willis and Coggeshall [174]. A schematic diagram showing the neurotransmitters and their receptors is shown in Fig. 4.

Glutamate. Glutamate mediates excitatory synaptic transmission between primary afferent nociceptors and dorsal horn neurons [130,131]. The role of spinal ionotropic glutamate receptors in hyperalgesia resulting from tissue injury has been well established [24]. In particular, N-methyl-D-aspartate (NMDA) glutamate receptors, calcium channels with a voltage-dependent Mg^{2+} block, are implicated in synaptic plasticity in a variety of systems including nociceptive transmission [25]. Spinal application of antagonists to NMDA glutamate receptors decreases hyperalgesia associated with hindpaw inflammation, joint inflammation, acid-induced muscle pain, formalin injection, and neuropathic pain models [13,28,93,116,138,148]. Blockade of spinal NMDA glutamate receptors prevents "wind-up" of both dorsal horn neurons and α-motor neurons resulting from repetitive conditioning stimuli of C-fiber strength [34,38,180]. Furthermore, the sensitization of dorsal horn neurons, including STT cells, that occurs after joint inflammation, formalin, capsaicin, or ultraviolet irradiation is prevented by NMDA-receptor antagonists [20,39,101].

American Physiological Society. (B) Recordings from a wide-dynamic-range neuron and a high-threshold neuron before and 3 hours after paw inflammation. Responses to innocuous brush and noxious pinch differentiated the two types of neurons. After paw inflammation there was an increase in response to all stimuli, innocuous brushing, moderate pressure, and noxious pinch for the wide-dynamic-range neuron. The high-threshold cell showed increases in moderate pressure and noxious pinch after paw inflammation. Reproduced from [90] with permission of Springer.

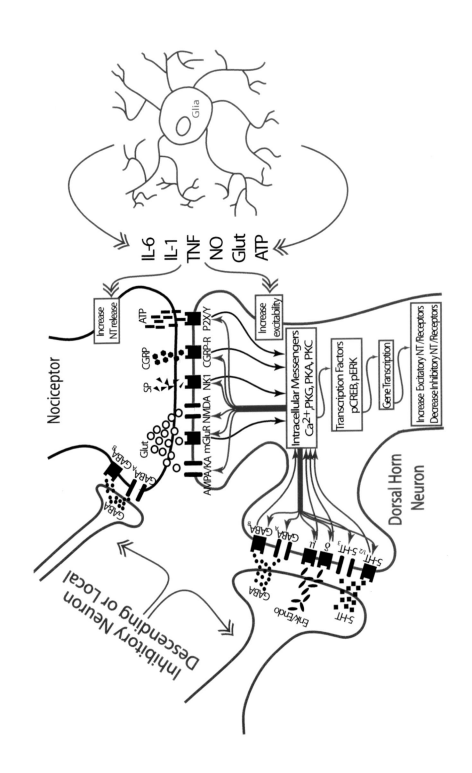

The non-NMDA ionotropic glutamate receptors—AMPA and kainite (AMPA/KA) receptors—form a complex with cation channels that allow passage of sodium ions, but some are also permeable to calcium, depending on subunit composition [70]. These AMPA/KA receptors are thought to mediate fast excitatory synaptic transmission between primary afferent fibers and dorsal horn neurons in response to noxious stimulation. Data are mixed on the role of AMPA/KA-receptor antagonists in the development and maintenance of hyperalgesia. AMPA/KA-receptor antagonists have no effect on hyperalgesia following carrageenan-induced paw inflammation, once developed [116,151]. In contrast, for knee joint inflammation, non-inflammatory muscle pain, peripheral neuropathy, and burn injury, hyperalgesia is reduced by spinal administration of AMPA/KA-receptor antagonists [93,138,141,148,151]. Lastly, Brennan and colleagues [185,186] showed that hyperalgesia associated with incision is preferentially reduced by AMPA/KA-receptor antagonists, but not by NMDA-glutamate receptor antagonists. Thus, several models and conditions are sensitive to AMPA/KA-receptor antagonists.

Although there are a number of selective NMDA-receptor antagonists, these agents cannot be used clinically because of adverse side effects. However, several clinically available drugs have NMDA-antagonist

← *Fig. 4.* Schematic representation of the dorsal horn. Glial cells can be activated by noxious stimuli and release inflammatory cytokines and neurotransmitters to act on the central terminals of nociceptors or dorsal horn neurons, increasing neurotransmitter release and excitability. Nociceptors release a number of neurotransmitters that act postsynaptically on their receptors to increase excitability. This increase in excitability can occur through activation of intracellular messengers that then phosphorylate cell surface receptors, or through phosphorylation of transcription factors. Phosphorylation of receptors can cause increased excitability or decreased inhibition to result in central sensitization. Changes in gene transcription can increase the production of excitatory neurotransmitters and receptors or decrease the production of inhibitory neurotransmitters and receptors, which would be manifested as central sensitization. Either local or descending inhibitory control can occur both presynaptically on nociceptors and postsynaptically on dorsal horn neurons and can again produce its effects directly on membrane currents, through phosphorylation of receptors, or through activation or inhibition of gene transcription. AMPA/KA = non-NMDA glutamate receptors; ATP = adenosine triphosphate; CGRP = calcitonin gene-related peptide; GABA = gamma-aminobutyric acid; Enk/Endo = Enkephalin/Endomorphin; Glut = glutamate; IL-1 = interleukin-1; IL-6 = interleukin-6; mGluR = metabotropic glutamate receptors; NK1 = neurokinin-1 receptor; NMDA = N-methyl-D-aspartate; NO = nitric oxide; SP = substance P; TNF-α = tumor necrosis factor alpha; NT = neurotransmitter; pCREB =; phosphorylated cAMP responsive element binding protein; pERK = phosphorylated extracellular signal-related kinases; PKA = protein kinase A; PKC = protein kinase C; PKG = protein kinase G.

activity, including ketamine, dextromethorphan, and memantine. These drugs are not selective antagonists but block the NMDA receptor non-competitively (see [171]). Clinically, Bell [9] showed in three case studies that low doses of the NMDA antagonist ketamine prevents the development of analgesic tolerance to opioids.

Neuropeptides. The neuropeptides substance P and calcitonin gene-related peptide (CGRP) are found in the central terminals of primary afferent fibers and are densely located in laminae I and II (for review see [97]). Substance P exerts its effects through activation of the neurokinin 1 (NK1) receptor in the superficial dorsal horn. Activation of the NK1 receptor produces nocifensive behaviors [172], increases the activity and responsiveness of dorsal horn neurons [111], and potentiates the NMDA glutamate receptor [41]. In contrast, blockade of neurokinin receptors reduces hyperalgesia associated with tissue injury and reduces sensitization of dorsal horn neurons [49,103,112,143,183]. Loss of NK1-containing neurons in the spinal cord similarly reduces hyperalgesia and sensitization of dorsal horn neurons following tissue injury [75,156]. Similarly, CGRP antagonists reduce sensitization of dorsal horn neurons [102]. In addition, CGRP slows the degradation of substance P in the spinal cord [127], resulting in a potentiation of the effects of substance P. Interactions between receptors can also potentiate responses. For example, spinal application of substance P in combination with CGRP greatly enhances the effects of either neuropeptide alone [177].

Adenosine. Adenosine is a neurotransmitter located in the dorsal horn of the spinal cord that exerts inhibitory actions through the A1 receptor. Spinal administration of adenosine, A1-receptor agonists, or drugs aimed at reducing the degradation of adenosine are analgesic and reduce hyperalgesia in inflammatory and neuropathic pain conditions [72,84,106,124,125]. In human subjects, modulation of adenosine in the spinal cord reduces neuropathic pain [44].

GABA. Gamma-aminobutyric acid (GABA) is an inhibitory neurotransmitter located in neuronal cells bodies of the dorsal horn. It exerts its actions through activation of the ionotropic receptor, $GABA_A$, and the metabotropic receptor, $GABA_B$. There is an upregulation of GABA following peripheral inflammation and a decrease in GABA following peripheral neuropathy [5,18], and activation of GABAergic receptors in the spinal cord reduces hyperalgesia and causes analgesia [61,155]. One potential mechanism that may contribute to hyperalgesia is a reduction in GABAergic inhibition. For example, STT cells show a reduced responsiveness to GABA agonists after induction of inflammation with capsaicin [88]. Clinically, several muscle relaxants (such as baclofen and benzodiazepines) exert their effects through activation of GABA receptors.

Intracellular messengers. Neurotransmitters acting on ionotropic receptors can increase calcium influx to activate calcium/calmodulin-dependent kinases and adenylate cyclases. Activation of G-protein-coupled receptors by various neurotransmitters leads to either activation or inhibition of second-messenger pathways, which in turn initiates or inhibits cellular events. Protein kinases mediate intracellular processes through the phosphorylation of receptors, cellular proteins, or transcription factors (Fig. 4). Phosphorylation of intracellular receptor proteins enhances the transport of these receptors to the cell membrane, thus making the cell more sensitive to ligands, whereas phosphorylation of transcription factors can initiate gene transcription and subsequently increase expression of nociception-related proteins.

In the spinal cord, activation of protein kinase A (PKA) or PKC produces mechanical hyperalgesia, sensitizes STT neurons, and phosphorylates transcription factors to enhance gene production [66,88,89,96,139,140,146,149]. Furthermore, blockade of PKA or PKC pathways in the spinal cord reverses mechanical hyperalgesia and dorsal horn neuron sensitization associated with deep tissue inflammation, repeated acid injections, or neuropathic pain [66,92,139,191,192]. Interestingly, PKC phosphorylates ionotropic channels, such as the NMDA and AMPA/KA receptors, which enhance glutamate-evoked currents on dorsal horn neurons [19]. This phosphorylation by PKC removes the Mg^{2+} block in the NMDA-receptor pore to increase the probability of the channel opening [22]. Thus, increased phosphorylation of glutamate receptors could enhance synaptic activity, resulting in increased excitation of nociceptive dorsal horn neurons.

Alternatively, activation of intracellular messengers can phosphorylate inhibitory neurotransmitter receptors to result in a decrease in efficacy of inhibitory neurotransmitters. For example, PKC reverses μ-opioid receptor inhibition in the spinal dorsal horn of rats, leading to decreased µ-opioid-receptor-mediated antinociception. PKC also decreases the ability of the inhibitory neurotransmitter GABA to inhibit STT cells [88]. Injection of capsaicin reduces the inhibition of STT neurons normally produced by electrical stimulation of the periaqueductal gray (PAG); this loss of inhibition is prevented by spinal blockade of PKC [87]. Thus, increased PKC activity reduces normal inhibition within the spinal cord, resulting in an overall increase in excitation.

Serotonin, norepinephrine, and opioids. Serotonin and norepinephrine (noradrenaline) are neurotransmitters found in descending projections from the brainstem, and endogenous opioids are also located in areas of descending inhibition (see the section below on descending inhibition).

Ascending Pathways

From the spinal cord, sensory information is conveyed to the brain by projection neurons that receive inputs from afferents directly, or indirectly through interneurons. Several ascending pathways transmit nociceptive information from somatic and visceral tissue [174,175]. The spinothalamic tract is the main pathway for transmission of nociceptive information (relayed through the thalamus) to higher centers involved in cortical processing and ultimately in the perception of pain (Fig. 1). The postsynaptic dorsal column pathway transmits nociceptive visceral stimuli to higher centers. The spinomesencephalic and spinoreticular pathways serve to integrate nociceptive information with areas involved in descending inhibition, descending facilitation, and autonomic responses associated with pain.

Spinothalamic Tract

The pathway considered by many to be most important for the transmission of nociceptive information, the STT, transmits information to neurons in the ventroposterior lateral (VPL) nucleus and medial thalamic nuclei, which include the central lateral, central medial, parafascicular, and medial dorsal nuclei and the posterior complex of the thalamus. The VPL projects to the primary (S1) and secondary (S2) somatosensory cortex, and this pathway is thought to be involved in the *sensory-discriminative* component of pain (i.e., its location, duration, quality, and intensity).

Neurons in the VPL receive convergent input from the dorsal column pathway that transmits information regarding touch sensation and from the STT conveying information regarding pain and temperature sensation [74,174,175]. The ascending projections from the medial thalamic nuclei and the posterior complex are more diffuse and include areas such as the anterior cingulate and insular cortices. This pathway is thought to be the basis for the *motivational-affective* component of pain (i.e., its unpleasantness).

Spinothalamic tract cells originate primarily in laminae I and V, with the majority crossing the midline to ascend in the contralateral anterolateral funiculus [174]. The STT cells from lamina I project via the lateral and dorsolateral funiculi to the medial thalamic nuclei. These cells respond almost exclusively to noxious thermal and mechanical stimuli and may play an important role in thermal nociception [31]. It has also been suggested that this pathway may be responsible for activating the body's own control systems to limit pain [114,164,175]. Several investigators support a role for WDR STT cells, particularly those in lamina V, which respond to both nociceptive and mechanoreceptive stimuli [176]. Sensitization of WDR neurons to innocuous mechanical stimuli may underlie allodynia, a painful response to an innocuous stimulus.

Spinomesencephalic and Spinoreticular Tracts

Cells of the spinomesencephalic tract originate in laminae I, IV, and V and send projections to the midbrain, particularly the PAG, the nucleus cuneiformis, and the pretectal nucleus [174,175]. These neurons are classified as high-threshold and WDR and have complex receptive fields. The projection to the PAG probably activates descending modulatory systems. The cells of origin of the spinoreticular pathways are located in the deep dorsal horn, laminae VII and VIII, and project to brainstem areas known to be involved in descending facilitation and inhibition of nociception. These nuclei include the nucleus gigantocellularis, nucleus paragigantocellularis lateralis, ventrolateral medulla, and parabrachial region. These neurons are nociceptive specific and are proposed to activate the endogenous analgesia system and signal homeostatic changes to brainstem autonomic centers.

Thalamus and Cortex

A number of studies show the importance of the thalamus and cortex in processing nociceptive transmission. These include studies recording and stimulating neurons in the human thalamus, recordings from thalamic and cortical neurons in animal models of pain, and imaging studies [58,59,67,81,113]. Stimulation of the principal sensory nucleus of the thalamus in humans can produce pain sensations, and thalamic neurons in humans respond to noxious thermal or mechanical stimuli [81]. Thus, the thalamus appears to integrate information regarding peripheral noxious stimuli. Recordings from neurons in animals show that nociceptive information is processed in the VPL of the thalamus as well as the somatosensory cortex, insular cortex, and anterior cingulate cortex [58,59]. Neurons in these thalamic and cortical areas become sensitized following inflammatory or neuropathic tissue injury.

Central processing of pain in humans has been assessed with imaging techniques, such as magnetic resonance imaging (MRI) and positron emission tomography (PET), that look at cerebral blood flow changes following specific stimuli. There is enhanced blood flow to an area with increased neuronal activity. These data indicate that the cortical regions most reliably activated by painful stimuli are S1 and S2 and the anterior cingulate cortex [29,67,113]. Bushnell and colleagues have elegantly examined the role of the somatosensory, cingulate, and insular cortices by using hypnotic suggestions to modulate the sensory-discriminative or motivational-affective component of pain [67,113]. These studies showed distinct brain sites for these two dimension of pain. Specifically, the primary and secondary somatosensory cortices are involved in discrimination and localization of a painful stimulus, i.e., the sensory-discriminative component, and the anterior insular and cingulate cortices mediate the unpleasantness of pain, i.e., the motivational-affective component.

Descending Modulation of Pain

Descending modulation of nociceptive information occurs through several nuclei, including the PAG, the rostral ventromedial medulla (RVM), and the lateral pontine tegmentum (Fig. 5). These sites were initially found to inhibit nociception through projections either directly or indirectly to the spinal cord [48,98]. Later studies showed a role for these structures in descending facilitation of nociception [108]. Anatomically, the PAG sends projections to the RVM and the lateral pontine tegmentum, but not directly to the spinal cord. The RVM and lateral pontine tegmentum then project to the spinal cord and modulate dorsal horn neuron activity and ultimately nociceptive information. It is generally thought that there is a balance between facilitation and inhibition from these descending

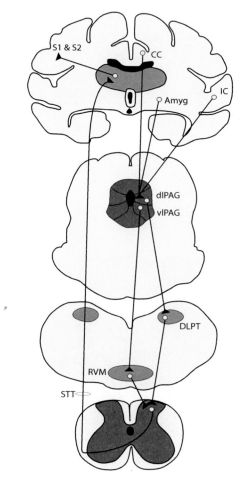

Fig. 5. Schematic representation of the descending inhibitory and facilitatory pathways and the spinothalamic tract. Amyg = amygdala; CC = cingulate cortex; dlPAG = dorsolateral periaqueductal gray; DLPT = dorsolateral pontine tegmentum; IC = insular cortex; RVM = rostroventromedial medulla; S1 and S2 = somatosensory cortex 1 and 2; STT = spinothalamic tract; vlPAG = ventrolateral periaqueductal gray.

modulatory pathways. This balance shifts after tissue injury in a time-dependent manner to result in a net output manifested as either increased facilitation or increased inhibition.

Descending Facilitation of Pain

Supraspinal centers can enhance nociception, resulting in referred pain, secondary hyperalgesia, and "mirror-image" or contralateral hyperalgesia [108]. Inactivation of the RVM completely blocks secondary hyperalgesia produced by knee joint inflammation, repeated acid injections, pancreatitis, or neuropathic injury [12,30,158,159,161,162]. Interestingly, these manipulations in the RVM do not affect the primary hyperalgesia produced by carrageenan injected into the plantar paw [161]. Similar to the findings observed for the spinal cord, increased glutamate release, phosphorylation of NMDA glutamate receptors, and increased numbers of NMDA glutamate receptors occur in the RVM after tissue injury [57,60,110,158,188]. More rostrally, the PAG, pontine nuclei, amygdala, and anterior cingulate cortex also play a role in descending facilitation [15,37,69,100]. The facilitation by many of these nuclei is most likely mediated through the RVM. Thus, supraspinal centers play a major role in the production and maintenance of hyperalgesia.

Descending Inhibition of Pain

The central inhibitory control of pain was initially discovered by Reynolds [118], who found that electrical stimulation of the *periaqueductal gray* (PAG) in the midbrain produces analgesia in rats. Early work focused primarily on two sites—the midbrain PAG and a site in the ventral medulla, the *nucleus raphe magnus* (NRM). Subsequent studies show that other nuclei in the *rostral ventromedial medulla* (RVM) are similarly involved in descending modulation of nociceptive information. These nuclei include the NRM, nucleus reticularis gigantocellularis pars alpha, and nucleus reticularis paragigantocellularis lateralis [7,48,65] (Fig. 5). Electrical or chemical stimulation of either the PAG or the RVM causes analgesia in rats, cats, and humans [42,46,52,85,118], and inhibits spinal neurons that respond to noxious stimuli [1,46,65,82,86,121,189]. The PAG does not project directly to the spinal cord, but rather projects to the RVM [16]. The RVM in turn projects to the spinal cord through axons running in the dorsolateral funiculus. Efferent projections from the RVM to the spinal cord are involved in inhibition of nociception, and some of the projections contain serotonin [74,137].

In addition to the PAG and RVM, other nuclei in the brain also inhibit pain and nociception when activated. These include the anterior pretectal nucleus, locus ceruleus/A7 cell groups, hypothalamus, somatosensory cortex, thalamus, red nucleus, medial habenula, parabrachial region, hypothalamus, prefrontal cortex, amygdala, reticulospinal tract, and rubrospinal tract [33,36,56,63,65,100,119,134,145,175]. Most of these sites relay either directly or indirectly through the RVM, which serves as the final common pathway to the spinal cord.

Three types of neurons located in the RVM play a role in descending nociceptive modulation, as described in rat studies using noxious heat applied to the tail: (1) ON cells, which increase their firing rate just before or at the time of tail flick; (2) OFF cells, which decrease their firing rate just before or at the time of tail flick; and (3) neutral cells, which do not respond consistently to noxious heat applied to the tail (Fig. 6) [47,65]. OFF cells are thought to be involved in descending inhibition, whereas ON cells are thought to be involved in descending facilitation of nociceptive information. Morphine, a μ-opioid agonist, excites OFF cells and reduces nocifensive behaviors when applied directly to neurons in the RVM or the PAG, or when administered systemically. Conversely, morphine or deltorphin, a δ-opioid agonist, will suppress ON-cell firing, thus attenuating nociceptive responsiveness (Fig. 6) [62,65]. Thus, activation of opioid receptors increases activity of OFF cells and decreases activity of ON cells to ultimately produce analgesia by increasing inhibition and decreasing excitation from the RVM.

The dorsolateral pontine tegmentum (DLPT) sends projections to the spinal cord primarily from the locus ceruleus and nucleus subceruleus. The DLPT uses norepinephrine as its neurotransmitter, and it is the primary source of norepinephrine in the spinal cord. Chemical or electrical stimulation of these nuclei causes antinociception, reduces hyperalgesia, and decreases activity in spinal neurons [73,83,160,187]. Norepinephrine may inhibit or facilitate nociceptive stimuli, depending on the activation of specific adrenergic receptors in the spinal cord (see the neurotransmitter section below).

In addition to receiving nociceptive input for the discrimination of pain, the somatosensory cortex also sends fibers that inhibit nociceptive transmission, either directly to the spinal cord via the corticospinal tract, or indirectly through the thalamus or PAG. Stimulation of the somatosensory cortex inhibits STT neurons [135,184] and causes primary afferent depolarization, resulting in presynaptic inhibition [17].

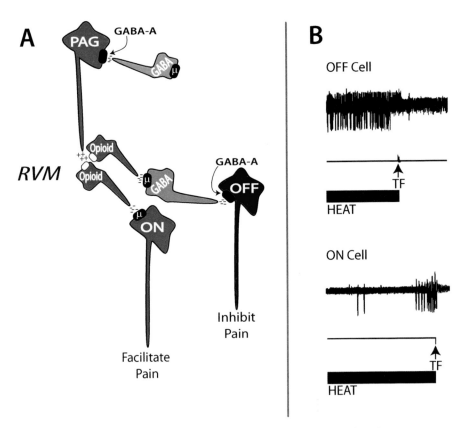

Fig. 6. (A) Schematic diagram of cells in the periaqueductal gray (PAG) and rostroventromedial medulla (RVM). Activation of OFF cells is thought to inhibit pain, while activation of ON cells is thought to facilitate pain. Projections from the PAG excite opioid cells in the RVM that activate μ-opioid receptors on ON cells, which inhibits these cells, thus decreasing facilitation. Some ON cells are GABAergic and tonically inhibit OFF cells. Activation of μ-opioid receptors on these GABAergic ON cells can then reduce the GABAergic inhibition of OFF cells, resulting in increased activity in OFF cells that would inhibit pain. (B) Representative recording of OFF cells and ON cells in response to noxious heat applied to the tail. The OFF cells stops firing in response to noxious heat, as measured by the tail flick (TF). The ON cell begins to fire immediately prior to the tail flick in response to noxious heat. Reprinted from [48], with permission from Elsevier.

Lesioning of the corticospinal tract blocks the primary afferent depolarization produced by stimulation of the somatosensory cortex, demonstrating that presynaptic inhibition of the central terminals of primary afferent fibers is mediated by activation of the corticospinal tract [17]. Thus, stimulation of the corticospinal tract (as with exercise) may reduce nociceptive input through the inhibition of spinal neurons or primary afferent fibers. Clinically, recent studies show that activation of the motor cortex with transcranial stimulation reduces pain in patients with neuropathic pain [80].

Diffuse noxious inhibitory controls (DNIC) is a term used to describe an innate pain modulatory system in which the application of noxious stimuli induces generalized analgesia. DNIC can be demonstrated experimentally by the application of painful stimuli to an extrasegmental site, which produces analgesia at the test site. For example, application of a noxious stimulus (heat or cold) to the arm increases the pressure pain threshold of the leg in normal subjects [163]. Activation of DNIC pathways reduces hyperalgesia and pain in both animals and human subjects, and it also reduces dorsal horn neuron activity [163]. The analgesia produced by DNIC is non-opioid and involves pathways outside the PAG-RVM pathway [163]. By mechanisms that are not fully understood, the subnucleus reticularis dorsalis in the medulla appears to mediate the analgesia produced by activating DNIC pathways [163]. Studies in people with chronic pain show less efficient DNIC, i.e., decreased inhibition to a noxious stimuli, in conditions such as temporomandibular disorder, chronic low back pain, fibromyalgia, osteoarthritis, chronic tension-type headache, and irritable bowel syndrome [11,76,77,79,107,122,173].

Neurotransmitters of Descending Systems

Opioids. After peripheral inflammation, in animals and human subjects, there is an upregulation of opioid receptors on the peripheral terminals of primary afferent fibers [91,153,154]. Additionally, macrophages, monocytes, and lymphocytes all contain opioid peptides, and the amount of endogenous opioid peptides in these cells increases in inflamed tissues [91,153]. Thus, there appears to be a peripheral endogenous mechanism to reduce pain in inflamed tissues. Opioid agonists, such as morphine, could produce their actions through activation of peripheral opioid receptors.

Opioid analgesia has been extensively studied in endogenous pain control mechanisms. The endogenous opioids include β-endorphins, methionine (met)- and leucine (leu)-enkephalin, endomorphin 1 and 2, and dynorphin A and B [48]. Each has a distinct anatomical distribution and activates specific receptors. There are three types of opioid receptors: μ, δ, and κ. Beta-endorphin and endomorphins activate μ-opioid receptors, the enkephalins activate δ-opioid receptors, and dynorphins activate κ-opioid receptors. Beta-endorphin is found in hypothalamic neurons and in the anterior and intermediate lobes of the pituitary [48]. Neurons located in the hypothalamus send β-endorphin-containing projections to the PAG and can "turn on" the endogenous analgesia system [170]. Release of β-endorphin from the pituitary occurs with exercise and stress, and there is an increase in measurable levels in the bloodstream [64,129,133]. Beta-endorphin does not readily cross the blood-brain barrier, and thus its role in stress-induced or exercise-induced analgesia is not known. However, one could postulate that β-endorphin in the bloodstream produces its analgesic effects peripherally by activating μ-opioid receptors on nociceptors, which are upregulated after tissue injury, to reduce peripheral sensitization.

Enkephalins, endomorphins, and dynorphins and their receptors are located in neurons in the brain and dorsal horn in areas known to be involved in analgesia such as the PAG, RVM, and the dorsal horn of the spinal cord [48,98]. Activation of opioid receptors with selective agonists, systemically or locally in the PAG, RVM, or spinal cord, produces analgesia and reduces hyperalgesia in a number of pain models including inflammatory pain, acid-induced muscle pain, and neuropathic pain [48,98,147,182].

Most of the clinically available opioids produce their effects through activation of μ-opioid receptors. Differences in effectiveness are based on potency of the drug. Clinically available opioids include morphine, codeine, tramadol, oxycodone, levorphanol, methadone, hydromorphone, buprenorphine, and fentanyl. Long-term clinical use of opioids is limited by the development of tolerance to their analgesic effects [132].

Serotonin. Serotonin is a neurotransmitter that is found in the RVM in neurons that send projections to the spinal cord, and in PAG neurons that project to the RVM [6,8,10]. Application of serotonin to the spinal cord decreases the activity of dorsal horn neurons and produces analgesia [98]. Thus, it appears that the PAG pathway produces analgesia using serotonin as its neurotransmitter in the spinal cord.

In the spinal cord, multiple families of serotonin receptors are present (5-HT_1, 5-HT_2, 5HT_3, 5-HT_4, 5-HT_5, 5-HT_6, and 5-HT_7) and have been extensively reviewed [98]. The role of individual serotonin receptors and receptor subtypes in nociceptive transmission is controversial, because 5-HT receptors have been implicated in both facilitation and inhibition of nociception. 5-HT_3 receptors, located on primary afferent fibers and dorsal horn neurons, are involved in descending inhibition from stimulation of the RVM, but not in descending facilitation [2,53]. 5-HT_{1A} receptors, on the other hand, are not found on primary afferent fibers; they mediate descending facilitation as well as inhibition [3,14,43]. 5-HT_2 receptors include a number of subtypes that appear to be involved in inhibition, but not in facilitation, of nociceptive responses [150].

Norepinephrine. Norepinephrine terminals in the spinal cord arise primarily from the DLPT [23,98]. Spinally, norepinephrine inhibits nociceptive stimuli through activation of α_2-adrenergic receptors [55,78,109]. On the other hand, activation of spinal dorsal horn α_1-adrenergic receptors mediates descending facilitation of nociception [104]. Thus, norepinephrine is involved in descending facilitatory and inhibitory nociceptive signaling, depending on receptor activation.

Tricyclic antidepressants, dual reuptake inhibitors, and selective serotonin reuptake inhibitors (SSRIs) are commonly used for chronic pain conditions. These inhibitors can be nonselective (amitryptiline, imipramine), exerting their effects by decreasing reuptake of norepinephrine and serotonin, or selective (fluoxetine, paroxetine, ritanserin, clomipramine), acting by decreasing reuptake of serotonin. A decrease in reuptake would result in greater neurotransmitter availability and increased inhibition of nociceptive information. Tricyclic antidepressants and SSRIs enhance antinociception and pain reduction in animals and humans [120,136,169]. Further, 5-HT_1 agonists such as sumatriptan, zolmitriptan, naratriptan, and rizatriptan are effective for treating migraine [54,99].

Potential Mechanisms of Central Sensitization

Sensitization of dorsal horn neurons can occur through multiple mechanisms, including those resulting in increased excitation or decreased inhibition. Short-term sensitization can result from increased release of excitatory neurotransmitters such as glutamate or substance P that consequently activate their receptor, depolarizing the neuron. Alternatively, decreased release of inhibitory neurotransmitters may also occur, which would result in an overall increase in excitability of nociceptive neurons. More long-term effects can occur through phosphorylation of receptors. For example, PKC phosphorylates the NMDA receptor to remove the magnesium block, resulting in a greater response to its agonist glutamate [21]. On the other hand, phosphorylation of GABA receptors results in a loss of inhibitory effect by GABA on STT cells [88]. Lastly, increased gene transcription could result in more long-term effects that include production of more excitatory neurotransmitters or receptors. Indeed, increased phosphorylation of transcription factors, increased activation of transcription factors, and an increased number of glutamate receptors occur in the spinal cord after tissue injury [45,66,96,190].

Correlation of Neuronal Changes with Pain Measures

Mechanisms underlying various pain types are distinctly different (see Table I). *Primary hyperalgesia* is thought to reflect increased sensitivity of nociceptors to noxious input, i.e., peripheral sensitization. Although sensitization occurs in the CNS within minutes after tissue injury, and central neurons show an enhanced response to application of noxious stimuli to the injured tissue, this central sensitization most likely reflects the increased activity of the nociceptors. However, repetitive electrical stimulation of C fibers with the same intensity of stimulation, in animals without tissue injury, results in a progressively increasing activity of dorsal horn neurons, termed "wind-up" [34]. Assessment of *temporal summation* in human subjects is thought to reflect wind-up of dorsal horn neurons and is used experimentally to assess the sensitivity of the CNS. Temporal summation is manifested as progressively increasing pain to

Table I
Behavioral responses and proposed mechanisms

Behavioral Manifestation	Definition	Proposed Site of Change	Proposed Mechanism of Change	Comments
Primary hyperalgesia	Increased pain sensitivity at the site of injury	PNS: nociceptors	Peripheral sensitization	Can manifest as decreased threshold to a noxious stimulus, or as increased pain to a suprathreshold stimulus
Referred pain	Spontaneous pain outside the area injury	CNS	Convergence-projection theory	Pain is perceived outside the area of injury; the term should not be used to describe increased sensitivity to painful stimuli (which is termed *hyperalgesia*)
Secondary hyperalgesia	Increased sensitivity outside the site of injury	CNS	Central sensitization to noxious stimuli	May involve changes in the nociceptive pathway anywhere from the spinal cord to the cortex
Allodynia	Painful response to non-nociceptive stimuli	CNS	Central sensitization to innocuous stimuli	This term should only be used when it is known that the test stimulus does not activate a nociceptor
Temporal summation	Progressively increasing pain to the same stimulus administered repetitively or over a long duration	CNS	Wind-up of dorsal horn neurons	This is an assessment used in clinical pain studies to analyze the sensitivity of the CNS
Pain	An unpleasant sensory and emotional experience associated with actual or potential tissue damage, or described in terms of such damage	CNS	N/A	Pain is a cortical evaluation of the response to noxious stimuli; i.e., pain only occurs when processed by the cortex

Abbreviations: CNS = central nervous system; PNS = peripheral nervous system.

repeated application of the same painful stimulus. Several pain conditions, including temporomandibular disorder, fibromyalgia, and tension-type headache, show enhanced temporal summation when compared to controls [4,123,152].

Referred pain is spontaneous pain felt outside the site of tissue injury. It is not evoked by noxious or innocuous stimuli, as is observed in hyperalgesia or allodynia. The *convergence-projection theory* is used to describe the mechanisms underlying referred pain. At the spinal level, neurons receive input from cutaneous as well as deep tissue such as muscles, joints, or viscera. The increased activity that results from injury to deep tissue is transmitted to the cortex, where it is misinterpreted as pain from the skin or another structure.

Secondary hyperalgesia could result from sensitization of dorsal horn neurons that occurs after tissue injury. Since central neurons have relatively large receptive fields that greatly expand after tissue injury, the increased response to noxious stimuli applied outside the site of injury is sent supraspinally. Alternatively, or in conjunction, activation of facilitatory pathways from supraspinal sites can result in enlarged receptive fields and increased sensitivity of dorsal horn neurons to noxious stimuli applied outside the area of injury. Thus, the cortex interprets this increased input as pain in response to noxious stimuli outside the area of injury, i.e., secondary hyperalgesia. *Allodynia* most likely results from the increased responsiveness of STT neurons to innocuous stimuli. Under normal conditions, the response to innocuous stimuli of WDR neurons does not reach the threshold for pain perception. However, after tissue injury, the responses to innocuous stimuli are increased and reach a threshold that is interpreted in the brain as pain.

References

[1] Aimone LD, Jones SL, Gebhart GF. Stimulation-produced descending inhibition from the periaqueductal gray and nucleus raphe magnus in the rat: mediation by spinal monoamines but not opioids. Pain 1987;31:123–36.
[2] Alhaider AA, Lei SZ, Wilcox GL. Spinal 5HT$_3$ receptor-mediated antinociception: possible release of GABA. J Neurosci 1991;11:1881–8.
[3] Alhaider AA, Wilcox GL. Differential roles of 5-hydroxytryptamine1A and 5-hydroxytryptamine1B receptor subtypes in modulating spinal nociceptive transmission in mice. J Pharmacol Exp Ther 1993;265:378–85.
[4] Ashina S, Bendtsen L, Ashina M, Magerl W, Jensen R. Generalized hyperalgesia in patients with chronic tension-type headache. Cephalalgia 2006;26:940–8.

[5] Baba H, Ji RR, Kohno T, Moore KA, Ataka T, Wakai A, Okamoto M, Woolf CJ. Removal of GABAergic inhibition facilitates polysynaptic A fiber-mediated excitatory transmission to the superficial spinal dorsal horn. Mol Cell Neurosci 2003;24:818–30.

[6] Basbaum AI. Descending control of pain transmission: possible serotonergic-enkephalinergic interactions. Adv Exp Med Biol 1981;133:177–89.

[7] Basbaum AI, Fields HL. The origin of descending pathways in the dorsolateral funiculus of the spinal cord of the cat and rat: further studies on the anatomy of pain modulation. J Comp Neurol 1979;187:513–32.

[8] Beitz AJ. The sites of origin of brainstem neurotensin and serotonin projections to the rodent nucleus raphe magnus. J Neurosci 1982;2:829–42.

[9] Bell RF. Low-dose subcutaneous ketamine infusion and morphine tolerance. Pain 1999;83:101–3.

[10] Bowker RM, Westlund KN, Coulter JD. Origins of serotonergic projections to the lumbar spinal cord in the monkey using a combined retrograde transport and immunocytochemical technique. Brain Res Bull 1982;9:271–8.

[11] Bragdon EE, Light KC, Costello NL, Sigurdsson A, Bunting S, Bhalang K, Maixner W. Group differences in pain modulation: pain-free women compared to pain-free men and to women with TMD. Pain 2002;96:227–37.

[12] Burgess SE, Gardell LR, Ossipov MH, Malan TP, Vanderah TW, Lai J, Porreca F. Time-dependent descending facilitation from the rostral ventromedial medulla maintains, but does not initiate, neuropathic pain. J Neurosci 2002;22:5129–36.

[13] Calcutt NA, Chaplan SR. Spinal pharmacology of tactile allodynia in diabetic rats. Br J Pharmacol 1997;122:1478–82.

[14] Calejesan AA, Chang MHC, Zhuo M. Spinal serotonergic receptors mediate facilitation of a nociceptive reflex by subcutaneous formalin injection into the hindpaw in rats. Brain Res 1998;798:46–54.

[15] Calejesan AA, Kim SJ, Zhuo M. Descending facilitatory modulation of a behavioral nociceptive response by stimulation in the adult rat anterior cingulate cortex. Eur J Pain 2000;4:83–96.

[16] Cameron AA, Khan IA, Westlund KN, Willis WD. The efferent projections of the periaqueductal gray in the rat: a *Phaseolus vulgaris*-leucoagglutinin study. II. Descending projections. J Comp Neurol 1995;351:585–601.

[17] Carpenter D, Lundberg A, Norrsell U. Primary afferent depolarization evoked from the sensorimotor cortex. Acta Physiol Scand 1963;59:126–42.

[18] Castro-Lopes JM, Tavares I, Tolle TR, Coito A, Coimbra A. Increase in GABAergic cells and GABA levels in the spinal-cord in unilateral inflammation of the hindlimb in the rat. Eur J Neurosci 1992;4:296–301.

[19] Cerne R, Jiang M, Randic M. Cyclic adenosine 3'5'-monophosphate potentiates excitatory amino acid and synaptic responses of rat spinal dorsal horn neurons. Brain Res 1992;596:111–23.

[20] Chapman V, Dickenson AH. Time-related roles of excitatory amino acid receptors during persistent noxiously evoked responses of rat dorsal horn neurones. Brain Res 1995;703:45–50.

[21] Chen L, Huang LYM. Sustained potentiation of NMDA-receptor-mediated glutamate responses through activation of protein kinase C by a μ-opioid. Neuron 1991;7:319–26.

[22] Chen L, Huang LYM. Protein-kinase-C reduces Mg^{2+} block of NMDA-receptor channels as a mechanism of modulation. Nature 1992;356:521–3.

[23] Clark FM, Proudfit HK. The projection of locus coeruleus neurons to the spinal cord in the rat determined by anterograde tracing combined with immunocytochemistry. Brain Res 1991;538:231–45.

[24] Coderre TJ, Fisher K, Fundytus ME. The role of ionotropic and metabotropic glutamate receptors in persistent nociception. In: Jensen TJ, Turner JA, Wiesenfeld-Hallin Z, editors. Proceedings of the 8th World Congress on Pain. Seattle: IASP Press; 1997. p. 259–75.

[25] Coderre TJ, Katz J, Vaccarino AL, Melzack R. Contribution of central neuroplasticity to pathological pain: review of clinical and experimental evidence. Pain 1993;52:259–85.

[26] Coderre TJ, Melzack R. Increased pain sensitivity following heat injury involves a central mechanism. Behav Brain Res 1985;15:259–62.

[27] Coderre TJ, Melzack R. Cutaneous hyperalgesia: contributions of the peripheral and central nervous systems to the increase in pain sensitivity after injury. Brain Res 1987;404:95–106.

[28] Coderre TJ, Melzack R. The role of NMDA receptor-operated calcium channels in persistent nociception after formalin-induced tissue injury. J Neurosci 1992;12:3671–5.

[29] Coghill RC, Talbot JD, Evans AC, Meyer E, Gjedde A, Bushnell MC, Duncan GH. Distributed processing of pain and vibration by the human brain. J Neurosci 1994;14:4095–108.

[30] Coutinho SV, Urban MO, Gebhart GF. Role of glutamate receptors and nitric oxide in the rostral ventromedial medulla in visceral hyperalgesia. Pain 1998;78:59–69.

[31] Craig AD, Bushnell MC, Zhang E-T, Blomqvist A. A thalamic nucleus specific for pain and temperature sensation. Nature 1994;372:770–-3.

[32] Craig AD, Hepplemann B, Schaible H-G. The projection of the medial and posterior articular nerves of the cat's knee to the spinal cord. J Comp Neurol 1988;276:279–88.

[33] Dafny N, Dong WQ, Prieto-Gomez C, Reyes-Vazquez C, Stanford J, Qiao JT. Lateral hypothalamus: site involved in pain modulation. Neuroscience 1996;70:449–60.

[34] Davies SN, Lodge D. Evidence for involvement of N-methylaspartate receptors in 'wind-up' of class 2 neurons in the dorsal horn of the rat. Brain Res 1987;424:402–6.

[35] DeLeo JA, Colburn RW, Nichols M, Malhotra A. Interleukin-6-mediated hyperalgesia/allodynia and increased spinal IL-6 expression in a rat mononeuropathy model. J Interferon Cytokine Res 1996;16:695–700.

[36] Desalles AF, Katayama Y, Becker MP, Hayes RL. Pain suppression induced by electrical stimulation of the pontine parabrachial region. J Neurosurg 1985;62:397–407.

[37] Desantana JM, Sluka KA. Blockade of the ventrolateral PAG prevents the effects of TENS. Neuroscience 2009; in press.

[38] Dickenson AH, Sullivan AF. Subcutaneous formalin-induced activity of dorsal horn neurones in the rat: differential response to an intrathecal opiate administered pre or post formalin. Pain 1987;30:349–60.

[39] Dougherty PM, Palecek J, Paleckova V, Sorkin LS, Willis WD. The role of NMDA and non-NMDA excitatory amino-acid receptors in the excitation of primate spinothalamic tract neurons by mechanical, chemical, thermal, and electrical stimuli. J Neurosci 1992;12:3025–41.

[40] Dougherty PM, Sluka KA, Sorkin LS, Westlund KN, Willis WD. Neural changes in acute arthritis in monkeys. I. Parallel enhancement of responses of spinothalamic tract neurons to mechanical stimulation and excitatory amino acids. Brain Res Rev 1992; 17:1-13.

[41] Dougherty PM, Willis WD. Enhancement of spinothalamic neuron responses to chemical and mechanical stimuli following combined micro-iontophoretic application of N-methyl-D-aspartic acid and substance-P. Pain 1991;47:85–93.

[42] Dubuisson D, Melzack R. Analgesic brain stimulation in the cat: effect of intraventricular serotonin, norepinephrine, and dopamine. Exp Neurol 1977;57:1059–66.

[43] Eide PK, Joly NM, Hole K. The role of spinal cord5-HT1A and 5-HT1B receptors in the modulation of a spinal nociceptive reflex. Brain Res 1990;536:195–200.

[44] Eisenach JC, Rauck RL, Curry R. Intrathecal, but not intravenous adenosine reduces allodynia in patients with neuropathic pain. Pain 2003;105:65–70.

[45] Fang L, Wu J, Lin Q, Willis WD. Protein kinases regulate the phosphorylation of the GluR1 subunit of AMPA receptors of spinal cord in rats following noxious stimulation. Mol Brain Res 2003;118:160–5.

[46] Fardin V, Oliveras JL, Besson JM. A reinvestigation of the analgesic effects induced by stimulation of the periaqueductal gray matter in the rat. II. Differential characteristics of the analgesia induced by ventral and dorsal PAG stimulation. Brain Res 1984;306:125–39.

[47] Fields HL, Basbaum AI. Central nervous system mechanisms of pain modulation. In: Wall PD, Melzack R, editors. Textbook of pain. New York: Churchill Livingstone; 1999. p. 243–57.

[48] Fields HL, Basbaum AI, Heinricher MM. Central nervous system mechanisms of pain modulation. In: McMahon SB, Koltzenburg M, editors. Textbook of pain. Philadelphia: Elsevier; 2006. p. 125–42.

[49] Fleetwood-Walker SM, Mitchell R, Hope PJ, El-Yassir N, Molony V, Bladon CM. The involvement of neurokinin receptor subtypes in somatosensory processing in the superficial dorsal horn of the cat. Brain Res 1990;519:169–82.

[50] Fu KY, Light AR, Matsushima GK, Maixner W. Microglial reactions after subcutaneous formalin injection into the rat hind paw. Brain Res 1999;825:59–67.

[51] Garrison CJ, Dougherty PM, Kajander KC, Carlton SM. Staining of glial fibrillary acidic protein (GFAP) in lumbar spinal cord increases following a sciatic nerve constriction injury. Brain Res 1991;565:1–7.

[52] Gebhart GF, Sandkuhler J, Thalhammer JG, Zimmermann M. Quantitative comparison of inhibition in spinal cord nociceptive information by stimulation in periaqueductal gray or nucleus raphe magnus of the cat. J Neurophysiol 1983;50:1433–45.

[53] Glaum SR, Proudfit HK, Anderson EG. 5-HT3 receptors modulate spinal nociceptive reflexes. Brain Res 1990;510:12–6.

[54] Goadsby PJ. Primary neurovascular headache. In: McMahon SB, Koltzenburg M, editors. Textbook of pain. Philadelphia: Elsevier; 2006. p. 851–74.

[55] Goldin SM, Subbarao K, Sharma R, Knapp AG, Fischer JB, Daly D, Durant GJ, Reddy NL, Hu L-Y, Magar S, et al. Neuroprotective use-dependent blockers of Na$^+$ and Ca^{2+} channels controlling presynaptic release of glutamate. Ann NY Acad Sci 1997;210–29.

[56] Gray BG, Dostrovsky JO. Red nucleus modulation of somatosensory responses of cat spinal cord dorsal horn neurons. Brain Res 1984;311:171–5.

[57] Guan Y, Guo W, Zou SP, Dubner R, Ren K. Inflammation-induced upregulation of AMPA receptor subunit expression in brain stem pain modulatory circuitry. Pain 2003;104:401–13.

[58] Guilbaud G, Benoist JM, Condes-Lara M, Gautron M. Further evidence for the involvement of SmI cortical neurons in nociception: their responsiveness at 24 hr after carrageenin-induced hyperalgesic inflammation in the rat. Somatosens Motor Res 1993;10:229–44.

[59] Guilbaud G, Kayser V, Benoist JM, Gautron M. Modifications in the responsiveness of rat ventrobasal thalamic neurons at different stages of carrageenin-produced inflammation. Brain Res 1986;385:86–98.

[60] Guo W, Zou S, Guan Y, Ikeda T, Tal M, Dubner R, Ren K. Tyrosine phosphorylation of the NR2B subunit of the NMDA receptor in the spinal cord during the development and maintenance of inflammatory hyperalgesia. J Neurosci 2002;22:6208–17.

[61] Hammond DL, Drower EJ. Effects of intrathecally administered THIP, baclofen, and muscimol on nociceptive threshold. Eur J Pharmacol 1984;103:121–5.

[62] Harasawa I, Fields HL, Meng ID. Delta opioid receptor mediated actions in the rostral ventromedial medulla on tail flick latency and nociceptive modulatory neurons. Pain 2000;85:255–62.

[63] Hardy SG. Analgesia elicited by prefrontal stimulation. Brain Res 1985;339:281–4.

[64] Harte JL, Eifert GH, Smith R. The effects of running and meditation on beta-endorphin, corticotropin-releasing hormone and cortisol in plasma, and on mood. Biol Psychol 1995;40:251–65.

[65] Heinricher MM. Organizational characteristics of supraspinally mediated responses to nociceptive input. In: Yaksh TL, editor. Anesthesia: biologic foundations. Philadelphia: Lippincott-Raven; 1997.

[66] Hoeger-Bement MK, Sluka KA. Phosphorylation of CREB and mechanical hyperalgesia is reversed by blockade of the cAMP pathway in a time-dependent manner after repeated intramuscular acid injections. J Neurosci 2003;23:5437–45.

[67] Hofbauer RK, Rainville P, Duncan GH, Bushnell MC. Cortical representation of the sensory dimension of pain. J Neurophysiol 2001;86:402–11.

[68] Hoheisel U, Mense S, Simons DG, Yu X-M. Appearance of new receptive fields in rat dorsal horn neurons following noxious stimulation of skeletal muscle: a model for referral of muscle pain? Neurosci Lett 1993;153:9–12.

[69] Holden JE, Schwartz EJ, Proudfit HK. Microinjection of morphine in the A7 catecholamine cell group produces opposing effects on nociception that are mediated by alpha-1 and alpha2-adrenoceptors. Neuroscience 1999;91:979–90.

[70] Hollmann M, Hartley M, Heinemann S. Ca2+ permeability of KA-AMPA-gated glutamate receptor channels depends on subunit composition. Science 1991;252:851–3.

[71] Hylden JLK, Nahin RL, Traub RJ, Dubner R. Expansion of receptive fields of spinal lamina I projection neurons in rats with unilateral adjuvant-induced inflammation: the contribution of dorsal horn mechanisms. Pain 1989;37:229–43.

[72] Jarvis MF, Mikusa J, Chu KL, Wismer CT, Honore P, Kowaluk EA, McGaraughty S. Comparison of the ability of adenosine kinase inhibitors and adenosine receptor agonists to attenuate thermal hyperalgesia and reduce motor performance in rats. Pharmacol Biochem Behav 2002;73:573–81.

[73] Jones SL, Gebhart GF. Spinal pathways mediating tonic, coeruleospinal, and raphe-spinal descending inhibition in the rat. J Neurophysiol 1987; 58:138-159.

[74] Jones SL, Light AR. Serotoninergic medullary raphespinal projection to the lumbar spinal-cord in the rat: a retrograde immunohistochemical study. J Comp Neurol 1992;322:599–610.

[75] Khasabov SG, Rogers SD, Ghilardi JR, Peters CM, Mantyh PW, Simone DA. Spinal neurons that possess the substance P receptor are required for the development of central sensitization. J Neurosci 2002;22:9086–98.

[76] Kosek E, Hansson P. Modulatory influence on somatosensory perception from vibration and heterotopic noxious conditioning stimulation (HNCS) in fibromyalgia patients and healthy subjects. Pain 1997;70:41–51.

[77] Kosek E, Ordeberg G. Lack of pressure pain modulation by heterotopic noxious conditioning stimulation in patients with painful osteoarthritis before, but not following, surgical pain relief. Pain 2000;88:69–78.

[78] Kuraishi Y, Hirota N, Sato Y, Satou M, Takagi H. Noradrenergic inhibition of the release of substance P from primary afferents in the rabbit spinal cord dorsal horn. Brain Res 1985;359:177–82.

[79] Lautenbacher S, Rollman GB. Possible deficiencies of pain modulation in fibromyalgia. Clin J Pain 1997;13:189–96.

[80] Lefaucheur JP, Drouot X, Menard-Lefaucheur I, Keravel Y, Nguyen JP. Motor cortex rTMS restores defective intracortical inhibition in chronic neuropathic pain. Neurology 2006;67:1568–74.

[81] Lenz FA, Lee JI, Garonzik IM, Rowland LH, Dougherty PM, Hua SE. Plasticity of pain-related neuronal activity in the human thalamus. Prog Brain Res 2000;129:259–73.

[82] Lewis VA, Gebhart GF. Morphine-induced and stimulation-produced analgesias at coincident periaqueductal central gray loci: evaluation of analgesic congruence, tolerance and cross-tolerance. Exp Neurol 1977;57:934–55.

[83] Li W, Zhao ZQ. Yohimbine reduces inhibition of lamina X neurones by stimulation of the locus coeruleus. Neuroreport 1993;4:751–3.

[84] Li X, Conklin D, Pan HL, Eisenach JC. Allosteric adenosine receptor modulation reduces hypersensitivity following peripheral inflammation by a central mechanism. J Pharmacol Exp Ther 2003;305:950–5.

[85] Liebeskind JC, Guilbaud G, Besson JM, Oliveras JL. Analgesia from electrical stimulation of periaqueductal grey matter in the cat: Behavioral observations and inhibitory effects on spinal cord interneurons. Brain Res 1973;50:441–6.

[86] Light AR, Casale EJ, Menetrey DM. The effects of focal stimulation in nucleus raphe magnus and periaqueductal gray on intracellularly recorded neurones in spinal lamina I and II. J Neurophysiol 1986;56:555–71.

[87] Lin Q, Peng YB, Willis WD. The inhibition of primate spinothalamic tract neurons produced by stimulation in periaqueductal gray is reduced by spinal bicuculline. Neurosci Abstracts 1994;20.1725.

[88] Lin Q, Peng YB, Willis WD. Inhibition of primate spinothalamic tract neurons by spinal glycine and GABA is reduced during central sensitization. J Neurophysiol 1996;76:1005–14.

[89] Lin Q, Peng YB, Willis WD. Possible role of protein kinase C in the sensitization of primate spinothalamic tract neurons. J Neurosci 1996;16:3026–34.

[90] Ma YT, Sluka KA. Reduction in inflammation-induced sensitization of dorsal horn neurons by transcutaneous electrical nerve stimulation in anesthetized rats. Exp Brain Res 2001;137:94–102.

[91] Machelska H, Stein C. Leukocyte-derived opioid peptides and inhibition of pain. J Neuroimmune Pharmacol 2006;1:90–7.

[92] Malmberg AB, Chen C, Tonegawa S, Basbaum AI. Preserved acute pain and reduced neuropathic pain in mice lacking PKCgamma. Science 1997;278:279–83.

[93] Mao J, Price DD, Hayes RL, Lu J, Mayer DJ. Differential roles of NMDA and non-NMDA receptor activation in induction and maintenance of thermal hyperalgesia in rats with painful peripheral mononeuropathy. Brain Res 1992;598:271–88.

[94] Mense S. Nociception from skeletal muscle in relation to clinical muscle pain. Pain 1993;54:241–89.

[95] Mense S, Craig AD. Spinal and supraspinal terminations of primary afferent fibers from the gastrocnemius-soleus muscle in the cat. Neuroscience 1988;26:1023–35.

[96] Miletic G, Pankratz MT, Miletic V. Increases in the phosphorylation of cyclic AMP response element binding protein (CREB) and decreases in the content of calcineurin accompany thermal hyperalgesia following chronic constriction injury in rats. Pain 2002;99:493–500.

[97] Millan MJ. The induction of pain: an integrative review. Prog Neurobiol 1999;57:1–164.

[98] Millan MJ. Descending control of pain. Prog Neurobiol 2002;66:355–474.

[99] Munglani R, Hill RG. Other drugs including sympathetic blockers. In: Wall PD, Melzack R, editors. Textbook of pain. New York: Churchill Livingstone; 1999. p. 1233–50.

[100] Neugebauer V, Li W. Differential sensitization of amygdala neurons to afferent inputs in a model of arthritic pain. J Neurophysiol 2003;89:716–27.

[101] Neugebauer V, Lucke T, Schaible HG. N-methyl-D-aspartate (NMDA) and non-NMDA receptor antagonists block the hyperexcitability of dorsal horn neurons during development of acute arthritis in rats knee joint. J Neurophysiol 1993;70:1365–77.

[102] Neugebauer V, Ruemenapp P, Schaible H-G. Calcitonin gene-related peptide is involved in the spinal processing of mechanosensory input from the rat's knee joint and in the generation and maintenance of hyperexcitability of dorsal horn neurons during development of acute inflammation. Neurosci 1996;71:1095–109.

[103] Neugebauer V, Weiretter F, Schaible H-G. Involvement of substance P and neurokinin-1 receptors in the hyperexcitability of dorsal horn neurons during development of acute arthritis in rat's knee joint. J Neurophysiol 1995; 73:1574–83.

[104] Nuseir K, Proudfit HK. Bidirectional modulation of nociception by GABA neurons in the dorsolateral pontine tegmentum that tonically inhibit spinally projecting noradrenergic A7 neurons. Neurosci 2000;96:773–83.

[105] Palecek J, Dougherty PM, Kim SH, Paleckova V, Lekan H, Chung JM, Carlton SM, Willis WD. Responses of spinothalamic tract neurons to mechanical and thermal stimuli in an experimental model of peripheral neuropathy in primates. J Neurophysiol 1992;68:1951–65.

[106] Pan HL, Xu Z, Leung E, Eisenach JC. Allosteric adenosine modulation to reduce allodynia. Anesthesiol 2001;95:416–20.

[107] Peters ML, Schmidt AJ, Van den Hout MA, Koopmans R, Sluijter ME. Chronic back pain, acute postoperative pain and the activation of diffuse noxious inhibitory controls (DNIC). Pain 1992;50:177–87.

[108] Porreca F, Ossipov MH, Gebhart GF. Chronic pain and medullary descending facilitation. Trends Neurosci 2002;25:319–25.

[109] Proudfit HK. Pharmacologic evidence for the modulation of nociception by noradrenergic neurons. Prog Brain Res 1988;77:357–70.

[110] Radhakrishnan R, Sluka KA. Increased glutamate and decreased glycine release in the rostroventromedial medulla during induction of a preclinical model of chronic widespread muscle pain. Neurosci Lett 2009; in press.

[111] Radhakrishnan V, Henry JL. Novel substance P antagonist, CP-96345, blocks responses of cat spinal dorsal horn neurons to noxious cutaneous stimulation and substance P. Neurosci Lett 1991;132:39–43.

[112] Radhakrishnan V, Henry JL. Antagonism of nociceptive responses of cat spinal dorsal horn neurons in vivo by the NK-1 receptor antagonists CP-96,345 and CP-99,994, but not by CP-96,344. Neuroscience 1995;64:943–58.

[113] Rainville P, Duncan GH, Price DD, Carrier B, Bushnell MC. Pain affect encoded in human anterior cingulate but not somatosensory cortex. Science 1997;277:968–71.

[114] Rees H, Roberts MHT. The anterior pretectal nucleus: a proposed role in sensory processing. Pain 1993;53:121–35.

[115] Reeve AJ, Patel S, Fox A, Walker K, Urban L. Intrathecally administered endotoxin or cytokines produce allodynia, hyperalgesia and changes in spinal cord neuronal responses to nociceptive stimuli in the rat. Eur J Pain 2000;4:247–57.

[116] Ren K, Williams GM, Hylden JLK, Ruda MA, Dubner R. The intrathecal administration of excitatory amino-acid receptor antagonists selectively attenuated carrageenan-induced behavioral hyperalgesia in rats. Eur J Pharmacol 1992;219:235–43.

[117] Rexed B. The cytoarchitectonic organization of the spinal cord in the rat. J Comp Neurol 1952;96:415–66.

[118] Reynolds DV. Surgery in the electrical analgesia induced by focal brain stimulation. Science 1969;164:444–5.

[119] Roberts MHT, Rees H. The antinociceptive effects of stimulating the pretectal nucleus of the rat. Pain 1986;25:83–93.

[120] Rosland JH, Hunskaar S, Hole K. Modification of the antinociceptive effect of morphine by acute and chronic administration of clomipramine in mice. Pain 1988;33:349–55.

[121] Rossi GC, Pasternak GW, Bodnar RJ. Mu and delta opioid synergy between the periaqueductal gray and the rostroventral medulla. Brain Res 1994;665:85–93.

[122] Sandrini G, Rossi P, Milanov I, Serrao M, Cecchini AP, Nappi G. Abnormal modulatory influence of diffuse noxious inhibitory controls in migraine and chronic tension-type headache patients. Cephalalgia 2006;26:782–9.

[123] Sarlani E, Garrett PH, Grace EG, Greenspan JD. Temporal summation of pain characterizes women but not men with temporomandibular disorders. J Orofac Pain 2007;21:309–17.

[124] Sawynok J, Reid A, Nance D. Spinal antinociception by adenosine analogs and morphine after intrathecal administration of the neurotoxins capsaicin, 6-hydroxydopamine and 5,7-dihydroxytryptamine. J Pharmacol Exp Ther 1991;258:370–80.

K.A. Sluka

[125] Sawynok J, Sweeney MI, White TD. Classification of adenosine receptors mediating antinociception in the rat spinal cord. Br J Pharmacol 1986;88:923–30.
[126] Schaible HG, Grubb BD. Afferent and spinal mechanisms of joint pain. Pain 1993;55:5–54.
[127] Schaible HG, Hope PJ, Lang CW, Duggan AW. Calcitonin gene-related peptide causes intraspinal spreading of substance P released by peripheral stimulation. Eur J Neurosci 1992;4:750–7.
[128] Schaible HG, Schmidt RF, Willis WD. Enhancement of the responses of ascending tract cells in the cat spinal cord by acute inflammation of the knee joint. Exp Brain Res 1987;66:489–99.
[129] Schedlowski M, Fluge T, Richter S, Tewes U, Schmidt RE, Wagner TO. Beta-endorphin, but not substance-P, is increased by acute stress in humans. Psychoneuroendocrinology 1995;20:103–10.
[130] Schneider SP, Perl ER. Selective excitation of neurons in the mammalian spinal dorsal horn by aspartate and glutamate in vitro: correlation with location and synaptic input. Brain Res 1985;360:339–43.
[131] Schneider SP, Perl ER. Comparison of primary afferent and glutamate excitation of neurons in the mammalian spinal dorsal horn. J Neurosci 1988;8:2062–73.
[132] Schug SA, Gandham N. Opioids: clinical use. In: McMahon SB, Koltzenburg M, editors. Textbook of pain. Philadelphia: Elsevier; 2006. p. 443–57.
[133] Schwarz L, Kindermann W. Changes in beta-endorphin levels in response to aerobic and anaerobic exercise. Sports Med 1992;13:25–36.
[134] Segal M, Sandberg D. Analgesia produced by electrical stimulation of catecholamine nuclei in the rat brain. Brain Res 1977;123:369–72.
[135] Senapati AK, Huntington PJ, LaGraize SC, Wilson HD, Fuchs PN, Peng YB. Electrical stimulation of the primary somatosensory cortex inhibits spinal dorsal horn neuron activity. Brain Res 2005;1057:134–40.
[136] Singh VP, Jain NK, Kulkarni SK. On the antinociceptive effect of fluoxetine, a selective serotonin reuptake inhibitor. Brain Res 2001;915:218–26.
[137] Skagerberg G, Bjorklund A. Topographic principles in the spinal projections of serotonergic and non-serotonergic brainstem neurons in the rat. Neuroscience 1985;15:445–80.
[138] Skyba DA, King EW, Sluka KA. Effects of NMDA and non-NMDA ionotropic glutamate receptor antagonists on the development and maintenance of hyperalgesia induced by repeated intramuscular injection of acidic saline. Pain 2002;98:69–78.
[139] Sluka KA. Stimulation of deep somatic tissue with capsaicin produces long-lasting mechanical allodynia and heat hypoalgesia that depends on early activation of the cAMP pathway. J Neurosci 2002;22:5687–93.
[140] Sluka KA, Audette KM. Activation of protein kinase C in the spinal cord produces mechanical hyperalgesia by activating glutamate receptors, but does not mediate chronic muscle-induced hyperalgesia. Mol Pain 2006;2:13.
[141] Sluka KA, Jordan HH, Westlund KN. Reduction in joint swelling and hyperalgesia following post-treatment with a non-NMDA glutamate receptor antagonist. Pain 1994;59:95–100.
[142] Sluka KA, Kalra A, Moore SA. Unilateral intramuscular injections of acidic saline produce a bilateral, long-lasting hyperalgesia. Muscle Nerve 2001;24:37–46.
[143] Sluka KA, Milton MA, Westlund KN, Willis WD. Differential roles of neurokinin 1 and neurokinin 2 receptors in the development and maintenance of heat hyperalgesia induced by acute inflammation. Br J Pharmacol 1997;120:1263–73.
[144] Sluka KA, Price MP, Wemmie JA, Welsh MJ. ASIC3, but not ASIC1, channels are involved in the development of chronic muscle pain. In: Dostrovsky JO, Carr DB, Koltzenburg M, editors. Proceedings of the 10th World Congress on Pain. Seattle: IASP Press; 2003. p. 71–9.
[145] Sluka KA, Rees H. The neuronal response to pain. Physiother Theory Pract 1997;13:3–22.
[146] Sluka KA, Rees H, Chen PS, Tsuruoka M, Willis WD. Inhibitors of G-proteins and protein kinases reduce the sensitization of spinothalamic tract neurons following intradermal injection of capsaicin in the primate. Exp Brain Res 1997;115:15–24.
[147] Sluka KA, Rohlwing JJ, Bussey RA, Eikenberry SA, Wilken JM. Chronic muscle pain induced by repeated acid injection is reversed by spinally administered μ and δ, but not κ, opioid receptor agonists. J Pharmacol Exp Ther 2002; 302:1146–50.
[148] Sluka KA, Westlund KN. Centrally administered non-NMDA but not NMDA receptor antagonists block peripheral knee joint inflammation. Pain 1993;55:217–25.
[149] Sluka KA, Willis WD. The effects of G-protein and protein kinase inhibitors on the behavioral responses of rats to intradermal injection of capsaicin. Pain 1997;71:165–78.

[150] Solomon RE, Gebhart GF. Mechanisms of effects of intrathecal serotonin on nociception and blood pressure in rats. J Pharmacol Exp Ther 1988;245:905–12.

[151] Sorkin LS, Yaksh TL, Doom CM. Pain models display differential sensitivity to Ca^{2+}-permeable non-NMDA glutamate receptor antagonists. Anesthesiology 2001;95:965–73.

[152] Staud R, Vierck CJ, Mauderli A, Cannon R. Abnormal temporal summation of second pain (wind-up) in patients with the fibromyalgia syndrome. Arthritis Rheum 1998;41:S353.

[153] Stein C. The control of pain in peripheral tissue by opioids. N Engl J Med 1995;332:1685–90.

[154] Stein C, Hassan AH, Przewlocki R, Gramsch C, Peter K, Herz A. Opioids from immunocytes interact with receptors on sensory nerves to inhibit nociception in inflammation. Proc Natl Acad Sci USA 1990;87:5935–9.

[155] Stewart PE, Hammond DL. Activation of spinal delta-1 or delta-2 opioid receptors reduces carrageenan-induced hyperalgesia in the rat. J Pharmacol Exp Ther 1994;268:701–8.

[156] Suzuki R, Morcuende S, Webber M, Hunt SP, Dickenson AH. Superficial NK1-expressing neurons control spinal excitability through activation of descending pathways. Nat Neurosci 2002;5:1319–26.

[157] Sweitzer SM, Colburn RW, Rutkowski M, DeLeo JA. Acute peripheral inflammation induces moderate glial activation and spinal IL-1beta expression that correlates with pain behavior in the rat. Brain Res 1999;829:209–21.

[158] Terayama R, Guan Y, Dubner R, Ren K. Activity-induced plasticity in brain stem pain modulatory circuitry after inflammation. Neuroreport 2000;11:1915–9.

[159] Tillu DV, Gebhart GF, Sluka KA. Descending facilitatory pathways from the RVM initiate and maintain bilateral hyperalgesia after muscle insult. Pain 2008;136:331–9.

[160] Tsuruoka M, Willis WD. Descending modulation from the region of the locus coeruleus on nociceptive sensitivity in a rat model of inflammatory hyperalgesia. Brain Res 1996;743:86–92.

[161] Urban MO, Zahn PK, Gebhart GF. Descending facilitatory influences from the rostral medial medulla mediate secondary, but not primary hyperalgesia in the rat. Neuroscience 1999;90:349–52.

[162] Vera-Portocarrero LP, Xie JY, Kowal J, Ossipov MH, King T, Porreca F. Descending facilitation from the rostral ventromedial medulla maintains visceral pain in rats with experimental pancreatitis. Gastroenterology 2006;130:2155–64.

[163] Villanueva L, Le BD. The activation of bulbo-spinal controls by peripheral nociceptive inputs: diffuse noxious inhibitory controls. Biol Res 1995;28:113–25.

[164] Wall PD. The biological function and dysfunction of different pain mechanisms. In: Sicuteri F, editor. Advances in pain research and therapy, Vol. 20. New York: Raven Press; 1992. p. 19–28.

[165] Wall PD, Woolf CJ. Muscle but not cutaneous C-afferent input produces prolonged increases in the excitability of the flexion reflex in the rat. J Physiol 1984;356:443–58.

[166] Watkins LR, Maier SF. Beyond neurons: evidence that immune and glial cells contribute to pathological pain states. Physiol Rev 2002;82:981–1011.

[167] Watkins LR, Martin D, Ulrich P, Tracey KJ, Maier SF. Evidence for the involvement of spinal cord glia in subcutaneous formalin induced hyperalgesia in the rat. Pain 1997;71:225–35.

[168] Watkins LR, Milligan ED, Maier SF. Glial activation: a driving force for pathological pain. Trends Neurosci 2001; 24:450–5.

[169] Watson CPN, Chipman ML, Monks RC. Antidepressant analgesics: a systematic review and comparative study. In: McMahon SB, Koltzenburg M, editors. Textbook of Pain. Philadelphia: Elsevier; 2006. p. 481–97.

[170] Watson SJ, Akil H. alpha-MSH in rat brain: occurrence within and outside of beta-endorphin neurons. Brain Res 1980; 182:217–23.

[171] Wiesenfeld-Hallin Z. Combined opioid-NMDA antagonist therapies. What advantages do they offer for the control of pain syndromes? Drugs 1998;55:1–4.

[172] Wilcox GL. Pharmacological studies of grooming and scratching behavior elicited by spinal substance P and excitatory amino acids. Ann NY Acad Sci 1988;525:228–36.

[173] Wilder-Smith CH, Schindler D, Lovblad K, Redmond SM, Nirkko A. Brain functional magnetic resonance imaging of rectal pain and activation of endogenous inhibitory mechanisms in irritable bowel syndrome patient subgroups and healthy controls. Gut 2004;53:1595–601.

[174] Willis WD, Coggeshall RE. Sensory mechanisms of the spinal cord. New York: Springer; 2004.

[175] Willis WD, Westlund KN. Neuroanatomy of the pain system and of the pathways that modulate pain. J Clin Neurophysiol 1997;14:2–31.

[176] Willis WD, Zhang X, Honda CN, Giesler GJ. A critical review of the role of the proposed VMpo nucleus in pain. J Pain 2002;3:79–94.

K.A. Sluka

[177] Woolf C, Wiesenfeld-Hallin Z. Substance P and calcitonin gene-related peptide synergistically modulate the gain of the nociceptive flexor withdrawal reflex in the rat. Neurosci Lett 1986;66:226–30.

[178] Woolf CJ. Evidence for a central component of post-injury pain hypersensitivity. Nature 1983;306:686–8.

[179] Woolf CJ, McMahon SB. Injury-induced plasticity of the flexor reflex in chronic decerebrate rats. Neuroscience 1985; 16:395–404.

[180] Woolf CJ, Thompson SW. The induction and maintenance of central sensitization is dependent on N-methyl-D-aspartic acid receptor activation; implications for the treatment of post injury pain hypersensitivity. Pain 1991;44:293–9.

[181] Woolf CJ, Wall PD. Relative effectiveness of C primary afferent fibers of different origins in evoking a prolonged facilitation of the flexor reflex in the rat. J Neurosci 1986;6:1433–42.

[182] Yaksh TL. Central pharmacology of nociceptive transmission. In: McMahon SB, Koltzenburg M, editors. Textbook of pain. Philadelphia: Elsevier; 2006. p. 371–414.

[183] Yashpal K, Radhakrishnan V, Coderre TJ, Henry JL. CP-96,345, but not its stereoisomer, CP,96,344, blocks the nociceptive responses to intrathecally administered substance P and to noxious thermal and chemical stimuli in the rat. Neuroscience 1993;52:1039–47.

[184] Yezierski RP, Gerhard KD, Shrock BJ, Willis WD. A further examination of effects of cortical stimulation on primate spinothalamic tract cells. J Neurophysiol 1983;49:424–41.

[185] Zahn PK, Brennan TJ. Lack of effect of intrathecally administered N-methyl-D-aspartate receptor antagonists in a rat model for postoperative pain. Anesthesiology 1998;88:143–56.

[186] Zahn PK, Umali E, Brennan TJ. Intrathecal non-NMDA excitatory amino acid receptor antagonists inhibit pain behaviors in a rat model of postoperative pain. Pain 1998;74:213–23.

[187] Zhao Z-Q, Duggan AW. Idazoxan blocks the action of noradrenaline but not spinal inhibition from electrical stimulation of the locus coeruleus and nucleus Kolliker-fuse of the cat. Neuroscience 1988;25:997–1005.

[188] Zhuo QQ, Imbe H, Zuo S, Dubner R, Ren K. Selective upregulation of the flip-flop splice variants of AMPA receptor subunits in the rat spinal cord after hindpaw inflammation. Mol Brain Res 2001;88:186–93.

[189] Zorman G, Belcher G, Adams JE, Fields HL. Lumbar intrathecal naloxone blocks analgesia produced by microstimulation of the ventromedial medulla in the rat. Brain Res 1982;236:77–84.

[190] Zou X, Lin Q, Willis WD. Enhanced phosphorylation of NMDA receptor 1 subunits in spinal cord dorsal horn and spinothalamic tract neurons after intradermal injection of capsaicin in rats. J Neurosci 2000;20:6989–97.

[191] Zou X, Lin Q, Willis WD. Role of protein kinase A in phosphorylation of NMDA receptor 1 subunits in dorsal horn and spinothalamic tract neurons after intradermal injection of capsaicin in rats. Neuroscience 2002;115:775–86.

[192] Zou XJ, Lin Q, Willis WD. Effect of protein kinase C blockade on phosphorylation of NR1 in dorsal horn and spinothalamic tract cells caused by intradermal capsaicin injection in rats. Brain Res 2004;1020:95–105

Correspondence to: Prof. Kathleen A. Sluka, PT, PhD, Graduate Program in Physical Therapy and Rehabilitation Science, The University of Iowa, 1-252 Medical Education Building, Iowa City, IA 52242-1190, USA. Tel: 319-335-9791; fax 319-335-9707; email: kathleen-sluka@uiowa.edu.

Individual Differences and Pain Variability

Laura Frey Law[a] and Steven Z. George[b]

[a]Graduate Program in Physical Therapy and Rehabilitation Science, The University of Iowa, Iowa City, Iowa, USA; [b]Center for Pain Research and Behavioral Health and Brooks Center for Rehabilitation Studies, Department of Physical Therapy, University of Florida, Gainesville, Florida, USA

Pain is both a diagnostic and prognostic indicator. For example, knee pain may be the first indication of osteoarthritis. However, the experience of pain can vary considerably among individuals with osteoarthritis. For example, severity of knee pain and osteoarthritic radiographic findings are not well correlated. Indeed, physical therapists commonly observe variability among individuals, finding that some patients are more or less sensitive to apparently similar pathology or painful stimuli. Individual differences in pain sensitivity result in variability in the pain experience at the group or population level. This chapter will explore selected clinically relevant factors that contribute to this interindividual variability.

Pain variability can be observed under clinical and experimental conditions, with each condition providing a unique perspective on the pain experience. Variability of pain in clinical pain conditions can be challenging to assess as it may be confounded by the duration of the disease process, the severity of the underlying injury, and the effects of previous treatment. Experimental conditions provide a means to study standard nociceptive stimuli across individuals to better delineate factors that contribute to pain variability. These models also allow for assessment of different components of the pain experience that are not readily available in clinical settings. For example, experimental pain models allow for the determination of threshold, tolerance, and responses to standard stimuli ranges. These properties allow investigators to make group comparisons, which may not be feasible in clinical settings. Several different pain models have been used in human subject studies, such as cold and heat pain, pressure or mechanical pain, infusion of algesic solutions, and ischemic or exercise-induced pain.

A specific example of interindividual pain variability from an experimental condition can be seen in Fig. 1, which depicts pain sensitivity, as determined by pain intensity ratings, for young, healthy subjects receiving a standard thermal stimulus at 49°C (S. George, unpublished data). The wide range of responses provides a clear indication of the variability of the pain experience, even under "ideal" circumstances involving healthy subjects receiving a controlled stimulus.

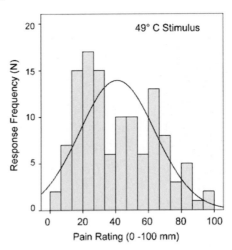

Fig. 1. Histogram of the distribution of cutaneous heat pain ratings (on a scale of 0–100) for 120 young, healthy subjects receiving a standard 49°C stimulus to the arm. Pain ratings showed extensive variability ranging from 0 to 100, with a mean of 41.1 (SD = 22.9).

As defined by the International Association for the Study of Pain, pain is an unpleasant sensory and emotional experience related to actual or potential tissue damage. It is readily accepted that pain sensitivity may depend on a myriad of factors (Fig. 2). Accordingly, a single factor is likely to explain only a small portion of the total variance in pain sensitivity. Further, these factors—sex, race, genetics, and psychological factors—are likely to interact in complex ways, making simple conclusions on the specific effect of a particular factor challenging. In this chapter we will highlight the current status of research on pain variability, acknowledging the inherent intricacies of the subject. We will discuss several sources of interindividual pain variability, considering studies of both clinical and experimental pain. We will focus on factors that have relevance to most clinical situations involving physical therapy: men versus women, ethnicity or race, psychological factors, age-related considerations, and heritability or genetics.

Pain sensitivity can be specific to the nature of the underlying stimulus; someone particularly sensitive to heat pain may not be sensitive to cold pain or deep-tissue pressure pain, and vice versa [29,33,42]. Additionally, pain sensitivity may depend on the specific pain measure; for example, pain threshold may vary considerably, whereas tolerance to the same the pain stimulus may be relatively consistent across individuals or vice versa. Thus, it is important to use caution when considering which factors influence pain sensitivity—they may be relevant only for specific nociceptive conditions and may not generalize across all situations.

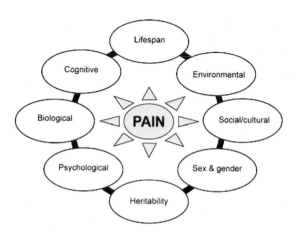

Fig. 2. Schematic representation of multiple interacting factors that may influence an individual's perception of pain. Modified and adapted from Berkley et al. [3].

Sex and Gender

Although the terms *sex* and *gender* are often used interchangeably, we will define sex as the biological distinction between males and females, whereas gender will be used to distinguish between social, cultural, or behavioral roles and expectations typically associated with men (e.g., masculinity) and women (e.g., femininity) [27,52]. While sex and gender are frequently correlated, they are not synonyms. Our discussion will include research that has investigated sex differences, as well as studies that have taken into consideration the underlying gender roles. Sex is one of the easiest individual differences to classify, and more information is available on differences in pain between men and women than on differences related to gender role.

Clinical Pain

Numerous clinical pain conditions are more prevalent in women, but there are also diagnoses that are more frequently seen in men (see Tables I, II) [2]. Several chronic musculoskeletal pain conditions commonly treated by physical therapists occur more frequently in women, such as fibromyalgia, osteoarthritis (after age 45), temporomandibular joint disorder, and carpal tunnel syndrome [2]. However, it is not well understood why these conditions may occur preferentially in women. It is not clear from clinical investigations whether women display greater pain sensitivity then men for similar diagnoses. In a review of multiple common recurrent pain conditions (headache, facial pain, back pain, musculoskeletal pain, and abdominal pain), women generally reported higher intensity, longer duration, and more frequent pain than men [62]. However, in more recent studies, no sex differences in pain intensity were reported in chronic musculoskeletal pain conditions [18,51], but women did report more widespread anatomical distribution of pain [18]. Further, no sex differences were noted in pain intensity ratings or medication use in cancer patients [61] or following oral surgery [33]. In fact, in a cohort of patients with acute and subacute low back pain, men reported higher pain intensity in comparison to women [19]. The mixed findings in observed clinical male-female differences may be related to differences in underlying pathology or tissue damage or in peripherally or centrally mediated pain signal processing, or they may result from biases in pain report and health care utilization.

Table I
Sex differences in prevalence of various painful disorders

Female Predominance	Male Predominance	No Sex Predominance
Migraine headache with aura	Migraine without aura	Acute tension headache
Chronic tension headache	Cluster headache	Cluster-tic syndrome
Post-dural puncture headache	Post-traumatic headache	"Jabs" and jolts" syndrome
Hemicrania continua	SUNCT syndrome	Secondary trigeminal neuralgia
Cervicogenic headache	Raeder's paratrigeminal syndrome	Neuralgia of nervus intermedius
Tic douloureux	Pancoast tumor	Painful ophthalmoplegia
Temporomandibular joint disorder	Thromboangiitis obliterans	Maxillary sinusitis
Occipital neuralgia	Brachial plexus avulsion	Toothache due to dentinoenamel defects
Periapical periodontitis and abscess	Pancreatic disease	Toothache due to pulpitis
Atypical odontalgia	Duodenal ulcer	Cracked tooth syndrome
Burning tongue	Abdominal migraine	Dry socket
Carotidynia	Lateral femoral cutaneous neuropathy	Vagus nerve neuralgia
Chronic paroxysmal hemicrania	Postherpetic neuralgia	Stylohyoid process syndrome
Temporal arteritis	Hemophilic arthropathy	Thoracic outlet syndrome
Carpal tunnel syndrome	Ankylosing spondylitis	Brachial plexus tumors
Raynaud's disease		Esophageal motility disorders
Chilblains		Chronic gastric ulcer
Causalgia		Crohn's disease
Reflex sympathetic dystrophy		Diverticular disease of colon
Hemicrania continua		Carcinoma of the colon
Chronic venous insufficiency		Familial Mediterranean fever
Fibromyalgia syndrome		Hereditary coproporphyria
Esophagitis		Acute herpes zoster
Reflux esophagitis with peptic ulcer		Burns
Slipping rib syndrome		
Twelfth rib syndrome		
Gallbladder disease		
Postcholecystectomy syndrome		
Irritable bowel syndrome		
Interstitial cystitis		
Acute intermittent porphyria		
Proctalgia fugax		
Chronic constipation		
Pyriformis syndrome		
Peroneal muscular atrophy		
Multiple sclerosis		
Rheumatoid arthritis		
Pain of psychological origin		

Source: Adapted from Greenspan et al. [27], with permission.
Abbreviations: SUNCT = short-lasting unilateral neuralgiform headache attacks with conjunctival injection and tearing.

Table II
Age-dependent sex differences in prevalence of various disorders

Female Predominance	Male Predominance
Gout (after age 60)	Gout (before age 60)
Osteoarthritis (after age 45)	Osteoarthritis (before age 45)
Livedo reticularis (after age 40)	Coronary artery disease (before age 65)
	Erythromelalgia (over age 50)

Source: Adapted from Greenspan et al. [27], with permission.

Experimental Pain

Results from human studies using experimental pain models are also mixed when it comes to sex differences. Pressure or mechanical pain most consistently results in male-female differences. In a meta-analysis of a total of 22 studies on sex differences in response to experimental stimuli, Riley et al. [47] found that females have lower pressure pain thresholds with a smaller effect size (Cohen's d = 0.59) and lower pressure pain tolerance with a larger effect size (d = 1.18). Women also display lower thresholds for thermal pain (d = 0.46), electrical pain (d = 0.59), and ischemic pain (d = 0.18) [47]. Tolerance measures are also typically lower for females, but the effect size varies more between stimuli. The largest effect size is observed for pressure pain, but smaller effect sizes have been observed for thermal pain (d = 0.09), electrical pain (d = 0.64), and ischemic pain (d = 0.16) [47]. More recently, Pool et al. [44] observed no sex differences in electrical pain threshold, but found that women had significantly lower pain tolerances.

Studies reporting pain ratings to a consistent algesic stimulus, such as pain with a thermal probe at a set temperature or exercise-induced pain, have observed both elevated [33,34] and equal [7,32,33] pain responses in women compared to men.

It has been suggested that women may exhibit greater centrally mediated pain responses. Women have consistently reported higher rates of temporal summation in response to thermal [15,18,53] and mechanical stimuli [54]. Temporal summation is the increased pain response to a consistent stimulus over time, believed to be related to the central processing of pain at the spinal cord level. Higher rates of temporal summation are indicative of "amplification" of pain and may be associated with the development of chronic pain syndromes. Referred pain, another form of centrally mediated pain, is also observed more frequently in women than men [16,46]. However, no sex differences in secondary hyperalgesia, also thought to be mediated centrally, have been noted with cutaneous heat and capsaicin pain models [32]. Collectively, these studies suggest that central processing of pain may differ between women and men, such that women have higher pain sensitivity and are more likely to amplify nociceptive signals.

Numerous studies have investigated the potential effect of the menstrual cycle in women on pain sensitivity. Contradictory reports reveal that this issue is far from well understood. In one meta-analysis of 16 studies, women were least sensitive (i.e., had the highest thresholds) to pressure pain, cold pain, thermal heat pain, and ischemic muscle pain during the follicular phase (days 6–11, immediately following the menstrual phase), with small to moderate effect sizes (Cohen's d = 0.34 to 0.48) [48]. However, in a more recent review by Sherman and LeResche [55], the addition of newer studies, coupled with inconsistencies in classifying menstrual phases in the prior studies, resulted in their conclusion that there is currently "little evidence" for menstrual cycle influences on experimentally evoked pain [55].

The experimental literature consistently suggests that women have higher pain sensitivity than men, suggesting differences in central processing. However, centrally mediated sex differences—such as differences in temporal summation, referred pain, and secondary hyperalgesia—may not be uniform across pain experiences. The studies outlined above, both clinical and experimental, do not account for gender, a potentially important confound.

Gender

Gender roles, which are influenced not only by the biological orientation of the individual, but also by social, cultural, and behavioral factors, have the potential to influence pain perception. Stereotypical gender roles suggest that men should have higher pain tolerance than women. This body of literature is much smaller than the previously reviewed literature related only to sex differences. However, there is some evidence to suggest that gender influences pain perception, independently of biological orientation.

Measurement of gender roles is not as simple as determining biological orientation, but self-report questionnaires can be used. Several approaches to measure gender roles have been reported specifically in relation to pain, such as the Gender Roles Expectations of Pain (GREP), a measure that considers the influence of socially learned responses to pain for men and women [52], and the Extended Personal Attributes Questionnaire, which includes a measure of perceived masculinity/femininity. Others have assessed how strongly individuals associate with their ideal gender group [44]. In several experimental pain models, gender roles and expectations mediate observed sex differences. Willingness to report pain (on the GREP questionnaire) was found to be more meaningful than sex differences in explaining differences between subjects in temporal summation [53]. This factor also added additional meaning to the sex differences in tolerance, threshold, and unpleasantness ratings to cold stimuli [69]. Similarly, masculinity/femininity scores partially mediated the sex differences observed in a cold pressor task [59]. Participants with a strong gender group identity displayed large male-female differences for both hypothetical and electrically stimulated pain tolerance ratings, whereas men and women with low gender group identity reported similar tolerances [44]. Finally, when gender roles are manipulated, men and women have equal tolerance to cold stimuli [50], which suggests that previously observed sex differences may be partially due to social expectations.

Gender roles have not been well explored in clinical settings. Women are more likely to seek medical attention and report health care complaints [37], although these results could be a result of either sex or gender differences. However, a large cross-cultural study of multiple health complaints in adolescents suggests that there are social gender roles contributing to these differences because they varied considerably between cultures [60]. The sex differences in recurring health complaints were generally small in 11-year-olds, but increased substantially by age 15 in some countries. This finding may be due to physiological changes with maturation, but it may also be evidence for increased influence of social roles and expectations. In summary, while gender roles are likely to influence clinical pain, the relationship is not well understood.

Ethnicity and Race

The terms *ethnicity* and *race* are often used interchangeably. However, for the purposes of this chapter we will define *ethnicity* as belonging to a group of people who share a common background related to social, cultural, language, and geographical factors [45]. In contrast, the term *race* will be used to describe group membership based on physical differences, although it is acknowledged that there is a strong social contribution to determination of race [36]. For example, the National Institutes of Health considers Caucasian, African American, and Asian to be races, whereas Hispanic is considered an ethnicity. Similar to sex and gender, both race and ethnicity can be confounded by additional complex social and cultural roles and expectations. Determination of ethnicity and race most commonly relies on subject self-report, and our discussion will focus on studies that used this methodology for identification, as opposed to genetic definitions using ancestry markers. Next to sex, ethnicity and race are probably the most common differences identified during clinical encounters.

Clinical Pain

Several studies have reported on ethnic and racial differences in the clinical pain experience, with varied results. For example, migraine headache is more prevalent in Caucasians than in either African Americans or Asians; however, African Americans report higher migraine pain intensities [56]. African Americans generally report greater pain than Caucasians across the lifespan and across various patient populations [11,26], but inconsistencies are also observed. African Americans, compared to Caucasians, report greater pain with temporomandibular disorders [68], greater postoperative pain after surgery to correct scoliosis [67], and higher pain with lower experimental pain tolerance with chronic pain conditions [11]. Conversely, in another study, similar pain intensities were reported in white and African American patients with a variety of chronic pain conditions [49].

Further complicating the issue, racial/ethnic associations with affective pain and disability ratings may differ from sensory-discriminative pain intensity ratings. For example, although African American subjects reported higher pain intensity from migraine headaches, their reports of pain disability were lower when compared to Caucasian subjects [56]. In another study, African Americans reported higher levels of pain unpleasantness, emotional distress, and pain behavior, despite similar pain intensities [49].

The inconsistency in these results may be due to other confounding factors such as sex, socioeconomic status, and pain location. When study participants are matched by sex, educational level, work status, duration of pain, and location of pain, similar levels of pain intensity, unpleasantness, and interference with activities are noted across racial and ethnic groups [13]. However, higher pain intensity occurs in African Americans even when investigators control for age and socioeconomic status [56]. Overall, racial disparities in pain reporting as well as in pain treatment have been consistently documented [26]. Accordingly, Green et al. suggest that greater education and training in racial and ethnic factors is warranted for all health care professionals [26].

Experimental Pain

The difficulty in comparing clinical pain conditions between ethnic and racial groups has led to interest in determining experimental pain sensitivities in both healthy and pain populations [5]. In a small sample of healthy college students, African American subjects had lower tolerance and higher ratings of unpleasantness to heat stimuli [12]. In a larger sample of college students, African American subjects had lower tolerance to heat, cold pressor, and ischemic pain when compared to Caucasians [5]. However, only for heat stimuli were the differences in pain intensity and unpleasantness ratings significantly higher for African Americans [5]. These results were largely supported in a follow-up study, with Hispanic subjects also exhibiting lower tolerance to heat and cold when compared to non-Hispanic Caucasian subjects [45]. Although relatively little information is available involving additional races, African Americans, Hispanics, and Asian Americans all had shorter withdrawal times and higher pain ratings than European Americans during the cold pressor task [33]. However, in a heat pain task, only Asian Americans displayed greater pain ratings at each temperature tested compared to African Americans, European Americans, and Hispanics [33].

Experimental pain variability varies between races and ethnicities with more consistency than is seen in clinical pain conditions. This statement is supported by an interesting study combining experimental and clinical pain models in patients seeking treatment for chronic pain. While African Americans reported both higher clinical pain intensity and disability ratings and lower experimental pain tolerance [11], the differences in clinical pain were smaller than the differences in experimental pain (tolerance). This finding suggests larger racial differences with experimentally induced pain as compared to clinical pain.

In addition to experimental pain sensitivity studies, racial and ethnic differences in endogenous pain inhibition have been reported. Diffuse noxious inhibitory control (DNIC; see Chapter 3) represents an endogenous descending inhibition system, in which the application of painful stimuli will evoke generalized analgesia and inhibit further pain. Using a DNIC protocol, one study found that non-Hispanic Caucasians had greater reduction in electrically induced pain following ischemic pain, when compared to African Americans, suggesting that Caucasians may have greater descending pain inhibition than African Americans [6].

Psychological Factors

Negative Emotionality, Pain Catastrophizing, and Fear of Pain

Various approaches have been used to investigate psychological traits (enduring dimensions of psychological individual differences) and states (temporary or transient dimensions of psychological individual differences). Trait individual differences can be classified in many ways, but hierarchical structures have been increasingly recognized. These include traditional higher-order personality dimensions, such as neuroticism and extraversion; trait and mood scales, such as negative or positive affect and state or trait anxiety; and various dispositional or vulnerability factors, including pain catastrophizing and pain-related fear. This section will focus on what we believe to be of most relevance for pain-related constructs— personality traits, negative emotionality, pain catastrophizing, and pain-related fear.

Personality traits have been characterized using several models, but the two most consistently described traits are neuroticism (also referred to as negative emotionality) and extraversion. Neuroticism is associated with anxious, worrisome, overly emotional, moody, and negative thoughts, feelings, and behaviors. Extraversion is associated with sociable, optimistic, excitement-craving, and easy-going traits. Neuroticism and extraversion are highly correlated with negative and positive affect, respectively; however, they are not opposites of each other [64]. For example, individuals can be high in both neuroticism and extraversion. Many personality assessment instruments are available, ranging from the 100-item Eysenck Personality Questionnaire to the 10-item Positive and Negative Affect Schedule [64].

Pain catastrophizing is a negative cognitive style, which at the extreme includes feelings and beliefs that the pain experienced is beyond the control of the individual and will inevitably result in the worst possible outcome. Pain catastrophizing is believed to be a multidimensional construct comprised of magnification, rumination, helplessness, and pessimism. The Pain Catastrophizing Scale is one example of a measure of pain catastrophizing [57]. Example statements include: "I feel I can't go on, it's awful and I feel that it overwhelms me, and I anxiously want the pain to go away."

Pain-related fear can also be measured in multiple ways. The Fear of Pain Questionnaire (FPQ) is a self-report measure of anticipated fear for hypothetical situations that assesses severe pain (e.g., "breaking your neck"), minor pain (e.g., "having a muscle cramp"), and medical (procedure-related) pain (e.g., "having a tooth pulled") [39]. A high score on the FPQ indicates a high level of pain-related fear. The Fear-Avoidance Beliefs Questionnaire (FABQ) assesses pain-related fear associated with clinical pain conditions, specifically addressing fear-avoidance beliefs of physical activity [63]. A practical example is an individual with an elevated FABQ score who is hesitant to resume therapeutic exercise in response to shoulder pain, believing such activity would result in re-injury. Pain-related fear may depend on an individual's prior pain experiences, present stress level, pain behavior, and certain personality traits.

Clinical Pain

Negative emotionality and its related facets have been associated with chronic pain perception, such that patients who express greater negative emotionality are more likely to report more health complaints and chronic pain conditions [25,40,65]. However, these studies are unable to clarify whether the poor health and chronic pain led to greater negative affect or vice versa. However, other prospective research suggests that pain-related fear and catastrophizing can predict poorer outcomes in patient populations. Fear-avoidance belief scores explained unique variance in 4-week disability scores and return-to-work status for patients with acute occupational low back pain [17]. Patients with elevated pain-related fear and catastrophizing measures at the acute stage of low back pain were more likely to have greater disability for up to 6 months [21]. Pain catastrophizing during acute low back pain was also predictive of self-reported disability at 6 months [43] and at 1 year [4]. However, elevated pain-related fear (as measured on the FABQ) was predictive of work status at 1 year when examined in isolation, but only pain centralization was predictive when several factors were considered simultaneously [66]. Collectively, these studies suggest a temporal relationship such that pain-related fear and pain catastrophizing at symptom onset are precursors to reports of chronic low back pain. Thus, they may be viewed as predictors of poor outcome and should be considered as possible risk factors for chronicity.

Experimental Pain

A large body of literature has compared psychosocial individual differences in relation to experimental cutaneous pain. Higher self-reports of negative emotionality, anxiety, pain catastrophizing, and fear of pain are associated with lower pain thresholds, lower pain tolerance, and higher pain sensory and affective ratings [10,28]. For example, fear of pain is a unique predictor of pain tolerance and intensity for the cold pressor task [19,31]. In patients with low back pain, fear-avoidance was related to initial heat pain ratings, while catastrophizing was related to temporal summation, i.e., the increase in pain ratings when the heat was maintained [23]. Fig. 3 shows an example of the association between fear of pain and heat pain ratings in an experimental pain condition. Higher pain ratings were positivity correlated with FPQ scores when a 49°C thermal stimuli was applied to the trunk in healthy individuals (S. George, unpublished data).

Although there are few studies involving experimental deep tissue pain, temporomandibular muscle pain responses were partially explained by negative affect during hypertonic saline infusion [70]. Further, fear of pain [21] and pain catastrophizing [22] are predictive of pain intensity, evoked pain, development of kinesiophobia, and shoulder disability in studies using the delayed-onset muscle soreness model.

In summary, both clinical and experimental studies consistently support the association between pain or disability outcomes and negative temperament, pain catastrophizing, and pain-related fear. Further, patients with low back pain respond differentially to rehabilitation based on their fear-avoidance beliefs [17,20], suggesting that patients' psychological traits may have important consequences on pain and disability and may affect the clinician's choice of treatment.

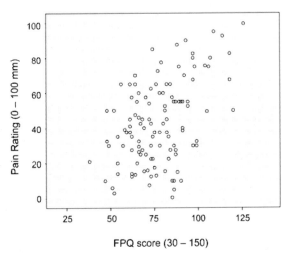

Fig. 3. Fear of pain is associated with experimental numerical pain ratings on a scale of 0–100 ($r = 0.47$, $P < 0.01$) in response to 49°C stimuli to the trunk. Fear of pain was measured with the Fear of Pain Questionnaire (FPQ).

Genetics and Heritability

Heritability has been traditionally investigated using twin studies or family-based studies to determine the underlying genetic versus environmental factors contributing to a disease. Although few twin studies have examined pain specifically, one study involving experimentally evoked pain (cold pressor and thermal heat) demonstrated that genetics accounted for roughly 60% of the variance in cold-pressor pain, but only 26% of the variance in heat pain [42]. This finding suggests that genetic factors can play an important role in pain sensitivity, but they may not influence different nociceptive stimuli equally.

While twin studies have been used for some time to investigate the general heritability of various conditions, the human genetic code was only mapped relatively recently. This advance has promoted rapidly evolving research on specific genetic variability as a contributing factor to various forms of pathology and disease. For example, 11% of the variance in a combined measure of overall pain sensitivity results from variations in a single gene [9]. Association studies are useful to investigate the links between specific genotype variations known as single nucleotide polymorphisms (SNPs) and pain phenotypes.

Genetic influences on phenotypes involve complex interactions between multiple genes and the environment. Accordingly, large samples are typically needed to determine significant associations between genotype and pain. To maximize statistical power and minimize false positives, multiple candidate pain genes have been identified and prioritized for use in association studies [1]. The criteria for prioritizing candidate pain genes for human association studies are: (1) adequate evidence supporting the gene's role in pain processing, (2) genetic variation frequent enough to affect clinical manifestation, and (3) a high likelihood that genetic variation affects protein function. Also gaining popularity are genome-wide association studies, which examine associations between phenotypes (e.g., pain) and SNPs sampled from across the entire human genome. Both approaches are likely to advance our understanding of the genetic influences on pain in the coming decades. Several lines of evidence now support the underlying hypothesis that genotype influences pain perception.

Three high-priority genes that have been successfully linked to pain perception in humans are the catecholamine-O-methyltransferase gene (*COMT*), the transient receptor potential subtype 1 gene (*TRPV1*), and the μ-opioid receptor gene (*OPRM1*). The *COMT* gene is important for the enzymatic breakdown of catecholamines—hormones released during physiological stress—such as epinephrine, norepinephrine, and dopamine. Thus, the COMT enzyme is probably involved in pain by altering the degradation of these substances. TRPV1, also known as the vanilloid receptor, is a membrane channel receptor found in both the peripheral and central nervous system. This receptor is activated by various nociceptive stimuli such as low pH, heat, and capsaicin (hot peppers), and thus it is likely to be involved in pain transmission. OPRM1 is a μ-opioid receptor that is involved in the analgesic response to opioid drugs. The OPRM1 gene is believed to be important in the variability of opioid response to medication and in the endogenous opioid mechanisms that serve to inhibit pain.

Clinical Pain

Genetic studies involving clinical pain patients are only beginning to emerge. In patients undergoing shoulder surgery, postsurgical pain at 3–5 months was associated with variations in the COMT gene [22]. The GCH1 gene (which governs the expression of guanosine triphosphate cyclohydrolase 1, an enzyme involved in catecholamine production) was associated with pain reports following diskectomy for radiculopathy [58]. As would be expected, the OPRM1 gene was associated with the morphine dose needed for pain control in patients with cancer pain [35].

Experimental Pain

In healthy subjects, COMT has been linked to pain perception and heterogeneity in studies using thermal, mechanical, and ischemic experimental pain stimuli [8,9]. A study of muscle pain using the hypertonic saline model found that COMT was associated with cortical imaging of μ-opioid receptor binding, suggesting that this gene plays an important role in pain perception [70]. Additionally, COMT inhibition activates the β-adrenergic receptors 2 and 3 (ADRB2 and ADRB3), which are also important in mediating catecholamine levels, ultimately influencing pain sensitivity [41]. The TRPV1 gene influences cold cutaneous pain but not noxious heat in humans [34]. The OPRM1 gene was associated with higher pressure pain thresholds [14] and with decreased event-related potentials from a pain stimulus [38] in healthy volunteers.

Age

The effect of age on pain variability can be difficult to assess because several of the previously discussed factors (physiological, psychological, and social) may vary from youth through adulthood, and potentially on into older adult years. While we have attempted to discuss several of these factors separately, considering them as a function of age has value for the clinician. A review of the literature including over 140 citations on age-related effects on pain concluded that thresholds were more frequently elevated (showing less sensitivity to pain) in older adults. However, the review found that age-related effects can vary with modality (thermal and mechanical more than electrical), location (distal more than proximal), and temporal/spatial characteristics [24]. However, it is less clear whether systematic changes in suprathreshold pain perception occur with aging. It is possible that older individuals may have a reduced region between pain awareness (threshold) and potential tissue injury. Advancing age may result in greater central sensitization, as determined by measures of temporal summation and secondary mechanical hyperalgesia, suggesting that older adults may experience greater pain sensitivity that may require more time to resolve than in younger adults [24].

Complexity

Each of the factors described above may interact in complex ways to influence pain. Although it is not yet clear how each of these interactions will ultimately affect diagnosis and treatment, it is important to realize that these factors may influence a patient's perception of pain. Current clinical practice considers this complexity by using selected demographic, clinical, and psychological factors to determine an individual's risk profile for developing chronic pain. These factors are readily available and allow for reasonable accuracy in predicting outcomes. Typically these factors are considered in isolation, which does not truly represent the complexity of the pain experience. However, recent studies have provided more complex risk assessment that allows clinicians to rate the relative risk of multiple factors [30]. Accuracy of future risk profiles will be improved by simultaneously considering many of the factors discussed in this chapter to determine the expected response to pain.

References

[1] Belfer I, Wu T, Kingman A, Krishnaraju RK, Goldman D, Max MB. Candidate gene studies of human pain mechanisms: methods for optimizing choice of polymorphisms and sample size. Anesthesiology 2004;100:1562–72.

[2] Berkley KJ. Sex differences in pain. Behav Brain Sci 1997;20:371–80.

[3] Berkley KJ, Zalcman SS, Simon VR. Sex and gender differences in pain and inflammation: a rapidly maturing field. Am J Physiol Regul Integr Comp Physiol 2006;291:R241–4.

[4] Burton AK, Tillotson KM, Main CJ, Hollis S. Psychosocial predictors of outcome in acute and subchronic low back trouble. Spine 1995;20:722–8.

[5] Campbell CM, Edwards RR, Fillingim RB. Ethnic differences in responses to multiple experimental pain stimuli. Pain 2005;113:20–6.

[6] Campbell CM, France CR, Robinson ME, Logan HL, Geffken GR, Fillingim RB. Ethnic differences in diffuse noxious inhibitory controls. J Pain 2008;9:759–66.

[7] Dannecker EA, Hausenblas HA, Kaminski TW, Robinson ME. Sex differences in delayed onset muscle pain. Clin J Pain 2005;21:120–6.

[8] Diatchenko L, Nackley AG, Slade GD, Bhalang K, Belfer I, Max MB, Goldman D, Maixner W. Catechol-O-methyltransferase gene polymorphisms are associated with multiple pain-evoking stimuli. Pain 2006;125:216–24.

[9] Diatchenko L, Slade GD, Nackley AG, Bhalang K, Sigurdsson A, Belfer I, Goldman D, Xu K, Shabalina SA, Shagin D, et al. Genetic basis for individual variations in pain perception and the development of a chronic pain condition. Hum Mol Genet 2005;14:135–43.

[10] Dixon KE, Thorn BE, Ward LC. An evaluation of sex differences in psychological and physiological responses to experimentally-induced pain: a path analytic description. Pain 2004;112:188–96.

[11] Edwards RR, Doleys DM, Fillingim RB, Lowery D. Ethnic differences in pain tolerance: clinical implications in a chronic pain population. Psychosom Med 2001;63:316–23.

[12] Edwards RR, Fillingim RB. Ethnic differences in thermal pain responses. Psychosom Med 1999;61:346–54.

[13] Edwards RR, Moric M, Husfeldt B, Buvanendran A, Ivankovich O. Ethnic similarities and differences in the chronic pain experience: a comparison of African American, Hispanic, and white patients. Pain Med 2005;6:88–98.

[14] Fillingim RB, Kaplan L, Staud R, Ness TJ, Glover TL, Campbell CM, Mogil JS, Wallace MR. The A118G single nucleotide polymorphism of the mu-opioid receptor gene (OPRM1) is associated with pressure pain sensitivity in humans. J Pain 2005;6:159–67.

[15] Fillingim RB, Maixner W, Kincaid S, Silva S. Sex differences in temporal summation but not sensory-discriminative processing of thermal pain. Pain 1998;75:121–7.

[16] Frey Law LA, Sluka KA, McMullen T, Lee J, Arendt-Nielsen L, Graven-Nielsen T. Acidic buffer induced muscle pain evokes referred pain and mechanical hyperalgesia. Pain 2008;140:254–64.

[17] Fritz JM, George SZ, Delitto A. The role of fear-avoidance beliefs in acute low back pain: relationships with current and future disability and work status. Pain 2001;94:7–15.

[18] George SZ, Bialosky JE, Wittmer VT, Robinson ME. Sex differences in pain drawing area for individuals with chronic musculoskeletal pain. J Orthop Sports Phys Ther 2007;37:115–21.

[19] George SZ, Dannecker EA, Robinson ME. Fear of pain, not pain catastrophizing, predicts acute pain intensity, but neither factor predicts tolerance or blood pressure reactivity: an experimental investigation in pain-free individuals. Eur J Pain 2006;10:457–65.

[20] George SZ, Fritz JM, Bialosky JE, Donald DA. The effect of a fear-avoidance-based physical therapy intervention for patients with acute low back pain: results of a randomized clinical trial. Spine 2003;28:2551–60.

[21] George SZ, Fritz JM, Childs JD. Investigation of elevated fear-avoidance beliefs for patients with low back pain: a secondary analysis involving patients enrolled in physical therapy clinical trials. J Orthop Sports Phys Ther 2008;38:50–8.

[22] George SZ, Wallace MR, Wright TW, Moser MW, Greenfield WH 3rd, Sack BK, Herbstman DM, Fillingim RB. Evidence for a biopsychosocial influence on shoulder pain: pain catastrophizing and catechol-O-methyltransferase (COMT) diplotype predict clinical pain ratings. Pain 2008;136:53–61.

[23] George SZ, Wittmer VT, Fillingim RB, Robinson ME. Sex and pain-related psychological variables are associated with thermal pain sensitivity for patients with chronic low back pain. J Pain 2007;8:2–10.

[24] Gibson SJ, Farrell M. A review of age differences in the neurophysiology of nociception and the perceptual experience of pain. Clin J Pain 2004;20:227–39.

[25] Goodwin RD, Castro M, Kovacs M. Major depression and allergy: does neuroticism explain the relationship? Psychosom Med 2006;68:94–8.

[26] Green CR, Anderson KO, Baker TA, Campbell LC, Decker S, Fillingim RB, Kalauokalani DA, Lasch KE, Myers C, Tait RC, et al. The unequal burden of pain: confronting racial and ethnic disparities in pain. Pain Med 2003;4:277–94.

[27] Greenspan JD, Craft RM, LeResche L, Arendt-Nielsen L, Berkley KJ, Fillingim RB, Gold MS, Holdcroft A, Lautenbacher S, et al. Studying sex and gender differences in pain and analgesia: a consensus report. Pain 2007;132:S26–45.

[28] Harkins SW, Price DD, Braith J. Effects of extraversion and neuroticism on experimental pain, clinical pain, and illness behavior. Pain 1989;36:209–18.

[29] Hastie BA, Riley JL 3rd, Robinson ME, Glover T, Campbell CM, Staud R, Fillingim RB. Cluster analysis of multiple experimental pain modalities. Pain 2005;116:227–37.

[30] Hill JC, Dunn KM, Lewis M, Mullis R, Main CJ, Foster NE, Hay EM. A primary care back pain screening tool: identifying patient subgroups for initial treatment. Arthritis Rheum 2008;59:632–41.

[31] Hirsh AT, George SZ, Bialosky JE, Robinson ME. Fear of pain, pain catastrophizing, and acute pain perception: relative prediction and timing of assessment. J Pain 2008;9:806–12.

[32] Jensen MT, Petersen KL. Gender differences in pain and secondary hyperalgesia after heat/capsaicin sensitization in healthy volunteers. J Pain 2006;7:211–7.

[33] Kim H, Neubert JK, Rowan JS, Brahim JS, Iadarola MJ, Dionne RA. Comparison of experimental and acute clinical pain responses in humans as pain phenotypes. J Pain 2004;5:377–84.

[34] Kim H, Neubert JK, San Miguel A, Xu K, Krishnaraju RK, Iadarola MJ, Goldman D, Dionne RA. Genetic influence on variability in human acute experimental pain sensitivity associated with gender, ethnicity and psychological temperament. Pain 2004;109:488–96.

[35] Klepstad P, Rakvag TT, Kaasa S, Holthe M, Dale O, Borchgrevink PC, Baar C, Vikan T, Krokan HE, Skorpen F. The 118 A > G polymorphism in the human mu-opioid receptor gene may increase morphine requirements in patients with pain caused by malignant disease. Acta Anaesthesiol Scand 2004;48:1232–9.

[36] LaViest T. Race, ethnicity, and health: a public health reader. San Francisco: Jossey-Bass; 2002.

[37] Lethbridge-Çejku M, Rose D, Vickerie J. Summary health statistics for U.S. Adults: National Health Interview Survey, 2004. National Center for Health Statistics. Vital Health Stat 2006;10:228.

[38] Lotsch J, Stuck B, Hummel T. The human mu-opioid receptor gene polymorphism 118A>G decreases cortical activation in response to specific nociceptive stimulation. Behav Neurosci 2006;120:1218–24.

[39] McNeil DW, Rainwater AJ 3rd. Development of the fear of pain questionnaire. III. J Behav Med 1998;21:389–410.

[40] Myrtek M, Fichtler A, Konig K, Brugner G, Muller W. Differences between patients with asymptomatic and symptomatic myocardial infarction: the relevance of psychological factors. Eur Heart J 1994;15:311–7.

[41] Nackley AG, Tan KS, Fecho K, Flood P, Diatchenko L, Maixner W. Catechol-O-methyltransferase inhibition increases pain sensitivity through activation of both beta2- and beta3-adrenergic receptors. Pain 2007;128:199–208.

[42] Nielsen CS, Stubhaug A, Price DD, Vassend O, Czajkowski N, Harris JR. Individual differences in pain sensitivity: genetic and environmental contributions. Pain 2008;136:21–9.

[43] Picavet HS, Vlaeyen JW, Schouten JS. Pain catastrophizing and kinosiophobia: predictors of chronic low back pain. Am J Epidemiol 2002;156:1028–34.

[44] Pool GJ, Schwegler AF, Theodore BR, Fuchs PN. Role of gender norms and group identification on hypothetical and experimental pain tolerance. Pain 2007;129:122–9.

[45] Rahim-Williams FB, Riley JL 3rd, Herrera D, Campbell CM, Hastie BA, Fillingim RB. Ethnic identity predicts experimental pain sensitivity in African Americans and Hispanics. Pain 2007;129:177–84.

[46] Reddy H, Arendt-Nielsen L, Staahl C, Pedersen J, Funch-Jensen P, Gregersen H, Drewes AM. Gender differences in pain and biomechanical responses after acid sensitization of the human esophagus. Dig Dis Sci 2005;50:2050–8.

[47] Riley JL 3rd, Robinson ME, Wise EA, Myers CD, Fillingim RB. Sex differences in the perception of noxious experimental stimuli: a meta-analysis. Pain 1998;74:181–7.

[48] Riley JL 3rd, Robinson ME, Wise EA, Price DD. A meta-analytic review of pain perception across the menstrual cycle. Pain 1999;8:225–35.

[49] Riley JL 3rd, Wade JB, Myers CD, Sheffield D, Papas RK, Price DD. Racial/ethnic differences in the experience of chronic pain. Pain 2002;100:291–8.

[50] Robinson ME, Gagnon CM, Dannecker EA, Brown JL, Jump RL, Price DD. Sex differences in common pain events: expectations and anchors. J Pain 2003;4:40–5.

[51] Robinson ME, Riley JL 3rd, Brown FF, Gremillion H. Sex differences in response to cutaneous anaesthesia: a double blind randomized study. Pain 1998;77:143–9.

[52] Robinson ME, Riley JL 3rd, Myers CD, Papas RK, Wise EA, Waxenberg LB, Fillingim RB. Gender role expectations of pain: relationship to sex differences in pain. J Pain 2001;2:251–7.

[53] Robinson ME, Wise EA, Gagnon C, Fillingim RB, Price DD. Influence of gender role and anxiety on sex differences in temporal summation of pain. J Pain 2004;5:77–82.

[54] Sarlani E, Greenspan JD. Gender differences in temporal summation of mechanically evoked pain. Pain 2002;97:163–9.

[55] Sherman JJ, LeResche L. Does experimental pain response vary across the menstrual cycle? A methodological review. Am J Physiol Regul Integr Comp Physiol 2006;291:R245–56.

[56] Stewart WF, Lipton RB, Liberman J. Variation in migraine prevalence by race. Neurology 1996;47:52–9.

[57] Sullivan MJ, Bishop S, Pivik J. Pain catastrophizing scale. Psychol Assess 1995;7:524–32.

[58] Tegeder I, Costigan M, Griffin RS, Abele A, Belfer I, Schmidt H, Ehnert C, Nejim J, Marian C, Scholz J, et al. GTP cyclohydrolase and tetrahydrobiopterin regulate pain sensitivity and persistence. Nat Med 2006;12:1269–77.

[59] Thorn BE, Clements KL, Ward LC, Dixon KE, Kersh BC, Boothby JL, Chaplin WF. Personality factors in the explanation of sex differences in pain catastrophizing and response to experimental pain. Clin J Pain 2004;20:275–82.

[60] Torsheim T, Ravens-Sieberer U, Hetland J, Valimaa R, Danielson M, Overpeck M. Cross-national variation of gender differences in adolescent subjective health in Europe and North America. Soc Sci Med 2006;62:815–27.

[61] Turk DC, Okifuji A. Does sex make a difference in the prescription of treatments and the adaptation to chronic pain by cancer and non-cancer patients? Pain 1999;82:139–48.

[62] Unruh AM. Gender variations in clinical pain experience. Pain 1996;65:123–67.

[63] Waddell G, Newton M, Henderson I, Somerville D, Main CJ. A Fear-avoidance beliefs questionnaire (FABQ) and the role of fear-avoidance beliefs in chronic low back pain and disability. Pain 1993;52:157–68.

[64] Watson D, Clark LA, Tellegen A. Development and validation of brief measures of positive and negative affect: the PANAS scales. J Pers Soc Psychol 1988;54:1063–70.

[65] Watson D, Pennebaker JW. Health complaints, stress, and distress: exploring the central role of negative affectivity. Psychol Rev1989;96:234–54.

[66] Werneke MW, Hart DL. Categorizing patients with occupational low back pain by use of the Quebec Task Force Classification system versus pain pattern classification procedures: discriminant and predictive validity. Phys Ther 2004;84:243–54.

[67] White SF, Asher MA, Lai SM, Burton DC. Patients' perceptions of overall function, pain, and appearance after primary posterior instrumentation and fusion for idiopathic scoliosis. Spine 1999;24:1693–9.

[68] Widmalm SE, Gunn SM, Christiansen RL, Hawley LM. Association between CMD signs and symptoms, oral parafunctions, race and sex, in 4–6-year-old African-American and Caucasian children. J Oral Rehabil 1995;22:95–100.

[69] Wise EA, Price DD, Myers CD, Heft MW, Robinson ME. Gender role expectations of pain: relationship to experimental pain perception. Pain 2002;96:335–42.

[70] Zubieta JK, Heitzeg MM, Smith YR, Bueller JA, Xu K, Xu Y, Koeppe RA, Stohler CS, Goldman D. COMT val158met genotype affects mu-opioid neurotransmitter responses to a pain stressor. Science 2003;299:1240–3.

Correspondence to: Laura A. Frey Law, PhD, PT, Graduate Program in Physical Therapy and Rehabilitation Science, The University of Iowa, 1-252 Medical Education Building, Iowa City, IA 52242-1190, USA. Tel: 1-319-335-9791; fax: 1-319-335-9707; email: laura-freylaw@uiowa.edu.

Section II

Physical Therapy Pain Management

Pain Assessment

5

Josimari M. DeSantana[a] and Kathleen A. Sluka[b]

[a]Department of Physical Therapy, Federal University of Sergipe, Aracaju, Sergipe, Brazil;
[b]Graduate Program in Physical Therapy and Rehabilitation Science,
The University of Iowa, Iowa City, Iowa, USA

Goals of Pain Assessment

The goal of pain assessment is to provide sufficient and accurate data to determine what treatment should be initiated. Accurate pain assessment is the first step in effective pain management. Information must be obtained about the nature of the pain, about the patient's physiological, behavioral, and emotional responses, and about the patient's previous experience with pain.

Pain is now considered the fifth vital sign by the American Pain Society and by the Joint Commission on Accreditation of Health Care Organizations, which has published regulations that require that pain should be assessed in all individuals [40]. Therefore, every patient must be checked for pain with every vital sign assessment. Assessment of pain is critical to understanding the nature of the pain and its meaning for the patient. Proper assessment of pain is important to aid in diagnosis, to guide the choice of therapy, and to help the clinician evaluate the progress and effectiveness of therapy [40].

Mechanisms and Management of Pain for the Physical Therapist
edited by Kathleen A. Sluka
IASP Press, Seattle, © 2009

95

The Joint Commission does not specify a particular tool or scale to use, but it does recommend that the practitioner consider age appropriateness when selecting a pain instrument. The guidelines of the United States Agency on Health Care Policy and Research (now the Agency on Health Care Research and Quality) also specify scheduled pain assessment and management and include specific infant recommendations [1]. Thus, pain should be routinely monitored, assessed, reassessed, and clearly documented to facilitate treatment and communication among clinicians [32].

Valid and reliable measurements of pain are needed to identify patients who require intervention and to evaluate the effectiveness of intervention. The two terms *pain assessment* and *pain measurement* are not interchangeable. They are widely used in the pain literature, but they have different meanings. Pain *assessment* connotes a more comprehensive and multifactorial concept, describing a complex process in which information about pain, its meaning, and its effect on the person is considered along with quantitative values. By contrast, pain *measurement* connotes the quantification of various aspects of the pain experience and is most commonly associated with the dimension of pain intensity [9,39,54].

This chapter will provide basic information about pain assessment and pain measurement, review the types of subjective questions that can be used to assess the nature of pain, compare specific instruments to measure pain, and discuss measures that evaluate the impact of pain on quality of life.

Memory for Pain

One thing to consider when assessing pain is that the capacity to remember pain intensity is poor. However, recall of activities reduced by pain is generally very good, as is recall of location of pain [23] (Fig. 1). As shown in Fig. 1A, people with low back pain were asked to recall their average pain intensity or to remember the least severe or most severe pain intensity. In this instance, people tended to overestimate their pain intensity upon recall when compared to measurements taken during the pain experience. However, Fig. 1B and C show that pain location and activities affected by pain are easily recalled with accuracy. Thus, assessments that rely on recall to measure pain intensity should be avoided. Further, common questions used by physical therapists such as "What is your pain at its worst?" or "What is your pain at the end of the day?" should be avoided.

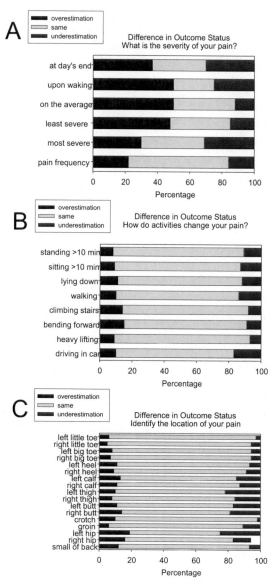

Fig. 1. Graphs A–C show the likelihood that someone would overestimate, underestimate, or correctly estimate three different parameters related to pain: (A) intensity, (B) activities that affect pain, and (C) location of pain. As can be seen, there is a lot of variability when people are asked to remember the intensity of pain, but substantially less when they are asked what activities can change their pain or the location of the pain. Reprinted from [23] with permission of Lippincott, Williams and Wilkins.

Memory of the intensity of pain is influenced by a number of factors. For the pain associated with a medical procedure, patients' judgment of total pain correlated strongly with the peak intensity of pain, but not with its duration [67]. Distinct factors determine the direction of pain memory: current pain intensity, emotion, expectation of pain, and peak intensity of previous pain [41]. Thus, it seems that the memory of pain is most strongly associated with pain intensity during the painful condition.

History of Pain

A thorough history to evaluate patients with pain includes the assessment of a number of variables that may play crucial roles in pain management. Patient characteristics such as age, gender, and ethnicity should never be missed in the assessment. Also, it is important to evaluate the presence or absence of depression, to assess how pain is affecting the patient's life, to obtain ratings of job satisfaction, and to find out about the support system available at home and at work. Listed below are important considerations to evaluate regarding the history of pain: (1) the pattern, intensity, location, and duration of the current episode of pain; (2) how and when the pain started; (3) previous episodes of pain and its treatment; (4) family history of similar pain conditions; (5) congenital problems since birth; (6) exacerbating and pain-relieving factors; (7) current mood and appetite; (8) quality of sleep; (9) presence or absence of fatigue; (10) previous accidents or injuries involving the area of pain; (11) activities of daily living; (12) work history; (13) sports and other leisure activities; (14) history of cancer and other chronic illnesses; (15) recent fever or unexplained weight loss; (16) history of hormonal disturbance; (17) use of medication, such as analgesics, anti-inflammatories, muscle relaxants, antidepressants, or corticosteroids; and (18) smoking and alcohol consumption history.

Techniques for Pain Assessment

Tools for pain measurement must have well-established reliability and validity, and they should have been used previously to assess pain outcomes. The types of assessments used will vary depending on the nature of the pain (acute or chronic) and on the practice setting of the therapist (in private practice, at a hospital, or in a multidisciplinary unit). In acute pain, the biomedical approach to pain assessment is frequently useful and adequate. However, in some acute pain situations, as well as in all chronic pain conditions, a biopsychosocial approach to pain assessment is required.

There are two main kinds of tools or scales for assessing pain: unidimensional and multidimensional. A unidimensional scale usually measures only one construct, such as pain intensity. A multidimensional scale simultaneously measures different constructs, whether or not it contains separate scales for each construct.

Pain measures are often classified as self-report, behavioral/observational, or physiological [85]. Self-report is the best method of assessing pain. Many validated self-report tools are available to help children and adults communicate their pain intensity. Patients unable to self-report pain must rely on others to recognize that they are in pain, assess the source of their pain, and then manage their pain accordingly.

Self-Report

Self-report measures are considered the "gold standard" and the most valid approach to pain measurement. Although self-report measures exist in verbal and nonverbal formats, both require the patient to have sufficient cognitive and language skills to understand the task and generate an accurate response [54,11]. Verbal self-report measures include structured interviews, questionnaires, self-rating scales, and pain adjective descriptors. Nonverbal measures include facial expression scales, visual analogue scales, and pain drawings [54,11].

Using a global rating scale, the therapist obtains a score of a patient's pain intensity. Tools such as numerical rating scales (NRS), visual analogue scales (VAS), and faces scales have been used as the foundation for global observational rating scales [13,17,18,29,81,83].

Facial expression seems to have an important role in the measurement of pain [21]. Most behavioral checklists and rating scales include items referring to the face. Facial expression scales are often used with young children to obtain a self-report of pain. All consist of a series of faces with varying expressions that range from neutral or smiling to distress or crying. The response requirement for young children is to point to the face that corresponds most closely to how much pain they have (pain intensity) [8,10,35], how the pain makes them feel (pain affect) [50], or both [88]. Facial expression scales are easy to administer, and most of them demonstrate adequate to excellent psychometric properties.

Behavior/Observation

In the absence of self-report, observation of behavior is a valid approach to pain assessment. Pain behaviors do not always mirror pain intensity accurately, and in some cases they indicate another physiological or emotional cause of distress [65]. The circumstances of the behavior and its potential sources must be considered when determining pain management. Consciousness of individual baseline behaviors and of changes that happen with discomfort is very useful in differentiating pain from other causes. A number of behavioral checklists and behavioral rating scales are available in the literature for assessing pain.

A behavior checklist provides a list of behaviors that are marked as either present (usually scored 1) or absent (usually scored 0), with no judgment of the intensity or frequency of the behavior [11,16]. The pain intensity score is defined as the number of items checked. The most common behavioral indices of pain in these scales include vocal, verbal, facial, postural, and motor behaviors. The instrument may or may not require observation for a specific period of time. Pain intensity is assumed to be greater if the observer notes a greater number of overt displays of pain.

Behavior rating scales incorporate a rating of the intensity, frequency, or duration of each behavior [2,27,50]. The most frequently used rating for individual behaviors is 0 (absent) to 2 (intense or frequent), but many other metrics have been used. In some such instruments, the metric chosen for each behavior may deliberately reflect the weight placed on that behavior as an index of pain; in other instruments, all items are arbitrarily weighted equally. Similarly, the number of items reflecting a particular domain of behavior may be chosen either according to evidence-based weighting, or more commonly arbitrarily, or based on the investigator's opinion. This approach allows for gradations in intensity or frequency of expressions of pain.

Observation of children's physical behaviors can be used to assess children's pain. These scales are used to infer pain in infants, in children who are unable to communicate, in children who are too young to comprehend the use of self-report scales, and in children with cognitive impairment or physical handicaps. Similarly, in cognitively impaired adults, behavioral observations are necessary to assess pain. Numerous behavioral scales have been developed that measure crying, facial expressions, verbal communication, and body movement as indicators of pain and distress [53,76].

Physiological Parameters

Physiological parameters such as heart rate, respiration rate, blood pressure, palmar sweating, cortisol levels, transcutaneous oxygen, vagal tone, and endorphin concentrations [22,78] have been tested as pain measures. Other physiological responses to pain include pupil dilation, flushing or pallor, nausea, and decreased oxygen saturation. However, physiological measures are not sensitive or specific as indicators of long-lasting pain and thus can only be used as a supplement to behavioral observations [28,79,89].

Physiological changes are seen primarily in the early stage of acute pain and usually subside with prolonged or chronic pain because of adaptation, making them unreliable indicators of persistent pain. Physiological responses match children's distress in a painful procedure or condition and mirror their global response to stress. There is not enough evidence to support any direct correlation between these physiological responses and pain. Thus, they are not optimal measures of pain experience. However, many of these parameters have been incorporated into behavioral scales to form a more comprehensive assessment, mainly in infants and nonverbal children.

Physiological parameters cannot be interpreted as a sign of pain in a number of situations because: (1) pain is a stressor, and changes in physiological parameters can occur as a response to either noxious stimuli or stress; and (2) those parameters have been used to investigate sharp pain of short duration, and there is a habituation of physiological responses to long-term pain [54,77]. Thus, physiological parameters should be used as a complementary measure to other more specific pain measures.

Pain Assessment in Adults

Pain Scales

Several rating scales are available to assess pain intensity. These scales have the advantage of being easy and quick to use, quantifiable, valid, and reliable. Furthermore, they are simple for the patient to understand and are sensitive to both pharmacological and nonpharmacological treatments. Pain scales such as the visual analogue scale (VAS), numerical rating scale (NRS), and verbal rating scale (VRS) have been commonly used to assess pain in adults in clinical practice as well as in clinical trials.

The VAS consists of a vertical or horizontal line, where the ends of the line represent the extreme limits of pain intensity (e.g., no pain or the worst pain imaginable) (Fig. 2B). Patients are asked to select a point or make a mark along the line to indicate the intensity of their pain. Many versions of visual analogue scales are found in the literature. Differences between scales include the anchor terminology, the presence or absence of divisions along the line, the units of measurement (e.g., centimeters or millimeters), the length of the scale (i.e., 10, 20, or 100 cm), and whether the scale is presented as a vertical or horizontal line [60]. The VAS is easy to administrate and reproduce and is applicable as a measure of pain in older children, adolescents, and adults [31].

Using the NRS, individuals are asked to rate the intensity of their pain on a scale of 0 (no pain) to 10 (worst pain). This scale is simple to administer, and the results are easily recorded. The NRS gives the most information when used in the sequential evaluation of pain and response to pain relief interventions [44] (Fig. 2A).

Some authors, recognizing the difficulty in discriminating pain intensity from pain unpleasantness and from other emotions such as fear, have adopted less specific terms such as "distress" or even "unpleasant" in place of "pain" in the title of their scale. Nevertheless, such scales may be treated by other researchers as predominantly or purely pain scales, and such "non-pain" scales are generally equally responsive to pain-producing or pain-relieving interventions compared to scales explicitly labeled as measures of pain. Few researchers have presented discriminant validity data showing that their observational scales can differentiate pain's intensity from its affective aspect or from other negative emotional states and reactions (Fig. 2C).

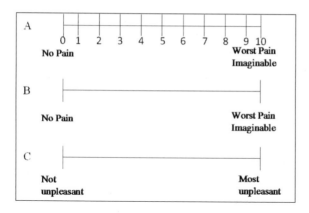

Fig. 2. (A) Numerical rating scale for pain. (B) Visual analogue scale for pain intensity. (C) Visual analogue scale for pain unpleasantness.

Body Diagrams

The use of a body diagram is a simple way to gain a graphical representation of the location of a patient's pain. The therapist simply asks the patient to draw the location of the pain on the diagram [75] (Fig. 3).

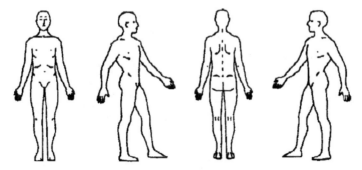

Fig. 3. Example of a body diagram in which the subject can draw the location of pain.

Multidimensional Pain Measures

As discussed in Chapter 1, pain is a multidimensional experience that results in multiple impairments, functional limitations, and disabilities. Thus, the measurement of pain should address not only the intensity of pain, but also the multidimensional nature of the pain experience as well as its impact on function and disability. Although unidimensional scales have been used successfully in recording pain intensity, they are not appropriate tools for collecting detailed information on either the affective component or other dimensions of the pain experience.

Pain Questionnaires

McGill Pain Questionnaire

Melzack and Casey [57] suggested that there are three major psychological dimensions of pain: sensory-discriminative, motivational-affective, and cognitive-evaluative. These dimensions interact with one another to provide quantitative and qualitative information on the components of pain. These dimensions formed the basis for the development of the McGill Pain Questionnaire (MPQ), which has become a tool for evaluating multidimensional aspects of the pain experience through the use of standard pain-related words. Evidence indicates that each pain condition is characterized by a distinctive group of words [72].

The MPQ offers a method to assess the sensory, affective, and evaluative components of pain. It is a self-administered measure consisting of four main parts [55] (Fig. 4). First, patients draw the location of their current pain on a body diagram. In the second part, which is the major component of the questionnaire, 78 pain descriptors are distributed across 20 subclasses, which are classified into five main classes. The subject is allowed to pick one word, or no words, from each subclass. The sensory class contains 10 subclasses (1–10), the affective class includes 5 subclasses (11–15), the evaluative class has 1 subclass (16), the miscellaneous class has 5 subclasses (17–20), and the total class contains all categories from 1 to 20. Further, each word from these categories has a rank value indicative of the relative intensity. Specifically, scoring is done by giving a number to the word chosen based on its location in the list so that the first number is given a 1, the second a 2, and so on. The maximal scores therefore for this part of the MPQ are 78 for the total, 42 for the sensory class, 14 for the affective class, and 5 for the evaluative class. The third part measures how the pain changes over time and lists the parameters that relieve or increase it. As a final point, the fourth part has a single measure of pain intensity that ranges from 1 to 5.

Different scores can be obtained from the MPQ, such as the Number of Words Chosen (NWC) (in part 2, with a range of 0–20), and Present Pain Intensity (PPI) in part 4, with a range of 1 (mild) to 5 (excruciating).

Patient's Name_____ Date_____ Time_____ am/pm Diagnosis_____

PRI: S_____ A_____ E_____ M_____ PRI(T)_____ PPI_____

Pain Rating Index: Circle the word or words that best describes your pain. You can only choose one word in any category. You may leave a category blank.

Mark your pain on the body diagram above.
E=External; I=Internal

1. Flickering Quivering Throbbing Pulsing Beating Pounding	11. Tiring Exhausting
	12. Sickening Suffocating
2. Jumping Flashing Shooting	13. Fearful Frightful Terrifying
3. Pricking Boring Drilling Stabbing Lancinating	14. Punishing Grueling Cruel Vicious Killing
4. Sharp Cutting Lacerating	15. Wretched Blinded
5. Pinching Pressing Gnawing Cramping Crushing	16. Annoying Troublesome Miserable Intense Unbearable
6. Tugging Pulling Wrenching	17. Spreading Radiating Penetrating Piercing
7. Hot Burning Scalding Searing	18. Tight Numb Drawing Squeezing Tearing
8. Tingling Itchy Smarting	19. Cool Cold Freezing
9. Dull Sore Hurting Aching Heavy	20. Nagging Nauseating Agonizing Dreadful Torturing
10. Tender Taut Rasping Splitting	

1. Which words would you use to describe the pattern of your pain?

1. Brief Transient Momentary	2. Rhythmic Periodic Intermittent	3. Continuous Steady Constant

2. What kind of things <u>relieve</u> your pain?

3. What kind of things make your pain <u>worse</u>?

People agree that the following 5 words represent pain of increasing intensity.
1 = mild 2 = discomforting 3 = distressing 4 = horrible 5 = excruciating
1. Which word describes your pain right now? _____
2. Which word describes your pain at its worst? _____
3. Which word describes your pain when it is least? _____
4. Which word describes the worst toothache you ever had? _____
5. Which word describes the worst headache you ever had? _____
6. Which word describes the worst stomach-ache you ever had? _____

Fig. 4. Reformatted from the original version of the McGill Pain Questionnaire (MPQ). The descriptors compose four major groups: sensory (S), 1–10; affective (A), 11–15; evaluative (E), 16; and miscellaneous (M), 17–20. The rank value for each descriptor is based on its position in the word set. The sum of the rank values is the pain rating index (PRI). The present pain intensity (PPI) is based on a scale of 0–5. Reprinted from [55] with permission of the IASP.

The rank values of the words chosen can be added to obtain a Pain Rating Index (PRI) for each category as well as a total PRI [59].

The MPQ has been shown to be a valid, objective, and reliable instrument [58]. It is one of the most widely used tests for pain assessment in both clinical and research settings and has been applied in diagnosis and research in a variety of pain problems. Its success has been further established by its translation or adaptation to many languages or cultures, including Dutch, French, German, Brazilian Portuguese, Norwegian, Swedish, Spanish, and Turkish.

Although the full MPQ takes only 5 minutes to administer, a short form of the MPQ (SF-MPQ) was developed to be used in situations in

Short Form of the McGill Pain Questionnaire

Patient's name:_____ Date:_____

		None	Mild	Moderate	Severe
1	Throbbing	0___	1___	2___	3___
2	Shooting	0___	1___	2___	3___
3	Stabbing	0___	1___	2___	3___
4	Sharp	0___	1___	2___	3___
5	Cramping	0___	1___	2___	3___
6	Gnawing	0___	1___	2___	3___
7	Hot-burning	0___	1___	2___	3___
8	Aching	0___	1___	2___	3___
9	Heavy	0___	1___	2___	3___
10	Tender	0___	1___	2___	3___
11	Splitting	0___	1___	2___	3___
12	Tiring-exhausting	0___	1___	2___	3___
13	Sickening	0___	1___	2___	3___
14	Fearful	0___	1___	2___	3___
15	Punishing-cruel	0___	1___	2___	3___

PPI
0   No Pain   _____
1   Mild   _____
2   Discomforting   _____
3   Distressing   _____
4   Horrible   _____
5   Excruciating   _____

VAS

├─────────────────────────────────────┤

     No   Worst
     Pain   Possible
                                     Pain

Fig. 5. The Short-Form of the McGill Pain Questionnaire. The sum of the rank values is the rating. Reprinted from [56] with permission of the IASP.

which administration of the complete questionnaire is too long (Fig. 5). The main component of the SF-MPQ consists of 15 descriptors (11 sensory and 4 affective) that are rated on an intensity scale from 0 to 3 (0 = none, 1 = mild, 2 = moderate, 3 = severe). Three pain scores are derived from the sum of the intensity rank values of the words chosen for sensory, affective, and total descriptors. The SF-MPQ still includes the PPI index of the standard MPQ and a VAS for pain intensity [56].

Brief Pain Inventory

Pain, mainly during its chronic stage, is often associated with physical and functional disabilities. The Brief Pain Inventory (BPI) is useful to assess the functional impact of pain (Fig. 6). The first part of the BPI measures pain severity using four different visual analogue scales anchored by 0 representing "no pain" and 10 being "pain as bad as you can imagine." The second part of the BPI measures how pain interferes with general activity, mood, walking, normal work, relationships with others, sleep, and enjoyment of life. Similar to the scale for pain severity, each functional item is ranked on an 11-point numeric scale, where 0 represents "does not interfere" and 10 denotes "completely interferes." The sum of the scores of the pain intensity items represents the intensity score, and the sum of the scores on the pain interference items represents the interference score [20]. Caution should be used because, as stated above, memory for pain intensity is poor, whereas memory for functional limitations as a result of pain is excellent.

Self-Efficacy Questionnaires

Numerous self-efficacy questionnaires are available to reveal the functional impact of pain on an individual. In general these questionnaires expand upon the BPI and use a VAS or NRS to assess the impact of pain on activities of daily living and social function. The use of a self-efficacy questionnaire is invaluable to understanding the pain experience. We have included two published and validated questionnaires that are used for people with chronic pain conditions as examples (Fig. 7 and Table I). The Pain Self-Efficacy Questionnaire (PSEQ) is a self-efficacy scale used for people with chronic pain that also asks the respondents to take pain into account when rating their self-efficacy beliefs (see items in Fig. 7). All

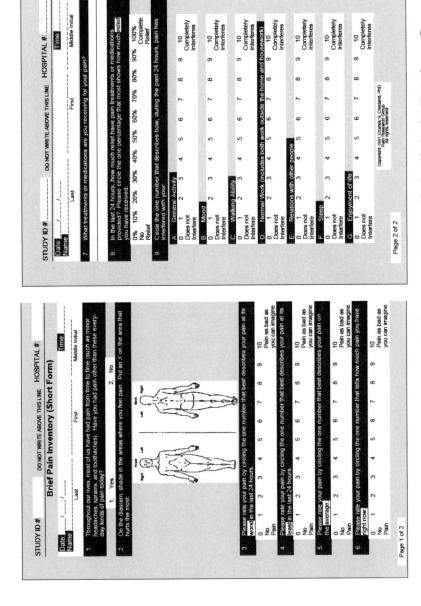

Fig. 6. The Brief Pain Inventory Form. Reprinted with permission from Dr. Charles Cleeland, MD Anderson Cancer Center.

PAIN S-E QUESTIONNAIRE (PSEQ)

NAME: _____ DATE: _____

Please note how **confident** you are that you can do the following things <u>at present,</u> **despite the pain.**
To indicate your answer, circle one of the numbers on the scale under each item, where 0= not at all
confident and 6 = completely confident.
For example:

   0 1 2 3 4 5 6
   Not at all   Completely
   confident   confident

Remember, this questionnaire is not asking whether or not you have been doing these things, but rather
how confident you are that you can do them at present, <u>despite the pain.</u>

---

1. I can enjoy things, despite the pain.
   0 1 2 3 4 5 6
   Not at all   Completely
   confident   confident
2. I can do most of the household chores (e.g., tidying up, washing dishes, etc.), despite the pain.
   0 1 2 3 4 5 6
   Not at all   Completely
   confident   confident
3. I can socialize with my friends or family members as often as I used to do, despite the pain.
   0 1 2 3 4 5 6
   Not at all   Completely
   confident   confident
4. I can copy with my pain in most situations.
   0 1 2 3 4 5 6
   Not at all   Completely
   confident   confident
5. I can do some form of work, despite the pain ("work" indicates housework, paid and unpaid
  work).
   0 1 2 3 4 5 6
   Not at all   Completely
   confident   confident
6. I can still do many of the things I enjoy doing, such as hobbies or leisure activity, despite the
  pain.
   0 1 2 3 4 5 6
   Not at all   Completely
   confident   confident
7. I can cope with my pain without medication.
   0 1 2 3 4 5 6
   Not at all   Completely
   confident   confident
8. I can still accomplish most of my goals in life, despite the pain.
   0 1 2 3 4 5 6
   Not at all   Completely
   confident   confident
9. I can live a normal lifestyle, despite the pain.
   0 1 2 3 4 5 6
   Not at all   Completely
   confident   confident
10. I can gradually become more active, despite the pain.
   0 1 2 3 4 5 6
   Not at all   Completely
   confident   confident

Fig. 7. The Pain Self-Efficacy Questionnaire. Reprinted from [62] with permission from Elsevier.

items include mention of performing the activities despite their pain, e.g., "I can do most of the household chores (e.g., tidying up, washing dishes), despite the pain" [62].

The Chronic Pain Self-Efficacy Scale (CPSS) (Table I) is designed to measure chronic pain patients' perceived ability to cope with its consequences. Each item in the CPSS is presented as a question by the examiner to the patient, e.g., "How certain are you that you can decrease your pain quite a bit?" [3]. The patient is then asked to respond on a 10-point Likert scale from 10 ("very uncertain") to 100 ("very certain"). Table I lists the questions for the CPSS, organized into three different domains: (1) pain management, (2) physical function, and (3) coping.

Fear-Avoidance Questionnaire

The Fear-Avoidance Beliefs Questionnaire (FABQ) is a self-report questionnaire of 16 items. This tool focuses on patients' beliefs about how physical activity and work affect their current low back pain. This questionnaire is based on fear theory and fear-avoidance cognitions, including beliefs about the seriousness of the illness and its effect on the patient's life, and on the concepts of somatic focusing and increased somatic awareness [84] (Table II). As will be seen in Chapter 16, this questionnaire has been used in physical therapy practice to screen patients with acute low back pain for placement into specific treatment programs.

Quality of Life Surveys

Pain is a central factor affecting the quality of life of those who have diseases characterized by chronic pain. The SF-36 Health Survey Questionnaire contains 36 items and takes about 5 minutes to complete. It measures health on eight multi-item dimensions, covering functional status (physical functioning, social functioning), role limitations (physical, emotional), well-being (mental health, vitality, pain), and overall evaluation of health (general health perception, health change). It is claimed that the SF-36 questionnaire is able to detect positive as well as negative states of health. In six of the eight dimensions, patients are asked to rate their responses on 3- or 6-point scales rather than simply responding yes or no (Table III). For each dimension, item scores are coded, summed, and transformed to

Table I
Chronic Pain Self-Efficacy Scale items

Self-Efficacy for Pain Management (PSE)

1. How certain are you that you can decrease you pain quite a bit?
2. How certain are you that you can continue most of your daily activities?
3. How certain are you that you can keep your pain from interfering with your sleep?
4. How certain are you that you can make a small-to-moderate reduction in your pain by using methods other than taking extra medication?
5. How certain are you that you can make a large reduction in your pain by using methods other than taking extra medications?

Self-Efficacy for Physical Function (PFE)

1. How certain are you that you can walk half a mile (0.8 km) on flat ground?
2. How certain are you that you can lift a 10-pound (4.5-kg) box?
3. How certain are you that you can perform a daily home exercise program?
4. How certain are you that you can perform your household chores?
5. How certain are you that you can shop for groceries or clothes?
6. How certain are you that you can engage in social activities?
7. How certain are you that you can engage in hobbies or recreational activities?
8. How certain are you that you can engage in family activities?
9. How certain are you that you can perform the work duties you had prior to the onset of chronic pain? (For homemakers, please consider your household activities as your work duties.)

Self-Efficacy for Coping with Symptoms (CSE)

1. How certain are you that you can control your fatigue?
2. How certain are you that you can regulate your activity so as to be active without aggravating your physical symptoms (e.g., fatigue, pain)?
3. How certain are you that you can do something to help yourself feel better if you are feeling blue?
4. As compared to other people with chronic medical problems like yours, how certain are you that you can manage your pain during your daily activities?
5. How certain are you that you can manage your physical symptoms so that you can do the things you enjoy doing?
6. How certain are you that you can deal with the frustration of chronic medical problems?
7. How certain are you that you can cope with mild to moderate pain?
8. How certain are you that you can cope with severe pain?

Source: Adapted from Appendix A of [3], with permission from IASP.

Note: Questionnaires are delivered to the subject, and the subject rates the response on a 10-point Likert scale from very uncertain to very certain.

a scale from 0 (worst health) to 100 (best health) [14]. Scores can also be transformed against population norms (set at 50). Negative health aspects would then show as <50 and positive health aspects as >50.

Another tool, proposed by the World Health Organization (WHO), is the WHO Quality of Life Assessment (WHOQOL). This

Table II
Fear-Avoidance Beliefs Questionnaire (FABQ)

Here are some of the things which other patients have told us about their pain.
For each statement, please circle a number from 0 to 6 to say how much physical
activities such as bending, lifting, walking or driving affect or would affect your
back pain.

	Completely disagree		Unsure		Completely agree	
1. My pain was caused by physical activity	0	1	2	3	4	5	6
2. Physical activity makes my pain worse	0	1	2	3	4	5	6
3. Physical activity might harm my back	0	1	2	3	4	5	6
4. I should not do physical activities which (might) make my pain worse	0	1	2	3	4	5	6
5. I cannot do physical activities which (might) make my pain worse	0	1	2	3	4	5	6

The following statements are about how your normal work affects or would affect
your back pain.

	Completely disagree		Unsure		Completely agree	
6. My pain was caused by my work or by an accident at work	0	1	2	3	4	5	6
7. My work aggravated my pain	0	1	2	3	4	5	6
8. I have a claim for compensation for my pain	0	1	2	3	4	5	6
9. My work is too heavy for me	0	1	2	3	4	5	6
10. My work makes or would make my pain worse	0	1	2	3	4	5	6
11. My work might harm my back	0	1	2	3	4	5	6
12. I should do my normal work with my present pain	0	1	2	3	4	5	6
13. I cannot do my normal work with my present pain	0	1	2	3	4	5	6
14. I cannot do my normal work till my pain is treated	0	1	2	3	4	5	6
15. I do not think that I will be back to my normal work within 3 months	0	1	2	3	4	5	6
16. I do not think that I will ever be able to go back to that work	0	1	2	3	4	5	6

Scoring

Scale 1: fear-avoidance beliefs about work: items 6, 7, 9, 10, 11, 12, 15.

Scale 2: fear-avoidance beliefs about physical activity: items 2, 3, 4, 5.

Source: Reprinted with permission from [84] with permission of the IASP.

Table III

Short Form-36 Quality of Life Questionnaire (Medical Outcomes Trust, 1992)

This survey asks for your views about your health. This information will help keep track of how you feel and how well you are able to do your usual activities. Please answer these questions by "check-marking" your choice. Please select only one choice for each item.			

1. In general, would you say your health is:
1. Excellent   2. Very good   3. Good   4. Fair   5. Poor

2. Compared to ONE YEAR AGO, how would you rate your health in general NOW?
1. MUCH BETTER than one year ago.
2. Somewhat BETTER now than one year ago.
3. About the SAME as one year ago.
4. Somewhat WORSE now than one year ago.
5. MUCH WORSE now than one year ago.

3. The following items are about activities you might do during a typical day. Does your health now limit you in these activities? If so, how much?

a) Vigorous activities, such as running, lifting heavy objects, participating in strenuous sports?	1. Yes, limited a lot	2. Yes, limited a little	3. No, not limited at all
b) Moderate activities, such as moving a table, pushing a vacuum cleaner, bowling, playing golf?	1. Yes, limited a lot	2. Yes, limited a little	3. No, not limited at all
c) Lifting or carrying groceries?	1. Yes, limited a lot	2. Yes, limited a little	3. No, not limited at all
d) Climbing several flights of stairs?	1. Yes, limited a lot	2. Yes, limited a little	3. No, not limited at all
e) Climbing one flight of stairs?	1. Yes, limited a lot	2. Yes, limited a little	3. No, not limited at all
f) Bending, kneeing or stooping?	1. Yes, limited a lot	2. Yes, limited a little	3. No, not limited at all
g) Walking more than a mile?	1. Yes, limited a lot	2. Yes, limited a little	3. No, not limited at all
h) Walking several blocks?	1. Yes, limited a lot	2. Yes, limited a little	3. No, not limited at all
i) Walking one block?	1. Yes, limited a lot	2. Yes, limited a little	3. No, not limited at all
j) Bathing or dressing yourself?	1. Yes, limited a lot	2. Yes, limited a little	3. No, not limited at all

4. During the past 4 weeks, have you had any of the following problems with your work or other regular activities as a result of your physical health?

a) Cut down on the amount of time you spent on work or other activities?	1. Yes	2. No
b) Accomplished less than you would like?	1. Yes	2. No
c) Were limited in the kind of work or other activities?	1. Yes	2. No
d) Had difficulty performing the work or other activities (for example it took extra effort)?	1. Yes	2. No

(Table III continues on next page)

(Table III, continued from previous page)

5. During the past 4 weeks, have you had any of the following problems with your work or other regular daily activities as a result of any emotional problems (such as feeling depressed or anxious)?		
a) Cut down on the amount of time you spent on work or other activities?	1. Yes	2. No
b) Accomplished less than you would like?	1. Yes	2. No
c) Didn't do work or other activities as carefully as usual?	1. Yes	2. No

6. During the past 4 weeks, to what extent has your physical health or emotional problems interfered with your normal social activities with family, friends, neighbors, or groups?
1. Not at all   2. Slightly   3. Moderately   4. Quite a bit   5. Extremely

7. How much bodily pain have you had during the past 4 weeks?
1. None   2. Very mild   3. Mild   4. Moderate   5. Severe   6. Very severe

8. During the past 4 weeks, how much did pain interfere with your normal work (including both work outside the home and housework)?
1. Not at all   2. A little bit   3. Moderately   4. Quite a bit   5. Extremely

9. These questions are about how you feel and how things have been with you during the past 4 weeks. For each question , please give the one answer that comes closest to the way you have been feeling. How much of the time during the past 4 weeks ...

	1. All of the time	2. Most of the time	3. A good bit of the time	4. Some of the time	5. A little of the time	6. None of the time
a) Did you feel full of pep?	1. All of the time	2. Most of the time	3. A good bit of the time	4. Some of the time	5. A little of the time	6. None of the time
b) Have you been a very nervous person?	1. All of the time	2. Most of the time	3. A good bit of the time	4. Some of the time	5. A little of the time	6. None of the time
c) Have you felt so down in the dumps that nothing could cheer you up?	1. All of the time	2. Most of the time	3. A good bit of the time	4. Some of the time	5. A little of the time	6. None of the time
d) Have you felt calm and peaceful?	1. All of the time	2. Most of the time	3. A good bit of the time	4. Some of the time	5. A little of the time	6. None of the time
e) Did you have a lot of energy?	1. All of the time	2. Most of the time	3. A good bit of the time	4. Some of the time	5. A little of the time	6. None of the time
f) Have you felt downhearted and blue?	1. All of the time	2. Most of the time	3. A good bit of the time	4. Some of the time	5. A little of the time	6. None of the time
g) Do you feel worn out?	1. All of the time	2. Most of the time	3. A good bit of the time	4. Some of the time	5. A little of the time	6. None of the time
h) Have you been a happy person?	1. All of the time	2. Most of the time	3. A good bit of the time	4. Some of the time	5. A little of the time	6. None of the time
i) Did you feel tired?	1. All of the time	2. Most of the time	3. A good bit of the time	4. Some of the time	5. A little of the time	6. None of the time

(Table III continues on next page)

(Table III, continued from previous page)

10. During the past 4 weeks, how much of the time has your physical health or emotional problems interfered with your social activities (like visiting with friends, relatives, etc.)? 1. All of the time 2. Most of the time. 3. Some of the time 4. A little of the time. 5. None of the time.					
11. How TRUE or FALSE is each of the following statements for you?					
a) I seem to get sick a little easier than other people.	1. Definitely true	2. Mostly true	3. Don't know	4. Mostly false	5. Definitely false
b) I am as healthy as anybody I know.	1. Definitely true	2. Mostly true	3. Don't know	4. Mostly false	5. Definitely false
c) I expect my health to get worse.	1. Definitely true	2. Mostly true	3. Don't know	4. Mostly false	5. Definitely false
d) My health is excellent.	1. Definitely true	2. Mostly true	3. Don't know	4. Mostly false	5. Definitely false

Source: Reprinted with permission from Medical Outcomes Trust and Quality Metric Inc.

generic quality-of-life instrument was designed to be applicable to people living in different circumstances, conditions, and cultures [86,87]. Two versions are available: the full version, WHOQOL-100 (100 items), and the short version, WHOQOL-BREF (26 items). The WHOQOL-100 produces scores relating to particular facets of quality of life (e.g., positive feelings, social support, financial resources), scores relating to larger domains (e.g., physical and psychological factors, social relationships), and a score relating to overall quality of life and general health. The WHOQOL-BREF produces domain scores, but not individual facet scores (Table IV). Regarding somatic diseases, the WHOQOL-100 has good to excellent validity and reliability [73]. It is based on a Likert-type scale and is scored from 1 to 5, with higher scores indicating a better quality of life.

Disease-Specific Questionnaires

Several disease-specific questionnaires have proven useful when evaluating particular diseases. These questionnaires include the Fibromyalgia Impact Questionnaire (FIQ, see Chapter14) [15], the Oswestry Disability Questionnaire [25], the Western Ontario and McMaster Universities Osteoarthritis Index (WOMAC, see Chapter 18) [6], and the Disabilities of the Arm, Shoulder and Hand (DASH) [5]. These questionnaires are commonly used in clinical trial research, and they are increasingly been used in clinical practice. In a diverse clinical practice, however, it is difficult to use a variety of disease-specific questionnaires, and therefore they are typically used in specialty clinics. However, in a chronic back pain clinic, the Oswestry Disability Questionnaire may prove more useful than the self-efficacy questionnaires listed above.

Table IV
The World Health Organization Quality of Life Survey (WHOQOL)

The following questions ask how you feel about your quality of life, health, or other areas of your life. I will read out each question to you, along with the response options. Please choose the answer that appears most appropriate. If you are unsure about which response to give to a question, the first response you think of is often the best one.

		Very poor	Poor	Neither poor nor good	Good	Very good
1.	How would you rate your quality of life?	1	2	3	4	5

		Very dis-satisfied	Dis-satisfied	Neither satisfied nor dis-satisfied	Satisfied	Very satisfied
2.	How satisfied are you with your health?	1	2	3	4	5

The following questions ask about how much you have experienced certain things in the last four weeks.

		Not at all	A little	A moderate amount	Very much	An extreme amount
3.	To what extent do you feel that physical pain prevents you from doing what you need to do?	5	4	3	2	1
4.	How much do you need any medical treatment to function in your daily life?	5	4	3	2	1
5.	How much do you enjoy life?	1	2	3	4	5
6.	To what extent do you feel your life to be meaningful?	1	2	3	4	5
7.	How well are you able to concentrate?	1	2	3	4	5
8.	How safe do you feel in your daily life?	1	2	3	4	5
9.	How healthy is your physical environment?	1	2	3	4	5

(Table IV continues on next page)

Table IV
Continued

The following questions ask about how completely you experience or were able to do certain things in the last four weeks.

		Not at all	A little	Mode-rately	Mostly	Com-pletely
10.	Do you have enough energy for everyday life?	1	2	3	4	5
11.	Are you able to accept your bodily appearance?	1	2	3	4	5
12.	Have you enough money to meet your needs?	1	2	3	4	5
13.	How available to you is the information that you need in your day-to-day life?	1	2	3	4	5
14.	To what extent do you have the opportunity for leisure activities?	1	2	3	4	5

		Very poor	Poor	Neither poor nor good	Good	Very good
15.	How well are you able to get around?	1	2	3	4	5

		Very dis-satisfied	Dis-satisfied	Neither satisfied nor dis-satisfied	Satisfied	Very satisfied
16.	How satisfied are you with your sleep?	1	2	3	4	5
17.	How satisfied are you with your ability to perform your daily living activities?	1	2	3	4	5
18.	How satisfied are you with your capacity for work?	1	2	3	4	5
19.	How satisfied are you with yourself?	1	2	3	4	5
20.	How satisfied are you with your personal relationships?	1	2	3	4	5
21.	How satisfied are you with your sex life?	1	2	3	4	5
22.	How satisfied are you with the support you get from your friends?	1	2	3	4	5
23.	How satisfied are you with the conditions of your living place?	1	2	3	4	5
24.	How satisfied are you with your access to health services?	1	2	3	4	5
25.	How satisfied are you with your transport?	1	2	3	4	5

(Table IV continues on next page)

Table IV
Continued

The following question refers to how often you have felt or experienced certain things in the last four weeks.

		Never	Seldom	Quite often	Very often	Always
26.	How often do you have negative feelings such as blue mood, despair, anxiety, depression?	5	4	3	2	1

Do you have any comments about the assessment?

[The following table should be completed after the interview is finished]

			Raw Score	Trans-formed Scores* 4–20	Trans-formed Scores* 0–100
		Equations for computing domain scores	Raw Score	4–20	0–100
27.	Domain 1	(6–Q3)+ (6–Q4) + Q10 + Q15 + Q16 + Q17 + Q18 ( ) + ( ) + ( ) + ( ) + ( ) + ( ) + ( )	a =	b:	c:
28.	Domain 2	Q5 + Q6 + Q7 + Q11 + Q19 + (6–Q26) ( ) + ( ) + ( ) + ( ) + ( ) + ( )	a =	b:	c:
29.	Domain 3	Q20 + Q21 + Q22 ( ) + ( ) + ( )	a =	b:	c:
30	Domain 4	Q8 + Q9 + Q12 + Q13 + Q14 + Q23 + Q24 + Q25 ( ) + ( ) + ( ) + ( ) + ( ) + ( ) + ( ) + ( )	a =	b:	c:

Source: Printed with permission from the World Health Organization.
*See Procedures Manual at WHOQOL Group Website.

Pain Assessment in Special Patient Populations

Most of the assessment measures described above have been used in cognitively intact adults, but some can also apply to other populations. This section outlines special considerations in pain assessment for newborns, children and adolescents, and neurologically or cognitively impaired patients.

Newborns

Assessment of the pain experience in infants and young children is regularly limited by their inability to verbalize pain or localize its source [36]. The infant, unless paralyzed or comatose, provides the health care practitioner with signals of pain through a variety of physiological and behavioral methods such as vocal expressions, including crying; facial expressions; rigid body posture; clenched hands or toes; body movements, such as withdrawal from a painful stimulus, or limpness or flaccidity in preterm or ill infants; altered sleep patterns; and inconsolability [26,74]. As can be seen, the use of these signals to rate pain is both indirect and inferential [36]. Parents play a crucial role when evaluating their infant's pain. Most parents can distinguish pain behaviors in their baby quite easily, so their evaluation should be included in pain assessment [17,42,61].

Many tools have been developed to assess infants' pain in several acute pain conditions. The Neonatal Facial Coding System (NFCS) is a systematic description of infant pain expression [33] (Table V). This coding system provides a detailed, anatomically based, and objective description of an infant's reaction to potentially painful events. The NFCS is used to score for the presence or absence (scored 0 or 1) of 10 discrete facial actions, namely brow bulge, eye squeeze, nasolabial furrow, open lips, vertical mouth stretch,

Table V
Systematic description of infant pain expression according
to the Neonatal Facial Coding System

Action	Description
Brow bulge	Bulging, creasing, and vertical furrows above and between the brows occurring as a result of the lowering and drawing together of the brows.
Eye squeeze	Identified by the squeezing or bulging of the eyelids. Bulging of the fatty pads about the infant's eyes is pronounced.
Nasolabial furrow	Primarily manifested by the pulling upward and deepening of the nasolabial furrow (a line or wrinkle that begins adjacent to the nostril wings and runs down and outward beyond the lip corners).
Open lips	Any separation of the lips is scored as open lips.
Stretch mouth (vertical)	Characterized by a tautness at the lip corners coupled with a pronounced downward pull on the jaw. Often, stretch mouth is seen when an already wide-open mouth is opened a fraction further by an extra pull at the jaw.
Stretch mouth (horizontal)	This appears as a distinct horizontal pull at the corners of the mouth.
Lip purse	The lips appear as if an "ooh" sound is being pronounced.
Taut tongue	Characterized by a raised, cupped tongue with sharp, tensed edges. The first occurrence of taut tongue is usually easy to see, often occurring with a wide-open mouth. After this first occurrence, the mouth may close slightly. Taut tongue is still scorable on the basis of the still-visible tongue edges.

Source: Adapted from [32], with permission of the IASP.
Note: If the action does not occur, 0 points are scored. If the action occurs, 1 point is scored. A score greater than 3 indicates pain.

horizontal mouth stretch, lip purse, taut tongue, tongue protrusion, and chin quiver. The NFCS has been validated and was recently used to study pain responses in children up to 18 months of age [45].

Another instrument that has been widely used for evaluating an infant's pain is the Neonatal Infant Pain Scale (NIPS), which quantifies the level of pain on a scale from 0 to 7 based on five behavioral characteristics: facial expressions, crying, movements of arms and legs, and state of arousal. In addition, breathing pattern is used as a physiological parameter [43]. The NIPS is very easy and quick to use (Table VI).

Table VI
Pain assessment on the Neonatal Infant Pain Scale

		Score
Facial Expression		
Relaxed muscles	Restful face, neutral expression	0
Grimace	Tight facial muscles; furrowed brow, chin, jaw (negative facial expression: nose, mouth, and brow)	1
Cry		
No cry	Quiet, no crying	0
Whimper	Mild moaning, intermittent	1
Vigorous cry	Loud scream; rising, shrill, continuous (Note: silent cry may be scored if baby is intubated by evidence of obvious mouth and facial movement)	2
Breathing Patterns		
Relaxed	Usual pattern for this infant	0
Change in breathing	Indrawing, irregular, faster than usual; gagging, breath holding	1
Arms		
Relaxed/restrained	No muscular rigidity; occasional random movement of arms	0
Flexed/extended	Tense, straight legs; rigid and/or rapid extension, flexion	1
Legs		
Relaxed/restrained	No muscular rigidity; occasional random movement of arms	0
Flexed/extended	Tense, straight legs; rigid and/or rapid extension, flexion	1
State of Arousal		
Sleeping/awake	Quiet, peaceful sleeping or alert random leg movement	0
Fussy	Alert, restless, and thrashing	1

Source: Printed with permission of Children's Hospital of Eastern Ontario.

Children and Adolescents

A number of tools or scales for assessing children's pain have been developed in the last three decades. They can be classified as physiological, behavioral/observational, or self-report, depending on the nature of the response that is measured [44]. Many factors can modify pain perception in children, including age, gender, cognitive level, previous experience with pain, family learning, and culture. These factors are usually stable in contrast to many cognitive, behavioral, and emotional factors, which vary depending on the situation, and they can greatly modify a child's perception and expression of pain [48,49].

Most 2-year-old children can report the presence and location of pain, but children do not have the cognitive skills needed to describe pain intensity until about 3 or 4 years of age. Generally, most 3-year-old children can use a three-level pain intensity scale with simple terms such as "no pain," "a little pain," or "a lot of pain." Four-year-old children can usually manage four- or five-item scales [19,30,35,37].

Probably the most commonly used assessment tool for children is the Faces Pain Scale. This scale consists of seven gender-neutral faces depicting "no pain" (neutral face) to "most pain possible" expressions, placed at equal intervals horizontally [10]. The children are instructed to point to the face that shows how much pain they feel. The faces are scored from 0 to 6. Variations of this scale, shown in Fig. 8, are the Wong-Baker FACES Pain Scale (Fig. 8A) [88] and the Faces Pain Scale-Revised [10] (Fig. 8B). These scales have been validated for use in both acute and chronic disease-related pain.

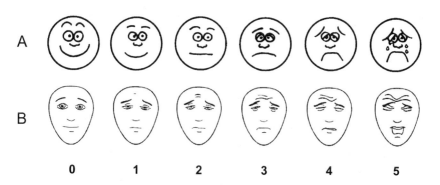

Fig. 8. (A) The Wong-Baker Faces Pain Scale, reprinted from [88] with permission. (B) The Faces Pain Scale-Revised, reprinted from [10] with permission of IASP.

When children are approximately 8 years of age, they are able to rate the quality of pain [51,69]. Thus, school-aged children and adolescents can also use verbal numerical rating scales, originally studied in adults to assess pain intensity.

Quantitative scales such as the visual analogue scale (VAS) [19], the Coloured Analogue Scale (CAS) [52], and numerical scales require more complex concepts and skills that generally emerge between 5 and 7 years. The CAS is similar to a VAS and was developed specifically for assessing pain in children. The CAS varies in three dimensions—color, width, and length—so that children can more easily understand that different scale positions reflect different values in pain intensity. A recent investigation showed that it has equivalent psychometric properties to a VAS [80]. This tool appears to be simple and easy to administer, making it practical for clinical use.

On the other hand, adolescents indicate preference for visual analogue and numerical rating scales [31].The Adolescent Pediatric Pain Tool (APPT) [69,70] and the Pediatric Pain Questionnaire (PPQ) [82] are examples of multidimensional pain measures used with older children and adolescents. The MPQ [55,56] is an example of an adult pain measure that has been used in clinical practice with older adolescents. In summary, there are many excellent pediatric self-report measures, and their clinical application requires careful consideration of age, developmental factors, and measurement issues [64].

Patients with Neurological or Cognitive Impairment

Unfortunately, some patients with dementia, patients with neurological disorders (affecting memory, language, or cognition), and critically ill or nonverbal children with serious cognitive problems are not able to offer an accurate evaluation about their own pain. Damage to the central nervous system affects the memory, language, and higher-order cognitive processing necessary to communicate the experience. Among older adults, despite changes in central nervous system functioning, persons with dementia or cognitive impairments still experience pain sensation to a degree similar to that of the cognitively intact individual [71]. Although self-report of pain is often possible in those with mild to moderate cognitive impairment, as dementia progresses, the ability to report pain decreases, and eventually self-report is no longer possible. Patients with severe dementia or neurological disorders are generally unable to report pain orally, in writing, or by other means [60,66]. Critiques of existing nonverbal pain assessment tools indicate that, although there are some tools with potential, there is no tool that has strong reliability and validity that can be recommended for broad adoption in clinical practice for persons with advanced dementia [34,76,90].

Facial expressions, verbalizations/vocalizations, body movements, changes in interpersonal interactions, alterations in activity patterns or routines, and changes in mental status have been identified as categories of potential pain indicators in older persons with dementia. Some behaviors are typically considered pain-related (e.g., facial grimacing, moaning, groaning, or rubbing a body part). Others are less obvious—agitation, restlessness, irritability, confusion, combativeness (particularly with care activities or treatments), or changes in appetite or activities—and require follow-up evaluation such as monitoring the response to analgesics. Tools for evaluating pain in patients with dementia are in varying stages of the development and validation process. Those with the strongest conceptual and psychometric support at this time, as well as clinical utility, are cited in Herr and colleagues' article [76], to which we refer the reader for additional information.

Physical and Functional Examination

In addition to the assessment of pain through pain scales and questionnaires, objective measures of hyperalgesia or function are useful. The patient's ability to engage in functional activities can be assessed by numerous self-report tools. These measures can assess the severity of pain during activities such as walking up and down stairs, sitting for a specific time, lifting specific weights, or performing activities of daily living. There is a good correspondence among self-reports, disease characteristics, physical therapists' or physicians' ratings of functional abilities, and objective functional performance [24,38].

Commonly used functional assessment scales are the Roland-Morris Disability Scale [68], the Functional Status Index [38], and the Oswestry Disability Scale [25]. A more extensive instrument, the Sickness

Impact Profile, includes over 150 questions to examine a range of physical activities and psychological features [7].

Range of Motion

Physical therapists routinely assess range of motion (ROM) of specific joints. Assessing active and passive ROM can give valuable information on limitations. To further clarify the nature of the pain, Maitland [47] suggests examining the point in the ROM when pain first becomes painful (P1) and the point when a person must stop due to pain (P2). This type of assessment can prove extremely valuable in understanding the nature and sensitivity of the pain so that the treatment plan can be individualized. For example, compare two patients with the same diagnosis, lateral epicondylalgia, who both have full passive ROM. In patient 1, P1 for elbow flexion is 10 degrees and P2 is 30 degrees. In patient 2, P1 for elbow flexion is 60 degrees and P2 is full ROM. Patient 1 is clearly limited in his abilities due to the pain, and his condition is highly sensitive. Patient 2 has full active ROM despite pain increasing at 60 degrees, and his condition is therefore not as sensitive as that of patient 1. Thus, the treatment approach for patient 1 should be geared toward pain reduction, and exercise should proceed more slowly. On the other hand, patient 2 can be treated more aggressively with active exercises and manual therapies as needed.

Strength

Assessment of strength and of the impact of pain on strength is a highly useful skill. Pain and strength are interrelated in several ways. First, strength can be limited as a result of pain. Full muscle contraction may not be possible because of pain. In this case, reducing pain will have an immediate effect on strength. On the other hand, a decrease in the strength of a particular muscle may result in abnormal function of the joint, and thus may result in pain. In this case, one must strengthen the weakened muscle to reduce pain, and thus relief of pain may be delayed. Third, long-standing disuse may result in a loss of strength in a particular muscle or muscle groups. In this case, strengthening of the muscle or muscle groups is necessary to return the patient to full functional status. However, there may be little direct impact of strengthening on the pain measure.

Hyperalgesia and Allodynia

Hyperalgesia to mechanical stimuli can be measured with a pressure algometer (Fig. 9A) by examining the pressure pain threshold both at the site of injury (primary hyperalgesia) and outside the site of injury (secondary hyperalgesia). These measures will give the therapist an understanding of the underlying mechanisms of the patient's pain condition. Primary hyperalgesia will indicate pain resulting from peripheral factors. However, if secondary hyperalgesia exists, a patient is likely to have alterations in the central processing of nociceptive stimuli.

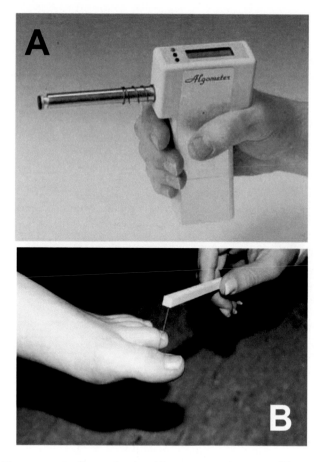

Fig. 9. (A) Measurement of hyperalgesia with a pressure algometer; (B) measurement of allodynia with a von Frey filament.

Allodynia, a painful response to nonpainful stimuli, particularly of the extremities (the hands and feet) is commonly measured using von Frey filaments (also known as Semmes Weinstein monofilaments) (Fig. 9B). This measure is extremely useful in patients with neuropathic pain, complex regional pain syndrome, or postoperative pain [4]. Using graded forces applied to the skin, the therapist can assess a threshold for pain response. Under normal conditions, only high forces will produce pain. However, after nerve injury, in complex regional pain syndrome, or post-operatively, the threshold decreases to a level that is considered indicative of allodynia. The therapist can also assess allodynia by brushing the skin with a cotton wisp or with sophisticated graded stimuli [46]. Patients with allodynia would clearly have a strong central component to their pain.

Functional Measures

Several functional tests are commonly used to assess the impact of pain on speed and function. In general these tests are timed. Functional tests have been found valuable for both acute and chronic pain. Novy and colleagues [63] analyzed several measures in people with low back pain and deter-mined that the functional factors tested fall into one of two categories: (1) speed and coordination or (2) endurance and strength. For speed and endurance, the "timed up and go" test (TUG) is commonly utilized. In this test the subject is asked to stand from sitting and walk a distance of 10 feet (3.048 meters), return, and sit back down. The time in which the subject performs this task is then recorded. Scores of 10 seconds or less are con-sidered within normal range [12]. Similar tests include the 50-foot walk test (the time it takes for a person to walk 50 feet [15.24 meters]; normally 8–9 seconds), the sit to stand test (the time it takes for a person to come from a sitting to a standing position five times; normally 7–8 seconds), and repeated trunk flexion (the time it takes to flex and extend the trunk five times; normally 14–16 seconds) [63]. All of these measures assess speed and coordination, and thus they do not all need to be performed in every patient.

For measures of endurance and strength, the 5-minute walk test measures the distance a person can walk in 5 minutes. The loaded reach task uses a standard weight, such as 5% body weight, and the patient holds the weight initially at shoulder height close to the body and then reaches forward as far as possible. The distance the person can reach is then recorded. These measures are particularly useful for documenting progress and effectiveness of treatment.

Summary

In summary, a battery of tests and measures should be used to assess both acute and chronic pain. Although generally acute pain is considered a symptom, it can have a huge impact on function and quality of life (see Chapter 1). Chronic pain clearly has a multidimensional nature and affects function and quality of life (see Chapter 1). Understanding the multidimensional nature of pain, the effect of pain on function, and the impact of pain on quality of life is vital to effective treatment. Furthermore, fear of pain and avoidance of activity are common in both acute and chronic pain conditions. Treatment of an individual who is afraid of re-injury will most likely involve a multidisciplinary approach using the biopsychosocial model. This approach is important for both acute and chronic pain conditions. However, for some people fear of pain is not a problem. For example, classical overachievers may constantly reinjure themselves. In this case, use of the biopsychosocial model may be inappropriate, and the biomedical model of treatment may be more important.

References

[1]   Acute Pain Management Guideline Panel. Acute pain management: operative or medical procedures and trauma. Clinical practice guideline. AHCPR publication 92–0032. Rockville: Agency for Health Care Policy and Research, Public Health Service, U.S. Department of Health and Human Services; 1992.

[2]   Ambuel B, Hamlett KW, Marx CM, Blumer JL. Assessing distress in pediatric intensive care environments: the COMFORT scale. J Pediatr Psychol 1992;17:95–109.

[3]   Anderson KO, Dowds BN, Pelletz RE, Edwards WT, Peeters-Asdourian C. Development and initial validation of a scale to measure self-efficacy beliefs in patients with chronic pain. Pain 1995;63:77–84.

[4]   Atherton DD, Taherzadeh O, Elliot D, Anand P. Age-dependent development of chronic neuropathic pain, allodynia and sensory recovery after upper limb nerve injury in children. J Hand Surg Eur 2008;33:186–91.

[5]   Beaton DE, Katz JN, Fossel AH, Wright JG, Tarasuk V, Bombardier C. Measuring the whole or the parts? Validity, reliability, and responsiveness of the Disabilities of the Arm, Shoulder and Hand outcome measure in different regions of the upper extremity. J Hand Ther 2001;14:128–46.

[6]   Bellamy N, Buchanan WW, Goldsmith CH, Campbell J, Stitt LW. Validation study of WOMAC: a health status instrument for measuring clinically important patient relevant outcomes to antirheumatic drug therapy in patients with osteoarthritis of the hip or knee. J Rheumatol 1988;15:1833–40.

[7]   Bergner M, Bobbitt RA, Carter WB, Gilson BS. The sickness impact profile: development and
      final revision of a health status measure. Med Care 1981;19:787–805.
[8]   Beyer JE, Ashley LC, Russell GA, DeGood DE. Pediatric pain after cardiac surgery: pharmaco-
      logic management. Dimens Crit Care Nurs 1984;3:326–34.
[9]   Beyer JE, Wells N. The assessment of pain in children. Pediatr Clin North Am 1989;36:837–54.
[10] Bieri D, Reeve RA, Champion GD, Addicoat L, Ziegler JB. The Faces Pain Scale for the self-
      assessment of the severity of pain experienced by children: development, initial validation, and
      preliminary investigation for ratio scale properties. Pain 1990;41:139–50.
[11] Boelen-van der Loo WJ, Scheffer E, de Haan RJ, de Groot CJ. Clinimetric evaluation of the pain
      observation scale for young children in children aged between 1 and 4 years after ear, nose, and
      throat surgery. J Dev Behav Pediatr 1999;20:222–7.
[12] Bohannon RW. Reference values for the timed up and go test: a descriptive meta-analysis. J
      Geriatr Phys Ther. 2006;29:64–8.
[13] Bosenberg A, Thomas J, Lopez T, Kokinsky E, Larsson LE. Validation of a six-graded faces scale
      for evaluation of postoperative pain in children. Pediatr Anaesth 2003;13:708–13.
[14] Brazier JE, Harper R, Jones NMB, O'Cathain A, Thomas KJ, Usherwood T, Westlake L. Val-
      idating the SF-36 health survey questionnaire: new outcome measure for primary care. BMJ
      1992;305:160–4.
[15] Burckhardt CS, Clark SR, Bennett RM. The fibromyalgia impact questionnaire: development and
      validation. J Rheumatol 1991;18:728–33.
[16] Chambers CT, Finley GA, McGrath PJ, Walsh TM. The parents' postoperative pain measure:
      replication and extension to 2–6-year-old children. Pain 2003;105:437–43.
[17] Chambers CT, Giesbrecht K, Craig KD, Bennett SM, Hunstsman E. A comparison on faces
      scales for measurement of pediatric pain: children's and parent's ratings. Pain 1999;83:25–35.
[18] Chambers CT, Hardial J, Craig KD, Court C, Montgomery C. Faces scales for the measurement
      of postoperative pain intensity in children following minor surgery. Clin J Pain 2005;21:277–85.
[19] Champion GD, Goodenough B, von Baeyer CL, Perrott D, Taplin JE, von Baeyer CL, Ziegler JB.
      Measurement of pain by self-report. Prog Pain Res Manage 1998;10:123–60.
[20] Craig KD. The facial expression of pain: better than a thousand words. Am Pain Soc J 1992;1:153–
      62.
[21] Craig KD, Grunau RVE. Neonatal pain perception and behavioral measurement. In: Anand KJS,
      McGrath PJ, editors. Pain in neonates. Amsterdam: Elsevier; 1993. p. 67–105.
[22] Dawson EG, Kanim LE, Sra P, Dorey FJ, Goldstein TB, Delamarter RB, Sandhu HS. Low back
      pain recollection versus concurrent accounts: outcomes analysis. Spine 2002;27:984–94.
[23] Deyo RA, Diehl AK. Measuring physical and psychosocial function in patients with low-back
      pain. Spine 1983;8:635–42.
[24] Fairbank JCT, Couper J, Davies JB, O'Brien JP. The Oswestry low back pain disability question-
      naire. Physiotherapy 1980;66:271–3.
[25] Franck LS, Greenberg CS, Stevens B. Pain assessment in infants and children. Pediatr Clin North
      Am 2000;47:487–512.
[26] Gauvain-Piquard A, Rodary C, Rezvani A, Serbouti S. The development of the DEGR(R): a scale
      to assess pain in young children with cancer. Eur J Pain 1999;3:165–76.
[27] Gedaly-Duff V. Palmar sweat index use with children in pain research. J Pediatr Nurs 1989;4:34.
[28] Gilbert CA, Lilley CM, Craig KD, McGrath PJ, Court CA, Bennett SM, Montgomery CJ. Postop-
      erative pain expression in preschool children: validation of the facial coding system. Clin J Pain
      1999;15:192–200.
[29] Goodenough B, Addicoat L, Champion GD, McInerney M, Young B, Juniper K, Ziegler JB. Pain
      in 4- to 6-year-old children receiving intramuscular injections: a comparison of the Faces Pain
      Scale with other self-report and behavioral measures. Clin J Pain 1997;13:60–73.
[30] Goodenough B, van Dongen K, Brouwer N, Abu-Saad HH, Champion GD. A comparison of
      the Faces Pain Scale and the Facial Affective Scale for children's estimates of the intensity and
      unpleasantness of needle pain during blood sampling. Eur J Pain 1999;3:301–15.
[31] Gordon DB, Dahl JL, Miaskowski C, McCarberg B, Todd KH, Paice JA, Lipman AG, Bookbinder
      M, Sanders SH, Turk DC, Carr DB. American Pain Society recommendations for improving
      the quality of acute and cancer pain management: American Pain Society Quality of Care Task
      Force. Arch Intern Med 2005;165:1574–80.
[32] Grunau RVE, Craig KD. Pain expression in neonates: facial action and cry. Pain 1987;28:395–
      410.

[33] Herr K, Coyne PJ, Manworren R, McCaffery M, Merkel S, Pelosi-Kelly J, Wild L. Pain assessment in the nonverbal patient: position statement with clinical practice recommendations. Pain Manage Nurs 2006;7:44–52.

[34] Hicks CL, von Baeyer CL, Spafford PA, van Korlaar I, Goodenough B. The Faces Pain Scale–revised: toward a common metric in pediatric pain measurement. Pain 2001;93:173–83.

[35] Hummel P, Puchalski M. Assessment and management of pain in infancy. Newb Infancy Nurs Rev 2001;1:114–21.

[36] Hunter M, McDowell L, Hennessy R, Cassey J. An evaluation of the Faces Pain Scale with young children. J Pain Symptom Manage 2000;20:122–9.

[37] Jette AM. The functional status index: reliability and validity of a self-report functional disability measure. J Rheumatol 1987;14:15–9.

[38] Johnston CC. Psychometric issues in the measurement of pain. In: Finley GA, McGrath PJ, editors. Measurement of pain in infants and children. Seattle: IASP Press; 1998. p. 5–20.

[39] Joint Commission on Accreditation of Healthcare Organizations. Implementing the new pain management standards. Oakbrook Terrace, IL: Joint Commission on Accreditation of Healthcare Organizations; 2000.

[40] Kalso E. Memory for pain. Acta Anaesthesiol Scand 1997;110:129–30.

[41] LaMontagne LL, Johnson BD, Hepworth JT. Children's ratings of postoperative pain compared to ratings by nurses and physicians. Issues Compr Pediatr Nurs 1991;14:241–7.

[42] Lawrence J, Alcock D, McGrath P, Kay J, MacMurray SB, Dulberg C. The development of a tool to assess neonatal pain. Neonatal Netw 1993;12:59–66.

[43] Leeland CS. Measurement of pain by subjective report. In: Chapman CR, Loeser JD, editors. Issues in pain management. Advances in pain research and therapy, Vol. 12. New York: Raven Press; 1989. p. 391–403.

[44] Liebelt EL. Assessing children's pan in the emergency department. Clin Ped Emerg Med 2000;1:260–9.

[45] Lilley CM, Craig KD, Grunau RE. The expression of pain in infants and toddlers: developmental changes in facial action. Pain 1997;72:161–70.

[46] Magerl W, Wilk SH, Treede RD. Secondary hyperalgesia and perceptual wind-up following intradermal injection of capsaicin in humans. Pain 1998;74:257–68.

[47] Maitland GD. Peripheral manipulation. London: Butterworth-Heinemann; 1990.

[48] McGrath PA. Pain assessment in children: a practical approach. Adv Pain Res Ther 1990;155–30.

[49] McGrath PA. Pain in the pediatric patient: practical aspects of assessment. Pediatr Ann 1995;24:126–38.

[50] McGrath PA, deVeber LL, Hearn MJ. Multidimensional pain assessment in children. In: Fields H, Dubner R, Cervero F, editors. Proceedings of the Fourth World Congress on Pain. New York: Raven Press; 1985. p. 387–93.

[51] McGrath PA, Gillespie J. Pain assessment in children and adolescents. In: Turk DC, Melzack R, editors. Handbook of pain assessment, 2nd ed. New York, NY: Guilford Press; 2001. p. 97–118.

[52] McGrath PA, Seifert CE, Speechley KN, Booth JC, Stitt L, Gibson MC. A new analogue scale for assessing children's pain: an initial validation study. Pain 1996;64:435–43.

[53] McGrath PJ. Behavioral measures of pain. Prog Pain Res Manage 1998;10:83–102.

[54] McGrath PJ, Unruh AM. Measurement and assessment of paediatric pain. In: Wall PD, Melzack R, editors. Textbook of pain, 4th ed. New York: Churchill Livingstone; 1999. p. 371–84.

[55] Melzack R. The McGill Pain Questionnaire: major properties and scoring methods. Pain 1975;1:277–99.

[56] Melzack R. The short-form McGill Pain Questionnaire. Pain 1987;30:191–7.

[57] Melzack R, Casey KL. Sensory, motivational, and central control determinants of pain: a new conceptual model. In: Kenshalo D, editor. The skin senses. Springfield, IL: Chas C. Thomas; 1968. p. 423–39.

[58] Melzack R, Katz J. The McGill Pain Questionnaire: appraisal and current status. In: Turk DC, Melzack R, editors. Handbook of pain assessment. New York: Guilford Press; 1992. p. 152–68.

[59] Melzack R, Torgerson WS. On the language of pain. Anesthesiology 1971;34:50–9.

[60] Merkel S. Pain assessment in infants and young children: the Finger Span Scale. Am J Nurs 2002;102:55–6.

[61] Miller D. Comparisons of pain rating from postoperative children, their mothers, and their nurses. J Pediatr Nurs 1996;22:145–9.

[62] Nicholas MK. The pain self-efficacy questionnaire: taking pain into account. Eur J Pain 2007;11:153–63.

[63] Novy DM, Simmonds MJ, Lee CE. Physical performance tasks: what are the underlying constructs? Arch Phys Med Rehab 2002;83:44–7.

[64] O'Rourke D. The measurement of pain in infants, children, and adolescents: from policy to practice. Phys Ther 2004;84:560–70.

[65] Pasero C, McCaffery M. No self-report means no pain-intensity rating. Am J Nurs 2005;105:50–3.

[66] Pasero C, McCaffery M. Pain in the critically ill. Am J Nurs 2002;102:59–60.

[67] Redelmeier DA, Kahneman D. Patients' memories of painful medical treatments: real-time and retrospective evaluations of two minimally invasive procedures. Pain 1996;66:3–8.

[68] Roland M, Morris RA. A study of the natural history of back pain. Part I: development of a reliable and sensitive measure of disability in low-back pain. Spine 1983;8:141–4.

[69] Savedra MC, Holzemer WL, Tesler MD, Wilkie DJ. Assessment of postoperation pain in children and adolescents using the adolescent pediatric pain tool. Nurs Res 1993;42:5–9.

[70] Savedra MC, Tesler MD, Holzemer WL, Wilkie DJ, Ward JA. Pain location, validity and reliability of body outline markings by hospitalized children and adolescents. Res Nurs Health 1989;12:307–14.

[71] Schuler M, Njoo N, Hestermann M, Oster P, Hauer K. Acute and chronic pain in geriatrics: clinical characteristics of pain and the influence of cognition. Pain Med 2004;5:53–262.

[72] Serlin RC, Mendoza TR, Nakamura Y, Edwards KR, Cleeland CS. When is cancer pain mild, moderate or severe? Grading pain severity by its interference with function. Pain 1995;61:277–84.

[73] Skevington SM, Carse MS, Williams AC. Validation of the WHOQOL-100: pain management improves quality of life for chronic pain patients. Clin J Pain 2001;17:264–75.

[74] Stevens B. Pain assessment in children: birth through adolescence. Child Adolesc Psychiatr Clin N Am 1997;6:725–43.

[75] Stinson JN, Kavanagh T, Yamada J, Gill N, Stevens B. Systematic review of the psychometric properties, interpretability and feasibility of self-report pain intensity measures for use in clinical trials in children and adolescents. Pain 2006;125:143–57.

[76] Stolee P, Hillier LM, Esbaugh J, Bol N, McKellar L, Gauthier N. Instruments for the assessment of pain in older persons with cognitive impairment. J Am Geriatr Soc 2005;53;319–26.

[77] Sweet SD, McGrath PJ. Physiological measures of pain. In: Finley GA, McGrath PJ, editors. Measurement of pain in infants and children. Seattle: IASP Press; 1998. p. 59–81.

[78] Szyfelbein SK, Osgood PF, Carr DB. The assessment of pain and plasma beta-endorphin immunoactivity in burned children. Pain 1985;22:173–82.

[79] Truog R, Anand KJS. Management of pain in the postoperative neonate. Clin Perinatol 1989;16:61–78.

[80] Tyler DC, Tu A, Douthit J, Chapman CR. Toward validation of pain measurement tools for children: a pilot study. Pain 1993;52:301–9.

[81] van Dijk M, Koot HM, Saad HH, Tibboel D, Passchier J. Observational visual analog scale in pediatric pain assessment: useful tool or good riddance? Clin J Pain 2002;18:310–16.

[82] Varni JW, Bernstein BH. Evaluation and management of pain in children with rheumatic diseases. Rheum Dis Clin North Am 1991;17:985–1000.

[83] Voepel-Lewis T, Merkel S, Tait AR, Trzcinka A, Malviya S. The reliability and validity of the face, legs, activity, cry, consolability observational tool as a measure of pain in children with cognitive impairment. Anesth Analg 2002;95:1224–49.

[84] Waddell G, Newton M, Henderson I, Somerville D, Main CJ. A fear-avoidance beliefs questionnaire (FABQ) and the role of fear-avoidance beliefs in chronic low back pain and disability. Pain 1993;52:157–68.

[85] Walco GA, Conte PM, Labay LE, Engel R, Zeltzer LK. Procedural distress in children with cancer: self-report, behavioral observations and physiological parameters. Clin J Pain 2005;21:484–90.

[86] WHOQOL Group. The World Health Organization Quality of Life Assessment (WHOQOL): development and general psychometric properties. Soc Sci Med 1998;46:1569–85.

[87] WHOQOL Group. The World Health Organization WHOQOL-BREF Quality of Life Assessment. Psychol Med 1998;28:551–8.

[88] Wong DL, Baker CM. Pain in children: comparison of assessment scales. Pediatr Nurs. 1988;14:9–17.

[89] Zeltzer I, Anderson CT, Schechter NL. Pediatric pain: current status and new directions. Curr Probl Pediatr 1990;20:415–86.
[90] Zwakhalen SM, Hamers JP, Abu-Saad HH, Berger MP. Pain in elderly people with severe dementia: a systematic review of behavioral pain assessment tools. BMC Geriatr 2006;6:3.

Correspondence to: Kathleen A. Sluka, PT, PhD, Graduate Program in Physical Therapy and Rehabilitation Science, The University of Iowa, 1-252 Medical Education Building, Iowa City, IA 52242-1190, USA. Tel: 1-319-335-9791; fax: 1-319-335-9707; email: kathleen-sluka@uiowa.edu.

General Principles of Physical Therapy Practice in Pain Management

Kathleen A. Sluka

*Graduate Program in Physical Therapy and Rehabilitation Science,
The University of Iowa, Iowa City, Iowa, USA*

Principles of Physical Therapy Practice

The practice of physical therapy involves providing service to patients who have impairments, functional limitations, disabilities, or changes in physical function and health status resulting from injury or disease [1]. Physical therapists interact and collaborate with other health professionals to provide health care to restore, maintain, and promote optimal physical function. With regard to pain, physical therapists are primarily involved in preventing the progression of impairments, functional limitations, and disabilities that may result either from the acute condition that produces pain or from the chronic pain condition itself. Specifically for chronic pain, restoration and promotion of optimal physical function to promote an improved quality of life is a critical role for physical therapists. For chronic pain, it is important to recognize that although the ultimate goal is a reduction in pain, pain relief may be minimal or may not be possible. However, physical function and quality of life may be greatly improved.

Mechanisms and Management of Pain for the Physical Therapist
edited by Kathleen A. Sluka
IASP Press, Seattle, © 2009

The evaluation process determines any impairments, functional limitations, disabilities, or changes in physical function. In pain management, restoration of function involves education and exercise, as well as a variety of manual therapies and other modalities. In acute pain management, the goals of therapy are aimed at reducing pain, decreasing peripheral inflammatory processes, and maintaining function. For chronic pain management, the goals of therapy are similarly aimed at reducing pain and improving function. Multiple treatment procedures are likely to be involved in this process. The physical therapist should make an educated treatment choice based on known mechanisms of action and clinical effectiveness.

The Guide to Physical Therapy Practice was developed by the American Physical Therapy Association to assist practicing physical therapists in their choice of tests and other evaluation measures, as well as treatments. The guide recommends that education, therapeutic exercise, and functional training form the core of physical therapy plans of care (Fig. 1). In addition, coordination of care with other health professionals, such as physicians and psychologists, should also be part of the initial treatment process. Other interventions should be added to a treatment plan as necessary to address findings in the evaluation procedure. For pain management, these other interventions include manual therapy, electrotherapy, and heat and cold therapy, which should be used in conjunction with education, exercise, and functional training.

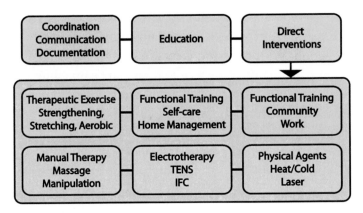

Fig 1. Diagrammatic representation of the general guidelines for physical therapy treatment from the Guide to Physical Therapy Practice [1].

Treatment of pain, either acute or chronic, involves a multidisciplinary approach that includes medical management, physical therapy, and psychological management. The goals for pain management, especially for chronic pain conditions, include the patient as an active participant. Specifically, physical therapy treatments should emphasize activity, with a focus on improved function rather than on impairments. All treatment plans should be based on evidence from both basic and clinical science.

Mechanisms of Action of Physical Therapy Treatments

Several theories have been proposed to explain the mechanisms of pain relief for physical therapy interventions. These include activation of gate control mechanisms, acting as a counterirritant, activation of endogenous opioids, and restoration of function to remove the peripheral irritant. The gate control theory generally states that activation of large-diameter afferents will reduce nociceptive activity in the dorsal horn of the spinal cord. Thus, any modality that activates these afferents could be explained by the gate control theory of pain. However, in some cases, we have more data on pharmacological mechanisms that expand upon the gate control theory. The counterirritant theory suggests that applying a painful stimulus will activate endogenous pain control mechanisms that reduce pain. For a modality to be a counterirritant, it would therefore need to be painful. Thus, hot packs and electrotherapy are probably not counterirritants. Activation of endogenous opioid pathways, such as the periaqueductal gray–rostroventromedial medulla (PAG–RVM) pathway, clearly mediates the effects of electrotherapy and aerobic exercise. Activation of such pathways would therefore result in decreased dorsal horn neuron activity and reduced input to higher brain centers. Lastly, exercise or manual therapies can increase range of motion and return normal function to a joint or tissue to eliminate a mechanical irritant.

Fig. 2 outlines the potential mechanisms by which physical therapy treatments can reduce pain. Treatments are generally aimed at treating the periphery and reducing peripheral sensitization of primary afferent fibers, or else they target the central nervous system in order to reduce central sensitization. In the periphery, removal of the peripheral mechanical or

chemical irritant causing sensitization of nociceptors would reduce input
to the spinal cord, thus reducing dorsal horn neuron sensitization. Alternatively, the activation of peripheral opioid receptors located on sensitized
nociceptors would reduce nociceptive input to the spinal dorsal horn, decreasing sensitization of dorsal horn neurons. Reducing the activation of
dorsal horn neurons reduces input to higher brain centers and thus relieves pain. Heat, cold, and manual therapy all have peripheral effects that
remove the mechanical or chemical irritant, while low-frequency transcutaneous electrical nerve stimulation (TENS) and possibly aerobic exercise activate peripheral opioid receptors. Centrally, therapies are aimed
at decreasing activation of spinal excitatory circuits or decreasing facilitation from supraspinal sites. Alternatively, physical therapy interventions
can increase local spinal inhibitory circuits or descending supraspinal
inhibition. Together, these approaches will reduce sensitization of dorsal
horn neurons, decreasing input to higher brain centers and lessening pain.

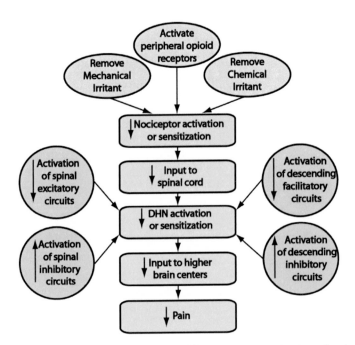

Fig. 2. Schematic diagram to explain potential basic science mechanisms for the actions
of physical therapy treatments to reduce pain. In general, treatments will have effects peripherally that will reduce nociceptor input and sensitization, or centrally that will decrease dorsal horn neuron activity and sensitization.

TENS, manual therapy, and exercise generally either reduce central excitation or increase central inhibition, or both.

Effective treatment of pain needs to be based on an adequate evaluation. The evaluation should be geared toward determining the peripheral and central components of the pain condition, and treatments should be selected that address these peripheral and central conditions. In addition, the evaluation should assess functional and activity limitations, and treatments should be aimed at improving these limitations. In recent years, there has been substantial research into the mechanisms by which physical therapy treatments reduce pain. These basic mechanisms will be elaborated on in the following chapters as they relate to a specific therapy.

All treatments for pain have a placebo effect. The placebo effect for pain is defined as a reduction in pain by the treatment's symbolic effect, rather than as a result of its specific therapeutic effect. The placebo effect is easily manipulated and can influence the effectiveness of treatment; it should always be taken into account in any assessment of the efficacy of treatment for pain. The placebo effect for pain relief, interestingly, is reversed by the opioid receptor antagonist, naloxone [6], suggesting activation of descending opioid inhibitory pathways. Neuroimaging studies confirm the activation of regions involved in opioid analgesia, including the prefrontal cortex, the anterior cingulate cortex, and the periaqueductal gray and medulla during a placebo treatment [6,9]. Thus, the placebo effect is real, it activates endogenous opioid pathways, and it should be utilized to enhance efficacy of treatment.

The control of supraspinal pathways over nociceptive activity can not only produce an enhanced analgesic effect, i.e., placebo, but can also produce decreased analgesic effectiveness or enhanced pain, termed nocebo. As with the placebo effect, there are known biological mechanisms underlying the nocebo effect. Blockade of cholecystokinin receptors with proglumide prevents the nocebo effect on pain relief [2,3,5]. Cholecystokinin is involved in opioid analgesia and tolerance, producing an anti-opioid effect when released [5]. Imaging studies show that the nocebo effect activates similar pathways to those subserving the placebo effect: the anterior cingulate, prefrontal, and insular cortices [5]. Thus, the nocebo also is real and uses anti-opioid mechanisms to enhance pain or reduce the effects of treatment. The clinician should also be careful not to produce a nocebo effect. Interactions with patients should, therefore, always be positive and encouraging to enhance the therapeutic efficacy of any given treatment and to avoid a negative effect on treatment.

As an example, George and colleagues recently investigated the effects of patient expectation on effectiveness of spinal manipulation [4]. In this study they gave instructions to different groups to suggest that the treatment was very effective, was ineffective, or had unknown effects. Pain threshold increased in the group that was instructed with a positive expectation, decreased in the group that was instructed with a negative expectation, and did not change in the group that received the neutral expectation. Thus, positive delivery of a treatment technique by the therapist is critical to obtain full effectiveness.

An Evidence-Based Approach for Physical Therapy

Several types of evidence can be used to make an educated decision on the choice of treatment. This evidence includes basic science mechanisms, effects in experimental pain models, randomized placebo-controlled trials, and systematic reviews or meta-analyses (Fig. 3). All types of evidence can be used to create an evidence-based treatment plan. The choice of therapy is stronger when there are multiple types of evidence to support the effectiveness of a given treatment.

Health care professionals, including physical therapists, need to make reliable treatment choices based on evidence. There is a wealth of information available that is difficult for the health care professional to read and synthesize. Reviews can be unscientific and biased in the way they collect data and summarize the information. Therefore, systematic reviews and meta-analyses attempt to minimize these biases and provide a reliable basis for clinical decision making. A hierarchy of evidence is often used, as outlined in Fig. 3B. At the top of the hierarchy are systematic reviews and meta-analyses, which analyze multiple randomized controlled trials in an attempt to allow health professionals to make evidence-based clinical decisions. If available, systematic reviews and meta-analyses would therefore provide the top level of evidence to support a particular treatment. However, caution should be used regarding negative results, given that these systematic reviews are based on the quality of the randomized controlled trials included.

The gold standard for clinical evidence is a randomized, double-blind, placebo-controlled trial. True double-blinding of the therapist and patient is difficult for many physical therapy treatments. For some therapies, such as hot packs or exercise, it is difficult to provide a placebo treatment. Many physical therapy treatments are thus compared against another therapy or medication to provide a means of assessing efficacy without a placebo treatment. Further, in many randomized controlled trials, the investigator examining the effects of treatment is blinded to the treatment allocation, which is difficult to achieve in the absence of a true placebo. At the bottom of the hierarchy of research evidence is typically evidence on basic science mechanisms or effects in experimental pain conditions. Subsequent chapters will describe the levels of evidence in terms of basic science mechanisms, randomized controlled trials, and where available systematic reviews from the Cochrane Library or meta-analyses. For recommendations on evidence-based practice, systematic reviews from the Cochrane Library will be used as the primary source, followed by systematic reviews and meta-analyses from the primary literature. If systematic reviews or meta-analyses of treatments are unavailable, randomized controlled trials will be described to support treatment recommendations.

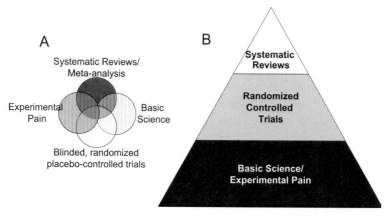

Fig. 3. Schematic diagram for the types of evidence that can be used to guide the choice of physical therapy treatments. The hierarchy includes basic science and experimental pain studies in human subjects, randomized controlled trials, and systematic reviews and meta-analyses of the clinical literature.

Ethical questions that routinely arise in the application of therapy are related to therapeutic efficacy of treatment. Should clinicians deliver and bill for a treatment that does not produce an analgesic effect above a placebo response? Should they deliver and bill for treatments that do not have clinical evidence to support their effectiveness? What is the minimal level of evidence required for a clinician to deliver and bill for treatment? Is it acceptable to use strong basic science evidence alone or in conjunction with nonrandomized controlled trials to support the choice of treatment? In a perfect world, where evidence is abundant and gives a clear positive or negative response for a treatment, the answer would be clear. If systematic reviews of high-quality evidence show a negative effect of treatment, then the clinician should not choose that treatment, unless as a last resort. On the other hand, if systematic reviews of the evidence show a positive effect of treatment for a given pain condition, that treatment should be included in the management plan. For example, strong evidence from systematic reviews supports the effectiveness of aerobic conditioning exercise for the treatment of fibromyalgia [4]. Therefore, any treatment plan for a patient with fibromyalgia should include an aerobic conditioning program.

Summary

The practice of physical therapy is typically aimed at finding and eliminating physical causes of pain, using a variety of techniques including exercises as well as manual therapies and modalities. For acute pain conditions associated with tissue damage and nociceptive pain, this biomedical approach to pain management is adequate and is likely to be successful. However, once pain becomes chronic, this model of practice needs modification and should always include an interdisciplinary approach to treatment. At this stage, physical therapy practice should shift to enhance the active involvement of the patient with education on activity modification and exercise, while minimizing passive treatments such as manual therapy and physical modalities. Manual therapy and physical modalities should only be used in chronic pain patients as an adjunct to the active exercise-oriented approach. Further, in some patients with acute pain, the pain is not proportional to the amount of tissue damage and thus is likely to involve significant central nervous system changes and psychosocial variables that need to be addressed.

References

[1] American Physical Therapy Association. Guide to physical therapy practice, 2nd ed. Phys Ther 2001;81:9–746.
[2] Benedetti F, Amanzio M, Casadio C, Oliaro A, Maggi G. Blockade of nocebo hyperalgesia by the cholecystokinin antagonist proglumide. Pain 1997;71:135–40.
[3] Benedetti F, Amanzio M, Vighetti S, Asteggiano G. The biochemical and neuroendocrine bases of the hyperalgesic nocebo effect. J Neurosci 2006;26:12014–22.
[4] Busch AJ, Barber KA, Overend TJ, Peloso PM, Schachter CL. Exercise for treating fibromyalgia syndrome. Cochrane Database Syst Rev 2007;CD003786.
[5] Colloca L, Benedetti F. Nocebo hyperalgesia: how anxiety is turned into pain. Curr Opin Anaesthesiol 2007;20:435–9.
[6] Levine JD, Gordon NC, Fields HL. The mechanism of placebo analgesia. Lancet 1978;2:654–7.

Correspondence to: Prof. Kathleen A. Sluka, PT, PhD, Graduate Program in Physical Therapy and Rehabilitation Science, The University of Iowa, 1-252 Medical Education Building, Iowa City, IA 52242-1190, USA. Tel: 1-319-335-9791; fax: 1-319-335-9707; email: kathleen-sluka@uiowa.edu.

Exercise-Induced Hypoalgesia: An Evidence-Based Review

Marie Hoeger Bement

Department of Physical Therapy, Marquette University, Milwaukee, Wisconsin, USA

Exercise is a necessary and important component in the management of pain. Physical therapists use different types of exercise to treat people with pain, including aerobic, strengthening, stretching, and range of motion exercises. The type of exercise prescribed, as well as the intensity and duration, vary widely and depend on a thorough evaluation, patient tolerance, and patient preference. Despite the frequent use of exercise in rehabilitation, the specifics regarding exercise prescription (intensity, duration, frequency, and type) and the mechanisms responsible for exercise-induced hypoalgesia (EIH) are not entirely clear. This confusion may be partly explained by the broad range of exercise parameters, including exercise type and dosage. For example, exercise interventions may incorporate aerobic activity, nonaerobic activity, or a combination of the two. Furthermore, exercise can be performed at different frequencies, intensities, and durations, which partially explains the current difficulty in providing specific dosage recommendations. The purpose of this chapter is to apply these parameters in the understanding of EIH, with a specific focus on their application to the rehabilitation setting. Research using healthy subjects will

Mechanisms and Management of Pain for the Physical Therapist
edited by Kathleen A. Sluka
IASP Press, Seattle, © 2009

be reviewed first as a comparison for research in individuals with a pain condition. Mechanisms will be explored at the end of the chapter to clarify how the prescription of exercise can relieve pain.

Both human and animal studies will be discussed. It is imperative to consider both types of research to understand all of the factors associated with EIH. Animal research permits better control over the variables that affect pain perception. Specifically, the affective-motivational component of pain is minimized, and it is easier to analyze peripheral and central mechanisms. Furthermore, with animal models the extent of injury, including the time course, is very well controlled. For example, investigators studying the role of exercise in managing chronic low back pain will have difficulty finding a large sample of human subjects with the same type of low back pain, and the likelihood that the subjects would experience the same psychosocial factors is slim. Moreover, the techniques used in animal studies frequently cannot be conducted in human subjects due to their invasive nature. Despite the frequent use of animal models, caution should be used when translating the findings to humans, which is why animal studies should be duplicated in humans, when possible.

Exercise-Induced Hypoalgesia in Healthy Subjects

Healthy human subjects typically do not experience ongoing pain, so to measure changes in pain perception after exercise a noxious stimulus is used to induce pain before and after exercise. Several types of experimental pain (ischemic, pressure, thermal, and electrical) may be used. Careful consideration should be given to the type of experimental pain stimulus used and the timing of stimulation. For example, greater hypoalgesia is reported *during* the performance of an isometric contraction compared to *after* the completion of the contraction [45]. Janal and colleagues report an acute decrease in ischemic pain 30 minutes after high-intensity aerobic exercise [34]. These changes in pain are dependent on the type of experimental pain. For example, unlike ischemic pain, the cold-pressor test is not associated with exercise-induced changes in pain perception. Similarly, pain decreases after 30 minutes of treadmill exercise at 75% of maximal oxygen uptake (VO_2max) with a pressure pain stimulus, but not with a thermal pain stimulus [32,56]. Thus, results after the same type of exercise may vary according to the choice of experimental pain stimulus and the timing of application. There is more variability in whether or not exercise produces a hypoalgesia response when a thermal experimental pain stimulus is used compared with mechanical or electrical stimuli; this variability may be related to exercise-induced changes in body temperature [38].

Another important parameter to consider in an analysis of the EIH literature is the pain measurement (i.e., threshold, intensity ratings, or tolerance). The majority of studies assess pain threshold, with fewer studies assessing pain intensity ratings and pain tolerance. The choice of outcome parameter may influence the interpretation of the ability of exercise to decrease pain. For example, after circuit training there is an increase in pain tolerance but not in pain threshold [3]. Likewise, after an 80% maximal voluntary contraction held to exhaustion, pain ratings decreased, but there was no change in pain threshold [5] (Fig. 1 G,H). Thus, it appears that EIH is more likely to occur when pain ratings or pain tolerance is measured compared with pain threshold.

The location of the noxious stimulus application is another consideration in the interpretation of the EIH literature. Exercise produces a systemic response because hypoalgesia is not localized to the body part performing the exercise [5,44,46]. Kosek and colleagues specifically assessed this issue and found that the magnitude of EIH is dependent on where the noxious stimulus is applied relative to the exercising body part [46]. Greater hypoalgesia is produced in the exercising limb compared with the contralateral limb and a distant resting muscle. There are no differences in the amount of EIH in the contralateral limb versus the distant resting muscle. This finding suggests that exercise does not have to be performed by the painful body part to achieve a decrease in pain, although greater decreases in pain are likely if the exercise is localized.

Most EIH research has been conducted using aerobic exercise in healthy individuals. Aerobic exercise most consistently produces a hypoalgesic response when performed at higher intensities ($\geq$200 watts or 60–75% VO_2max) [38]. However, percentage of maximum heart rate and self-selected measures are less reliable for gauging the necessary intensity [38]. Thus, the magnitude and quantification of intensity are important determinants in EIH.

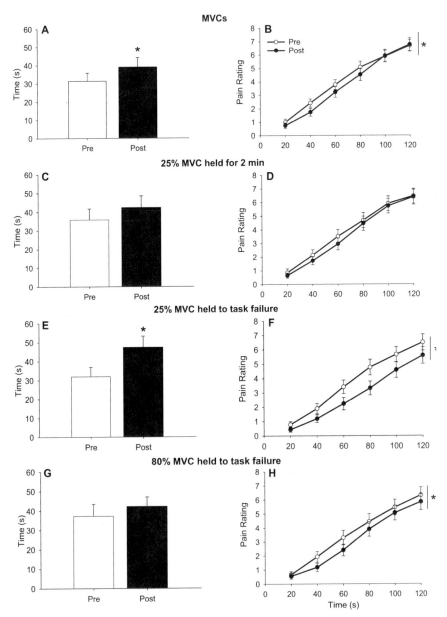

Fig 1. The magnitude of exercise-induced hypoalgesia following the performance of an isometric contraction is dependent on intensity and duration. Pain threshold increased and pain ratings decreased after the performance of three maximal voluntary contractions (MVCs) (A,B) and after a 25% MVC was held to task failure (E,F). Pain ratings decreased, but there was no change in pain threshold, after an 80% MVC was held to task failure (G,H). There was no change in pain threshold or pain ratings following the 25% MVC held to task failure (C,D). Data are represented as the mean ± SEM [5].

Duration is also important because there appears to be an interaction between intensity and duration of exercise [32,38]. For example, Hoffman and colleagues measured pain perception after treadmill running for 10 minutes at 75% of VO$_2$max, 30 minutes at 50% of VO$_2$max, and 30 minutes at 75% of VO$_2$max [32]. Pain ratings decreased only after the high-intensity and longer-duration exercise (75% of VO$_2$max for 30 minutes) (Fig. 2). In nonhuman subjects, the increase in pain threshold following 3 weeks of spontaneous running correlates with the amount of exercise activity; animals that run more have higher thresholds compared with the animals that run less [61]. These findings indicate that EIH following aerobic exercise is dependent on the intensity and duration of the exercise.

Less research has been conducted on nonaerobic activity or strengthening exercises. In contrast to aerobic exercise, both low- and high-intensity nonaerobic exercise protocols produce hypoalgesia. Typically, low-intensity contractions are held until the point of exhaustion,

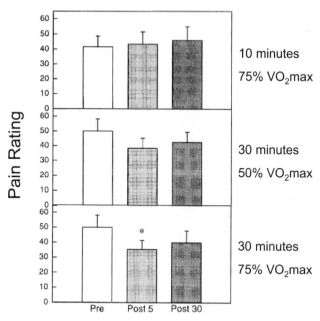

Fig 2. Exercise-induced hypoalgesia following aerobic exercise is dependent on intensity and duration. Pain ratings do not change after aerobic exercise performed either at 75% of maximal oxygen uptake (VO$_2$max) for 10 minutes or at 50% of VO$_2$max for 30 minutes. Pain ratings decrease after aerobic exercise performed at 75% of VO$_2$max for 30 minutes (i.e., high intensity, longer duration) [32]. Reprinted with permission from Elsevier.

although this is not required to produce hypoalgesia [5,42]. Koltyn and colleagues reported decreases in pain after a 40–50% maximal voluntary contraction held for 2 minutes [42]. Furthermore, the magnitude of exercise-induced analgesia following an isometric contraction is dependent on both the intensity and duration. For example, the greatest decrease in pain occurred after a low-intensity and long-duration isometric contraction (25% maximal voluntary contraction held to task failure) compared with high- and low-intensity contractions of shorter duration [5] (Fig. 1). For lower-intensity contractions to produce hypoalgesia, they must be held for a longer duration.

When a low-intensity isometric contraction is held until task failure, it produces a significant amount of fatigue (i.e., exercise-induced decrease in force). Despite this finding, fatigue is not required for EIH. Force did not decline during the performance of three maximal voluntary contractions, although there was an increase in pain threshold and decrease in pain ratings (Fig. 1) [5]. Thus, it appears that strengthening exercises can be performed at a lower intensity than aerobic exercise to produce hypoalgesia.

Interestingly, a small but significant body of EIH literature suggests that there are sex differences. Specifically, women may experience greater EIH than men, which is not dependent on the type of exercise. Following aerobic exercise (treadmill running for 10 minutes at 85% maximal heart rate), women, but not men, experience a decrease in pain [65]. Likewise, following maximal isometric contractions, women report increases in pain threshold and decreases in pain ratings, whereas men experience only decreases in pain ratings [42]. After the performance of submaximal isometric contractions, women show increases in pain threshold and decreases in pain ratings, whereas men show no changes [42]. Thus, it would appear that sex differences are greater following submaximal isometric contractions, with changes in both pain threshold and pain ratings, or perhaps pain threshold is a more sensitive measurement of sex differences. The fact that this phenomenon has only recently emerged may be related to the issue that the majority of early EIH research was conducted in male subjects [37]. Considerably more research, in which both men and women are included as subjects, is necessary before conclusions can be made on the existence of sex differences in EIH.

Exercise-Induced Hypoalgesia in Subjects with Pain

Exercise is frequently used in the rehabilitation setting as part of a pain management program. Compared with the EIH literature pertaining to healthy adults, much less is known regarding exercise in people with pain. Despite the limited amount of high-quality research, most studies indicate that exercise is beneficial and has very few detrimental effects (Table I). Systematic reviews, outlined in Table I, show that exercise is beneficial for a variety of pain conditions including neck pain, chronic low back pain, pelvic pain, osteoarthritis, patellofemoral pain, intermittent claudication, fibromyalgia, rheumatoid arthritis, and tendonitis. However, a few systematic reviews have concluded that exercise is not beneficial, including a review on the use of exercise in the management of acute low back pain that found that the incorporation of exercise was similar to no treatment [26]. Similarly, reviews on the role of exercise in juvenile idiopathic arthritis and on the use of stretching for delayed-onset muscle soreness found that no effect on pain was associated with the exercise intervention [29,66].

One of the issues in interpreting the EIH literature is the difficulty in extrapolating data from healthy individuals and applying it to individuals with a pain condition. Caution should be used because pain will influence how subjects respond to exercise and affect their ability to perform certain types of exercise. For example, women with fibromyalgia reported a decrease in pain threshold (i.e. hyperalgesia) during an isometric contraction of the lower extremity, whereas women without fibromyalgia reported an increase in pain threshold (i.e. hypoalgesia) [45] (Fig. 3). Furthermore, many individuals cannot tolerate the high-intensity protocols that produce hypoalgesia in healthy adults due to difficulty with physical exertion. Consequently, low-intensity programs such as walking are frequently recommended for these individuals.

The ability to cull specific recommendations from EIH research is difficult. For example, the response to a single exercise session may not be reflective of the long-term changes in pain that occur with increasing exercise frequency. Individuals with chronic neck muscle pain (trapezius myalgia) who participated in a strength training protocol

Table I

Table of evidence for exercise-induced hypoalgesia

Disease/Pain Condition	Ref.	Review Type	No. Studies	Results
Mechanical neck disorders	[57]	Systematic review	16	(+) Strong evidence for proprioceptive exercises and dynamic resisted strengthening exercises for chronic neck disorders; moderate evidence for early mobilizing exercises in patients with acute whiplash
Mechanical neck disorders	[36]	Cochrane review	31	(+)
Back and neck pain	[58]	Cochrane review	18	(+) Physical conditioning programs that include cognitive-behavioral approach; reduction in sick days for workers with chronic back pain; no evidence for acute back pain
Low back pain	[25]	Cochrane review	61	(+) Strong evidence for chronic low back pain
Chronic low back pain	[27]	Systematic review	43	(+) Supervised individually designed programs with stretching component; high dose more effective than low dose
Chronic low back pain	[62]	Systematic review	6	(+) Nonloaded movement exercise compared with no treatment; comparable to other types, including strengthening and stabilization
Chronic low back pain	[64]	Systematic review	3	Lumbar stabilization exercises (+); comparable to other exercise programs
Chronic low back pain	[50]	Systematic review	12	Lumbar extensor strengthening (+); comparable to other exercise programs
Spinal and pelvic pain	[20]	Systematic review	13	Stabilization exercise (+) for chronic but not acute low back pain, cervicogenic headache and associated neck pain, pelvic pain, and in reducing recurrence of acute low back pain
Pelvic and back pain in pregnancy	[54]	Cochrane review	8	Strengthening, sitting pelvic tilt exercises, and/or water gymnastics (+)

Condition	Ref	Type	N	Findings
Osteoarthritis (hip or knee)	[22]	Cochrane review	19	Land-based (+) for knee osteoarthritis; not enough studies to assess hip osteoarthritis
Osteoarthritis (knee)	[9]	Cochrane review	1	Aerobic (+); high and low intensity equally effective
Osteoarthritis (hip and/or knee)	[2]	Cochrane review	6	Aquatics (+) short-term; no long-term effects documented
Osteoarthritis	[53]	Systematic review	26	Strengthening (+); general physical activity (+)
Osteoarthritis (hip or knee)	[55]	Systematic review	11	Acute benefits of exercise therapy not sustained long-term (more than 6 months post-treatment); benefits associated with booster sessions post-treatment
Patellofemoral pain syndrome	[28]	Cochrane review	3	Quadriceps strengthening exercises (+); open and closed kinetic exercises equally effective
Intermittent claudication	[6]	Cochrane review	8	Supervised exercise (+) with increase in maximal treadmill walking distance compared with nonsupervised exercise
Intermittent claudication	[47]	Cochrane review	10	(+) with increase in maximal walking time
Fibromyalgia	[12]	Cochrane review	34	Supervised aerobic (+); strength and flexibility are under-evaluated
Fibromyalgia	[10]	Systematic review	5	Strengthening (+)
Rheumatoid arthritis	[52]	Systematic review	15	(+)
Juvenile idiopathic arthritis	[66]	Cochrane review	3	Exercise not beneficial
Delayed-onset muscle soreness in young adults	[29]	Cochrane review	10	Stretching not beneficial
Lower-extremity tendinosis	[67]	Systematic review	11	Eccentric exercise (+); unclear if more effective than other forms of therapeutic exercise

reported prolonged decreases in their worst pain score throughout the 10-week program, although initially they experienced an immediate increase in pain [1]. In contrast, individuals who participated in a general fitness program reported immediate decreases in pain that lasted less than 2 hours [1]. Thus, acute changes in pain perception at the initiation of an exercise program do not predict the long-term response from regular participation.

Research is lacking in regard to long-term benefits, including guidelines for exercise progression [2,12,50]. For example, it is not clear whether people should follow the same EIH training protocol over time or if gradual progression should be prescribed to accommodate increases in cardiovascular fitness and to continue to produce exercise-induced benefits. A systematic review on osteoarthritis found that the benefits from an acute exercise program are not sustained over the long term (≥6 months) [55]. However, individuals who participated in booster sessions after treatment did obtain long-term pain benefits, a finding that was

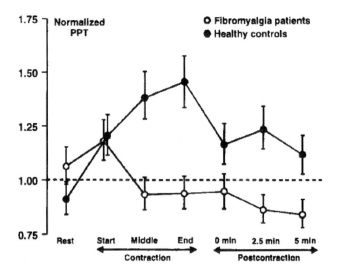

Fig 3. Individuals with and without a pain condition have differing pain responses during and after the performance of an isometric contraction (22% maximal voluntary contraction held to exhaustion). Women without fibromyalgia (healthy controls) experience an increase in pain threshold starting at the initiation of the isometric contraction, whereas women with fibromyalgia report a decrease in threshold in the middle of the isometric contraction that remains decreased after the contraction [45]. Reprinted with permission from the International Association for the Study of Pain.

probably related to exercise adherence [55]. Thus, the traditional rehabilitation approach in which patients receive supervised exercise therapy for a finite period may be less beneficial than scheduling patients for periodic evaluations over a longer period of time.

As indicated earlier, low-intensity exercise programs are frequently recommended for individuals with a pain condition, especially for those with chronic pain, partly because of the pain management benefits. For example, older adults with various painful conditions experience decreases in pain following low-intensity activities such as walking, light resistance exercise, and Tai Chi [39]. This does not mean that high-intensity exercise is not effective, only that additional research needs to be conducted in order to determine whether EIH in people with a pain condition is dependent on intensity. For example, high-intensity aerobic exercise is not typically recommended for the treatment of low back pain. Hoffman and colleagues report, however, that individuals with chronic low back pain show decreases in pressure pain perception following high-intensity cycle ergometry [31]. Similarly, individuals with chronic low back pain report decreases in pain after a high-intensity aerobic training protocol [15]. A systematic review on the treatment of osteoarthritis concluded that high- and low-intensity forms of aerobic exercise are equally effective [9]. Thus, the role of exercise intensity in EIH for people with a pain condition is incompletely understood and may be dependent on the type of pain condition.

In addition to intensity, exercise type is an important factor in prescription. Andersen and colleagues examined two types of physical exercise, localized strength training versus general fitness training (leg bicycling), for 10 weeks in the management of chronic neck muscle pain [1]. The strength training sessions initially led to an acute increase in pain, which transitioned to a decrease in pain over the 10-week period. In contrast, individuals in the general fitness program showed an acute and transient decrease in pain. Thus, for the management of chronic neck muscle pain, strength training is more clinically relevant than general fitness training. General fitness training may be used early in rehabilitation, however, to produce short-term pain relief, especially for those individuals who may have difficulty tolerating strength training due to pain.

With most pain conditions, there is a lack of research to distinguish whether one type of exercise is better than another. Frequently, one exercise tends to be emphasized over others. In relation to chronic back pain, Liddle and colleagues reviewed 16 randomized controlled trials (RCTs) and found that the majority (12 trials) contained a strengthening component [48]. Specific to fibromyalgia, a systematic review concluded that supervised aerobic exercise provides benefits and that both strength and flexibility exercises were insufficiently evaluated [12]. A later review concluded that strengthening exercises are beneficial [10]. The importance of exercise type in EIH is not clear, but the best type of exercise is probably dependent on the pain condition.

A review of exercise studies in the management of osteoarthritis pain concluded that many different types of exercise are beneficial in the management of pain [38]. These include stretching, strengthening, walking, aquatics, cycling, and Tai Chi [53]. Whether one type of exercise is more effective than another is not known. Two systematic reviews on chronic low back pain found that lumbar stabilization exercises and lumbar extensor strengthening are beneficial, with both types of exercise showing results comparable to those of other exercise programs [50,64]. Perhaps EIH, at least in the management of osteoarthritis pain and chronic low back pain, is less dependent on exercise type than on increasing overall general activity.

Reviews of the EIH literature for people with pain conditions show that high-quality research studies are necessary to guide specific recommendations regarding exercise prescription [12,26,48,53]. For example, in a review of RCTs on the effect of exercise in the management of chronic low back pain, only 10 out of a possible 51 were rated as high quality [48]. Future research should address the role of exercise dosage (i.e. intensity, duration, and frequency), type (aerobic versus nonaerobic), progression, and long-term effects. Researchers should evaluate these variables for each pain condition because someone with low back pain may not have the same exercise response as someone with fibromyalgia. Furthermore, there is likely to be variability within the same pain condition. In a study of individuals with myofascial pain of the jaw, Dao and colleagues were able to define subgroups based on response to exercise [18].

Compliance

Regardless of the pain condition or whether or not pain is present, compliance is a big issue [38]. Exercise research tends to have high attrition and low compliance rates. This problem increases over time, especially in chronic pain conditions such as fibromyalgia. Lack of compliance may explain some of the contradictory results of EIH in patients given the same exercise dosage, because if compliance is low, then exercise may be erroneously concluded to be ineffective.

As previously indicated, people tend to be less compliant over time, such as when they are discharged from rehabilitation and are no longer being supervised. Supervised home exercise programs, which may be related to increases in exercise compliance, are frequently recommended for various pain conditions [6,7,12,27]. Unfortunately, Liddle and colleagues found that exercise supervision and follow-up advice were underutilized in the management of chronic low back pain [49].

Even when exercise produces notable changes in pain reports, compliance is still difficult. An exercise study in individuals with fibromyalgia found that greater improvements were reported with cardiovascular training compared with stress management [68]. Despite the increased benefits demonstrated with cardiovascular training, more people were likely to continue with stress management. Similarly, Buckelew and colleagues found that the benefits associated with exercise and relaxation training were best maintained over a 2-year period when the two interventions were combined [11]. These two studies indicate that exercise should be prescribed in conjunction with some type of behavioral training.

Exercise delivery was addressed by Carroll and colleagues in a systematic review regarding exercise promotion in underserved populations [14]. The authors' specific recommendations were to provide a brief counseling session that incorporates the patient's goals and a written handout. These goals should be individualized to assist with exercise promotion and compliance. For example, if a patient wants to transition from standing to sitting on the floor, without pain, to play with his or her grandchildren, then the exercises should promote this activity. The activity may be broken down into separate activities, such as squatting exercises, with a thorough explanation about the benefits of each exercise. Personalizing exercise prescription to meet each patient's individualized goals will help the therapist to build rapport with patients while helping them to understand the importance of the exercises and thus promoting better compliance.

In a study of individuals with knee osteoarthritis, compliance was associated with patients' ability to integrate the exercise into everyday life, with their perception of the effectiveness of exercise, and with their perception of their symptoms [13]. These issues can be addressed in the rehabilitation setting through patient education. For example, to help with integration into everyday life, exercises may be performed during activities of daily living. For example, posture exercises can be done every morning in the shower or while brushing one's teeth. Furthermore, patients should have a thorough understanding of the expected effectiveness of their efforts, such as the impact of regular exercise on pain management. Patients should realize that pain relief may occur gradually, with possible slight increases in pain initially, and should understand that these slight increases do not mean that they are hurting themselves but rather that the body is adapting to exercise [49].

In relation to the perception of symptoms, regular exercisers tend to experience greater improvements in mood after an exercise session than non-exercisers [30]. Thus, people who are inactive may have a more difficult time in obtaining exercise-induced psychological changes than those who exercise regularly. This difference may change how some patients perceive pain and affect their motivation to continue exercising. The perception of symptoms may also dictate compliance, because decreases in pain may result in exercise cessation due to completion of the pain management goals. For instance, patients tend to stop exercising when they feel good and to start again once symptoms reappear. Therapists need to education patients on the benefits of regular exercise, including the ability of exercise to prevent or decrease the recurrence of pain while also improving mood.

Mechanisms of Exercise-Induced Hypoalgesia

Opioid Mechanisms

Several mechanisms modulate changes in pain perception following exercise. The most studied mechanism is activation of the opioid system. Research shows that EIH produces systemic effects in that hypoalgesia is not localized to the exercising body part, which suggests that exercise is mediated by changes in the central nervous system or by circulating substances acting on peripheral neurons. Activation of the opioid system could explain both of these events.

Specifically, exercise-induced activation of the opioid system may influence both the peripheral and central nervous systems. In regard to the involvement of the peripheral nervous system, several studies show increases in β-endorphin levels in the plasma [19,34,59] (reviewed by [23]). These endogenous opioids, which are released by the pituitary, do not cross the blood-brain barrier. Thus, increases in plasma β-endorphins would be expected to influence the peripheral, but not central, nervous system.

Less is known regarding exercise-induced central activation of the opioid system. In the central nervous system, β-endorphins are released via the hypothalamus, which has projections to the periaqueductal gray and can thus activate descending inhibitory pathways. Most of our knowledge concerning central activation is from animal models. Voluntary exercise of long duration (5–6 weeks of voluntary wheel running) increased β-endorphin levels in the cerebrospinal fluid in hypertensive animals [33]. These levels remained elevated for up to 2 days after exercise termination. Central increases in β-endorphin levels were also found in female rats that performed a high-intensity fatigue protocol [8]. Thus, exercise-induced activation of the opioid system has both peripheral and central mechanisms of action.

Several factors are involved in whether or not exercise activates the opioid system. For instance, the release of β-endorphins is dependent on both exercise intensity and duration, although the duration of the exercise may be of less importance than its intensity [23,60]. Moderately high-intensity exercise consistently alters plasma β-endorphin levels, with increases reported 15–60 minutes after a single exercise session in healthy individuals [60]. Despite the pervasive view that opioids are the main mechanism responsible for EIH, very few exercise studies have assessed both changes in plasma β-endorphin levels and pain perception. These studies show that the increase in β-endorphin levels and the decrease in pain are not correlated and that the timing is different between the peak release of β-endorphins and the decrease in pain; moreover, the majority of subjects are young, active males [19,34]. Thus, the exact role of the opioid system in EIH is not clear.

Specific to patient populations, the importance of exercise intensity in activation of the opioid system is probably different when pain is present. In a chronic muscle pain model, *low-intensity* exercise produces hypoalgesia through activation of the opioid system [4]. Thus, activation of the opioid system appears to be less dependent on exercise intensity when chronic pain is present. Additional research, such as whether β-endorphin levels increase following exercise in people with a pain condition, needs to be conducted before definitive conclusions can be made. Preliminary results suggest that similar mechanisms may be responsible for EIH in people with and without pain, though the exercise protocol required to activate these mechanisms may be different if pain is present.

In addition to exercise intensity, opioid activation may depend on the type of exercise. For example, data on β-endorphin release following resistance training are inconclusive, with different studies reporting increases, decreases, and no changes [23]. These differences may be dependent on the training status of the participants, the intensity of the exercise, and the timing of the measurement [23]. In contrast to resistance exercise, considerably more research has been conducted on aerobic exercise, which consistently shows increases in β-endorphin levels after exercise of moderate to high intensity [23] (Fig. 4). Because both resistance training and aerobic exercise produce hypoalgesia, the type of exercise may dictate whether opioid or non-opioid mechanisms are involved.

Due to sex differences in pain perception, men and women may also respond differently to pain management interventions. Specific differences have been noted in that women tend to experience greater opioid analgesia than men [16]. This finding may help explain the EIH research in which women experience hypoalgesia to a greater degree than men. Goldfarb and colleagues found that men and women have similar increases in β-endorphin levels following high-intensity cycling [24] (Fig. 4). Whether or not women experience greater analgesia given the same degree of β-endorphin release is not known because pain was not assessed in this study.

Given that exercise results in activation of the endogenous opioid system, another important issue is the development of withdrawal

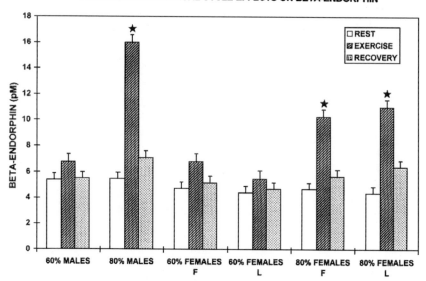

Fig 4. Plasma β-endorphin release is dependent on exercise intensity, with increased levels noted following high-intensity (80% VO$_2$max), but not low-intensity (60% VO$_2$max), aerobic exercise. The increase in β-endorphin levels is similar between men and women, and in women the increase is not dependent on the phase of the menstrual cycle (L = luteal; F = follicular) [24]. Reprinted with permission from Wolters Kluwer Health.

symptoms or tolerance, similar to the consequences of exogenous activation of the opioid system. In animal models, long-term voluntary exercise produces a cross-tolerance to exogenous opioids. Specifically, chronically exercised animals show a decreased analgesic response to opioid agonists compared with sedentary animals [35]. This decreased response to opioid drugs does not occur after a short bout of exercise. Similarly, physical withdrawal symptoms have been demonstrated after naloxone treatment in exercising animals, but not in sedentary animals [63]. In humans, data on the effect of training on EIH and activation of the opioid system are inconclusive [23]. The possibility of exercise-induced tolerance to opioid activation should be a consideration in exercise prescription because it may have implications for the long-term effectiveness of the intervention.

Non-Opioid Mechanisms

Several non-opioid mechanisms have been implicated in EIH. Specifically, exercise therapy has the potential to influence several variables in how an individual perceives pain. For example, exercise may impact all three aspects of the biopsychosocial model. As discussed in Chapter 1, this model is used to understand the various factors involved in the pain experience.

"Bio" refers to the biological factors involved in the pain experience. Disease activity and overall physical condition are two biological factors that exercise can modify. For example, exercise may slow the disease activity or improve someone's overall physical condition, thereby decreasing pain. In particular, instability and poor alignment may produce mechanical abnormalities that activate nociceptors. Exercise can improve body mechanics and thus remove mechanical irritation of nociceptors.

"Psycho" refers to the psychological factors that influence pain reports. These factors include a person's emotional status and pain coping skills. Exercise improves the affective-motivational component of pain, as demonstrated by the contemporary term "runner's high," which refers to the elevation in mood that frequently accompanies higher-intensity exercise [34]. In a review on exercise and mood elevation, Hoffman and Hoffman indicate that exercise of moderate intensity is the most likely to produce an enhanced mood, which lasts for 3–24 hours following exercise [30].

"Social" refers to the social factors that affect how an individual experiences pain. Social support and response of one's spouse are included in these factors. Damush and colleagues assessed motivational factors for individuals with knee osteoarthritis in relation to exercise compliance and found that social support from family members, friends, and medical professionals was beneficial, as was having an exercise partner [17]. Accordingly, social support may be incorporated by exercising in an exercise facility or with other people, including family members. Thus, therapists need to take the biopsychosocial model into account when prescribing exercise to help achieve the maximal amount of pain relief.

Other theories on pain mechanisms may also relate to EIH. One such theory is the gate control theory. In accordance with this theory, it could be said that exercise activates large afferent fibers, producing hypoalgesia by inhibiting pain signals in the spinal cord from ascending to supraspinal structures. The gate control theory would apply to virtually all types of exercise and supports the idea that even general increases in physical activity can improve pain.

An alternate theory suggests that exercise activates the cortico-spinal tract to reduce pain. As discussed in Chapter 3, activation of the corticospinal tract decreases spinothalamic tract neuron responsiveness in the dorsal horn of the spinal cord and produces presynaptic inhibition. Thus, any form of active exercise (aerobic exercise such as walking or bicycling, active range of motion exercises, or strengthening) could increase the activity of the corticospinal tract to decrease sensitization of dorsal horn neurons and consequently reduce pain.

Another theory incorporates the idea of exercise as a stressor in that EIH may be a form of stress-induced analgesia. Specifically, changes in anxiety levels have been implicated in modulating levels of pain [21,51]. Previous research on exercise-induced anxiety levels has produced mixed results, showing no change [40,41], decreases [42], and increases [5]. Despite the varied response of anxiety after exercise, all of the previous studies reported a decrease in pain, indicating that changes in anxiety levels alone do not explain exercise-induced analgesia.

The cardiovascular response associated with exercise suggests that change in blood pressure may be another possible mechanism for EIH. Koltyn and Umeda wrote a review regarding the interaction between EIH and blood pressure [43]. Typically, exercise produces an increase in blood pressure concurrent with a decrease in pain perception [43]. The fact that EIH is partially dependent on higher intensity of exercise further supports the role of blood pressure due to the greater increases associated with more strenuous activity. Additionally, exercise may alter the blood pressure response during a noxious stimulus. Koltyn and colleagues found that exercise blunted the blood pressure increase during an experimental pain stimulus [40,41,43]. As with the majority of the EIH mechanisms, the influence of blood pressure changes is not entirely clear.

Overall, the EIH literature suggests that there is an interaction between opioid and non-opioid mechanisms. The exact nature of this interaction is not known. It is likely that specific protocols such as high-intensity aerobic exercise in healthy adults are modulated by the opioid system, but changes in the intensity, duration, or frequency of exercise or the presence of pain may affect the mechanisms involved. Through improved understanding of the mechanisms of EIH, the prescription of exercise can be better applied to the rehabilitation setting.

Summary

A review of the literature on EIH specific to individuals without a pain condition indicates that hypoalgesia after aerobic exercise is dependent on both intensity and duration. Hypoalgesia is more likely to occur with higher intensities of longer duration. In contrast, EIH following isometric contractions occurs with both low and high intensities and is not dependent on the presence of fatigue. For lower-intensity contractions to produce hypoalgesia, they need to be performed for a longer duration, with the greatest increase in hypoalgesia associated with lower-intensity contractions held until the point of exhaustion.

Compared with EIH in healthy individuals, much less is known regarding EIH in people with a pain condition. Typically, lower-intensity exercise protocols are prescribed to address the tolerance issue associated with higher-intensity exercise. However, recent studies show that individuals with chronic pain may experience a decrease in pain following high-intensity aerobic activity. Thus, the role of intensity is not clear in people with a pain condition. Furthermore, the change in pain after a single exercise session is not predictive of long-term pain adaptations, which may be related to the exercise type. For example, as described above, individuals may experience initial increases in pain with resistive exercise, followed by decreases in pain with regular exercise participation.

In regard to the mechanisms responsible for EIH in healthy individuals, activation of the opioid system has received the most study. The role of the opioid system is not clear because few studies have assessed the exercise-induced changes in β-endorphin levels and pain, which are not correlated and may occur at different times. Most research has assessed β-endorphin levels in the plasma, which indicates involvement of the peripheral nervous system. However, animal studies demonstrate central activation in addition to peripheral involvement. This activation of the endogenous opioid system is dependent on exercise dosage as well as type, with increases most consistently occurring following aerobic activity of higher intensity.

Activation of the opioid system may be at least partially responsible for EIH in people with a pain condition, but the exercise dosage required for activation is likely to differ. Unlike the situation with healthy individuals, low-intensity exercise can produce hypoalgesia due to opioid activation in an animal model of chronic pain. In addition to the opioid system, there are non-opioid mechanisms for EIH. These mechanisms are less well known and include exercise-induced modulation of the biopsychosocial model of pain, spinal gating mechanisms as proposed in the gate control theory, and the cardiovascular response. The interaction and activation of the opioid and non-opioids mechanisms are not clear.

Throughout the literature, the necessity for high-quality research is apparent. Several areas need further study, including the most effective exercise dosage required to produce hypoalgesia in people with a pain condition. It is clear that exercise recommendations should take into account the type of exercise as well as the pain condition. The mechanisms of how exercise relieves pain need to be studied in order to guide the most effective exercise prescription, because by understanding how something works we can better apply it. Future research may lead to a protocol in which exercise is prescribed to *prevent* the development of chronic pain.

References

[1]   Andersen LL, Kjaer M, Sogaard K, Hansen L, Kryger AI, Sjogaard G. Effect of two contrasting types of physical exercise on chronic neck muscle pain. Arthritis Rheum 2008;59:84–91.
[2]   Bartels EM, Lund H, Hagen KB, Dagfinrud H, Christensen R, Danneskiold-Samsoe B. Aquatic exercise for the treatment of knee and hip osteoarthritis. Cochrane Database Syst Rev 2007:CD005523.
[3]   Bartholomew JB, Lewis BP, Linder DE, Cook DB. Post-exercise analgesia: replication and extension. J Sports Sci 1996;14:329–34.
[4]   Bement MK, Sluka KA. Low-intensity exercise reverses chronic muscle pain in the rat in a naloxone-dependent manner. Arch Phys Med Rehabil 2005;86:1736–40.
[5]   Bement MKH, DiCapo J, Rasiarmos R, Hunter SK. Dose response of isometric contractions on pain perception in healthy adults. Med Sci Sports Exerc 2009;40:1880–9.
[6]   Bendermacher BL, Willigendael EM, Teijink JA, Prins MH. Supervised exercise therapy versus non-supervised exercise therapy for intermittent claudication. Cochrane Database Syst Rev 2006:CD005263.
[7]   Bennell K, Hinman R. Exercise as a treatment for osteoarthritis. Curr Opin Rheumatol 2005;17:634–40.
[8]   Blake MJ, Stein EA, Vomachka AJ. Effects of exercise training on brain opioid peptides and serum LH in female rats. Peptides 1984;5:953–8.
[9]   Brosseau L, MacLeay L, Robinson V, Wells G, Tugwell P. Intensity of exercise for the treatment of osteoarthritis. Cochrane Database Syst Rev 2003:CD004259.
[10] Brosseau L, Wells GA, Tugwell P, Egan M, Wilson KG, Dubouloz CJ, Casimiro L, Robinson VA, McGowan J, Busch A, et al. Ottawa Panel evidence-based clinical practice guidelines for strengthening exercises in the management of fibromyalgia: part 2. Phys Ther 2008;88:873–86.
[11] Buckelew SP, Conway R, Parker J, Deuser WE, Read J, Witty TE, Hewett JE, Minor M, Johnson JC, Van Male L, et al. Biofeedback/relaxation training and exercise interventions for fibromyalgia: a prospective trial. Arthritis Care Res 1998;11:196–209.

[12] Busch AJ, Barber KA, Overend TJ, Peloso PM, Schachter CL. Exercise for treating fibromyalgia syndrome. Cochrane Database Syst Rev 2007;CD003786.

[13] Campbell R, Evans M, Tucker M, Quilty B, Dieppe P, Donovan JL. Why don't patients do their exercises? Understanding non-compliance with physiotherapy in patients with osteoarthritis of the knee. J Epidemiol Community Health 2001;55:132–8.

[14] Carroll JK, Fiscella K, Epstein RM, Jean-Pierre P, Figueroa-Moseley C, Williams GC, Mustian KM, Morrow GR. Getting patients to exercise more: a systematic review of underserved populations. J Fam Pract 2008;57:170–6.

[15] Chatzitheodorou D, Kabitsis C, Malliou P, Mougios V. A pilot study of the effects of high-intensity aerobic exercise versus passive interventions on pain, disability, psychological strain, and serum cortisol concentrations in people with chronic low back pain. Phys Ther 2007;87:304–12.

[16] Craft RM. Sex differences in drug- and non-drug-induced analgesia. Life Sci 2003;72:2675–88.

[17] Damush TM, Perkins SM, Mikesky AE, Roberts M, O'Dea J. Motivational factors influencing older adults diagnosed with knee osteoarthritis to join and maintain an exercise program. J Aging Phys Act 2005;13:45–60.

[18] Dao TT, Lund JP, Lavigne GJ. Pain responses to experimental chewing in myofascial pain patients. J Dent Res 1994;73:1163–7.

[19] Droste C, Greenlee MW, Schreck M, Roskamm H. Experimental pain thresholds and plasma beta-endorphin levels during exercise. Med Sci Sports Exerc 1991;23:334–42.

[20] Ferreira PH, Ferreira ML, Maher CG, Herbert RD, Refshauge K. Specific stabilisation exercise for spinal and pelvic pain: a systematic review. Aust J Physiother 2006;52:79–88.

[21] Fox E, O'Boyle C, Barry H, McCreary C. Repressive coping style and anxiety in stressful dental surgery. Br J Med Psychol 1989;62:371–80.

[22] Fransen M, McConnell S, Bell M. Exercise for osteoarthritis of the hip or knee. Cochrane Database Syst Rev 2003:CD004286.

[23] Goldfarb AH, Jamurtas AZ. Beta-endorphin response to exercise. An update. Sports Med 1997;24:8–16.

[24] Goldfarb AH, Jamurtas AZ, Kamimori GH, Hegde S, Otterstetter R, Brown DA. Gender effect on beta-endorphin response to exercise. Med Sci Sports Exerc 1998;30:1672–6.

[25] Hayden JA, van Tulder MW, Malmivaara A, Koes BW. Exercise therapy for treatment of non-specific low back pain. Cochrane Database Syst Rev 2005:CD000335.

[26] Hayden JA, van Tulder MW, Malmivaara AV, Koes BW. Meta-analysis: exercise therapy for non-specific low back pain. Ann Intern Med 2005;142:765–75.

[27] Hayden JA, van Tulder MW, Tomlinson G. Systematic review: strategies for using exercise therapy to improve outcomes in chronic low back pain. Ann Intern Med 2005;142:776–85.

[28] Heintjes E, Berger MY, Bierma-Zeinstra SM, Bernsen RM, Verhaar JA, Koes BW. Exercise therapy for patellofemoral pain syndrome. Cochrane Database Syst Rev 2003:CD003472.

[29] Herbert RD, de Noronha M. Stretching to prevent or reduce muscle soreness after exercise. Cochrane Database Syst Rev 2007:CD004577.

[30] Hoffman MD, Hoffman DR. Exercisers achieve greater acute exercise-induced mood enhancement than nonexercisers. Arch Phys Med Rehabil 2008;89:358–63.

[31] Hoffman MD, Shepanski MA, Mackenzie SP, Clifford PS. Experimentally induced pain perception is acutely reduced by aerobic exercise in people with chronic low back pain. J Rehabil Res Dev 2005;42:183–90.

[32] Hoffman MD, Shepanski MA, Ruble SB, Valic Z, Buckwalter JB, Clifford PS. Intensity and duration threshold for aerobic exercise-induced analgesia to pressure pain. Arch Phys Med Rehabil 2004;85:1183–7.

[33] Hoffmann P, Terenius L, Thoren P. Cerebrospinal fluid immunoreactive beta-endorphin concentration is increased by voluntary exercise in the spontaneously hypertensive rat. Regul Pept 1990;28:233–9.

[34] Janal MN, Colt EW, Clark WC, Glusman M. Pain sensitivity, mood and plasma endocrine levels in man following long-distance running: effects of naloxone. Pain 1984;19:13–25.

[35] Kanarek RB, Gerstein AV, Wildman RP, Mathes WF, D'Anci KE. Chronic running-wheel activity decreases sensitivity to morphine-induced analgesia in male and female rats. Pharmacol Biochem Behav 1998;61:19–27.

[36] Kay TM, Gross A, Goldsmith C, Santaguida PL, Hoving J, Bronfort G. Exercises for mechanical neck disorders. Cochrane Database Syst Rev 2005:CD004250.

[37] Koltyn KF. Analgesia following exercise: a review. Sports Med 2000;29:85–98.

[38] Koltyn KF. Exercise-induced hypoalgesia and intensity of exercise. Sports Med 2002;32:477–87.

[39] Koltyn KF. Using physical activity to manage pain in older adults. J Aging Phys Act 2002;10:226–39.

[40] Koltyn KF, Arbogast RW. Perception of pain after resistance exercise. Br J Sports Med 1998;32:20–4.

[41] Koltyn KF, Garvin AW, Gardiner RL, Nelson TF. Perception of pain following aerobic exercise. Med Sci Sports Exerc 1996;28:1418–21.

[42] Koltyn KF, Trine MR, Stegner AJ, Tobar DA. Effect of isometric exercise on pain perception and blood pressure in men and women. Med Sci Sports Exerc 2001;33:282–90.

[43] Koltyn KF, Umeda M. Exercise, hypoalgesia and blood pressure. Sports Med 2006;36:207–14.

[44] Koltyn KF, Umeda M. Contralateral attenuation of pain after short-duration submaximal isometric exercise. J Pain 2007;8:887–92.

[45] Kosek E, Ekholm J, Hansson P. Modulation of pressure pain thresholds during and following isometric contraction in patients with fibromyalgia and in healthy controls. Pain 1996;64:415–23.

[46] Kosek E, Lundberg L. Segmental and plurisegmental modulation of pressure pain thresholds during static muscle contractions in healthy individuals. Eur J Pain 2003;7:251–8.

[47] Leng GC, Fowler B, Ernst E. Exercise for intermittent claudication. Cochrane Database Syst Rev 2000:CD000990.

[48] Liddle SD, Baxter GD, Gracey JH. Exercise and chronic low back pain: what works? Pain 2004;107:176–90.

[49] Liddle SD, David Baxter G, Gracey JH. Physiotherapists' use of advice and exercise for the management of chronic low back pain: a national survey. Man Ther 2009:14:189–96.

[50] Mayer J, Mooney V, Dagenais S. Evidence-informed management of chronic low back pain with lumbar extensor strengthening exercises. Spine J 2008;8:96–113.

[51] Okawa K, Ichinohe T, Kaneko Y. Anxiety may enhance pain during dental treatment. Bull Tokyo Dent Coll 2005;46:51–8.

[52] Ottawa Panel. Evidence-based clinical practice guidelines for therapeutic exercises in the management of rheumatoid arthritis in adults. Phys Ther 2004;84:934–72.

[53] Ottawa Panel. Evidence-based clinical practice guidelines for therapeutic exercises and manual therapy in the management of osteoarthritis. Phys Ther 2005;85:907–71.

[54] Pennick VE, Young G. Interventions for preventing and treating pelvic and back pain in pregnancy. Cochrane Database Syst Rev 2007:CD001139.

[55] Pisters MF, Veenhof C, van Meeteren NL, Ostelo RW, de Bakker DH, Schellevis FG, Dekker J. Long-term effectiveness of exercise therapy in patients with osteoarthritis of the hip or knee: a systematic review. Arthritis Rheum 2007;57:1245–53.

[56] Ruble SB, Hoffman MD, Shepanski MA, Valic Z, Buckwalter JB, Clifford PS. Thermal pain perception after aerobic exercise. Arch Phys Med Rehabil 2005;86:1019–23.

[57] Sarig-Bahat H. Evidence for exercise therapy in mechanical neck disorders. Man Ther 2003;8:10–20.

[58] Schonstein E, Kenny DT, Keating J, Koes BW. Work conditioning, work hardening and functional restoration for workers with back and neck pain. Cochrane Database Syst Rev 2003:CD001822.

[59] Schwarz L, Kindermann W. Beta-endorphin, catecholamines, and cortisol during exhaustive endurance exercise. Int J Sports Med 1989;10:324–8.

[60] Sforzo GA. Opioids and exercise. An update. Sports Med 1989;7:109–24.

[61] Shyu BC, Andersson SA, Thoren P. Endorphin mediated increase in pain threshold induced by long-lasting exercise in rats. Life Sci 1982;30:833–40.

[62] Slade SC, Keating JL. Unloaded movement facilitation exercise compared to no exercise or alternative therapy on outcomes for people with nonspecific chronic low back pain: a systematic review. J Manipulative Physiol Ther 2007;30:301–11.

[63] Smith MA, Yancey DL. Sensitivity to the effects of opioids in rats with free access to exercise wheels: mu-opioid tolerance and physical dependence. Psychopharmacology 2003;168:426–34.

[64] Standaert CJ, Weinstein SM, Rumpeltes J. Evidence-informed management of chronic low back pain with lumbar stabilization exercises. Spine J 2008;8:114–20.

[65] Sternberg WF, Bokat C, Kass L, Alboyadjian A, Gracely RH. Sex-dependent components of the analgesia produced by athletic competition. J Pain 2001;2:65–74.

[66] Takken T, van Brussel M, Engelbert RH, Van der Net J, Kuis W, Helders PJ. Exercise therapy in juvenile idiopathic arthritis. Cochrane Database Syst Rev 2008:CD005954.

[67] Wasielewski NJ, Kotsko KM. Does eccentric exercise reduce pain and improve strength in physically active adults with symptomatic lower extremity tendinosis? A systematic review. J Athl Train 2007;42:409–21.

[68] Wigers SH, Stiles TC, Vogel PA. Effects of aerobic exercise versus stress management treatment in fibromyalgia. A 4.5 year prospective study. Scand J Rheumatol 1996;25:77–86.

Correspondence to: Marie Hoeger Bement, PT, PhD, Assistant Professor, Department of Physical Therapy, Marquette University, P.O. Box 1881, Milwaukee, WI, 53201-1881, USA. Tel: 1-414-288-6738; fax: 1-414-288-5987; email: marie-hoeger.bement@marquette.edu.

Transcutaneous Electrical Nerve Stimulation and Interferential Therapy

Kathleen A. Sluka[a] and Deirdre M. Walsh[b]

[a]Graduate Program in Physical Therapy and Rehabilitation Science, The University of Iowa, Iowa City, Iowa, USA; [b]Health and Rehabilitation Sciences Research Institute, University of Ulster, Newtownabbey, Northern Ireland, United Kingdom

In the field of electrotherapy, the term "transcutaneous electrical nerve stimulation" (TENS) can be used to describe a range of electrical currents, including neuromuscular electrical stimulation and interferential therapy (IFT). However, for the purposes of this chapter, TENS will refer only to those devices that are used to apply low-voltage electrical currents to the skin primarily for the purposes of pain relief (Fig. 1). TENS is a safe, non-invasive treatment with relatively few contraindications that can be either self-administered or therapist-administered. Although early prototypes of TENS units were available from the late 1800s [90], a theoretical foundation for electroanalgesia did not emerge until Melzack and Wall's gate control theory of pain was published in 1965 [51]. After the theory was published, clinical studies began reporting the success of *percutaneous* electrical stimulation for pain relief [89]. At that time, Norman Shealy began using an early TENS model as a screening device for his chronic pain patients who were being considered for dorsal column stimulation [74]. Shealy discovered that some patients responded better to TENS than to dorsal column stimulation; subsequently *transcutaneous* electrical nerve stimulation emerged as a viable modality in the field of pain management. Since the 1970s, advances in technology have produced a range of electrodes and TENS units for clinicians to choose from.

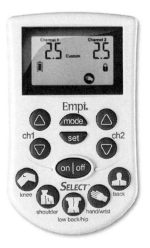

Fig. 1. SELECT TENS Unit (Empi, United States).

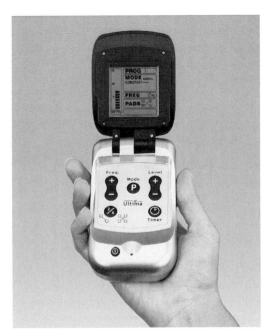

Fig. 2. Ultima IF4160 Portable Interferential Unit (TensCare, United Kingdom).

Interferential therapy involves the application to the skin of two medium-frequency currents (in the range of 2,000–4,000 Hz) in order to produce an amplitude-modulated low-frequency effect within the tissues [57]. With the development of small portable devices, IFT can now be either self-administered or therapist-administered (Fig. 2). The basic concept behind IFT is that skin impedance (resistance) is inversely proportional to the frequency of an applied current; therefore, there is less skin resistance to a frequency of 2,000 Hz than to a frequency of 200 Hz. It has been claimed that IFT can be used to treat deeper tissues because lower pulse amplitude is required to overcome the associated skin resistance. The two medium-frequency currents "interfere" within the tissues and produce an amplitude-modulated beat frequency, which is calculated as the difference between the values of the two currents applied. For example, if 4,000-Hz and 4,150-Hz medium-frequency currents are applied to the skin, the resultant beat frequency within the tissues is 150 Hz (see Fig. 3). However, there is little scientific evidence behind the principle of IFT producing a low-frequency current within the tissues with a greater depth of penetration. IFT has been used clinically since the 1950s, but despite its popularity in physical therapy departments [18,25,58], limited data are available on its mechanisms of action and indeed its clinical efficacy [55].

The objective of this chapter is to provide an overview of the pertinent research relating to the theory and clinical application of TENS and

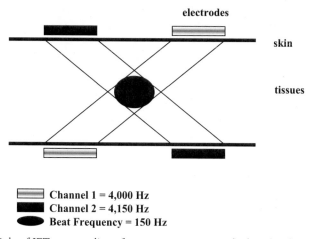

Fig. 3. Principle of IFT: two medium-frequency currents applied to the skin to produce a low beat frequency within the tissues.

IFT. Most of the basic science and clinical literature focuses on TENS of both low and high frequency. However, some literature is emerging to support the use of IFT for pain relief.

TENS and IFT Parameters

A typical TENS unit allows the parameters of pulse duration, frequency, pulse amplitude, and type of output (constant, burst, or modulated) to be manipulated. *Pulse duration* is the length of each pulse (usually in microseconds or milliseconds). *Frequency* is the number of pulses delivered per second (usually in hertz). *Pulse amplitude* refers to the strength of the output and is measured in milliamperes or volts, depending on whether the device provides a constant current or constant voltage. *Type of output* describes the pattern in which the pulses are delivered (see Fig. 4). A constant output produces pulses in a constant pattern over time. A burst output produces trains (or bursts) of pulses delivered at a low frequency, while the internal frequency of the train is high. A modulated output means that the pulses are delivered in a pattern in which one or several of the parameters (e.g., amplitude) are varied in a cyclical fashion.

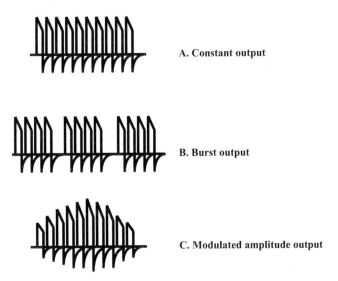

A. Constant output

B. Burst output

C. Modulated amplitude output

Fig. 4. Type of TENS output.

The most common modes of TENS used in clinical practice are described as conventional or high-frequency TENS (>50 Hz) and acupuncture-like or low-frequency TENS (1–10 Hz). Original TENS units used a carbon rubber and gel application, whereas most units today come with a supply of self-adhesive electrodes. Electrodes are typically placed at the site of injury or pain, proximal to the injury over a nerve supplying the affected area, or spinally at the appropriate segmental level.

In an IFT unit, the parameters that can be manipulated are beat frequency, sweep frequency, and pulse amplitude. The *beat frequency* is selected by manipulating the frequency of the two medium-frequency currents and ranges between 1 and 150 Hz. For example, to produce a beat frequency of 100 Hz, one channel is set at 4,000 Hz and the second is set at 4,100 Hz. IFT can be applied using two or four electrodes with the same choice of electrode placement as for TENS, described above. In a four-electrode arrangement, a low-frequency effect is believed to be produced in the tissues, as illustrated in Fig. 3. In a two-electrode arrangement, it is suggested that the medium-frequency currents mix within the unit, and therefore a low-frequency "premodulated" current is delivered to the skin. Ozcan et al. [57] compared sensory, motor, and pain thresholds using premodulated IFT and "true" IFT in a group of healthy adults. They also compared crossed currents and parallel currents for each type of IFT. Their study concluded that "true" IFT had no measurable advantage over premodulated IFT in terms of depth efficiency (as assessed by thresholds), torque production, or comfort.

Manipulation of the *sweep frequency* allows the therapist to move the beat frequency through a selected range, e.g., 100–120 Hz, during the treatment time. The pattern in which the beat frequency changes from highest to lowest levels can also be altered. For example, typical sweep patterns involve increasing the frequency over a 6-second interval and then decreasing it over a 6-second interval (written as 6^6).

Theories of TENS Analgesia

Two theories are commonly used to support the use of TENS. The gate control theory of pain is most commonly used to explain the inhibition of pain by TENS. According to the theory, stimulation of large-diameter afferents by TENS inhibits nociceptive-fiber-evoked responses in the dorsal horn. Much more detailed data are now available on the mechanisms of action of TENS with regard to anatomical pathways, neurotransmitters and their receptors, and the types of neurons involved in inhibition (Table I). Release of endogenous opioids also has been suggested to explain the actions of TENS, particularly with low-frequency stimulation. Recent data support this theory for both low- and high-frequency TENS stimulation [40,81].

Table I
Summary of basic science mechanisms for low- and high-frequency TENS

Mechanism	Low-Frequency	High-Frequency
Reduces primary hyperalgesia	+	+
Reduces secondary hyperalgesia	+	+
Reduces central sensitization	+	+
Activates PAG	+	+
Activates RVM	+	+
Activates spinal inhibitory mechanisms	+	+
Activates peripheral inhibitory mechanisms	+	–
Uses opioids	+ μ (RVM, SC, P)	+ δ (RVM, SC)
Uses serotonin	+ 5-HT$_2$, 5-HT$_3$ (SC)	– (SC)
Uses norepinephrine centrally	– (SC)	– (SC)
Uses α_{2A} adrenergic receptors	+ (P)	+ (P)
Uses GABA	+ (SC)	+ (SC)
Uses acetylcholine (activates muscarinic receptors)	+ M1, M3 (SC)	+ M1, M3 (SC)
Reduces glutamate release	–	+ (SC)
Reduces substance P release/content	?	+ (SC, P)
Activates autonomic nervous system	+ (P)	+ (P)

Abbreviations and symbols: +, involved in analgesia; –, not involved in analgesia; ?, unknown if involved in analgesia; GABA = gamma-aminobutyric acid; 5-HT = 5-hydroxytryptophan; M1, M3 = muscarinic receptors; μ = mu-opioid receptors; P = periphery; PAG = periaqueductal gray; RVM = rostral ventromedial medulla; SC = spinal cord; TENS = transcutaneous electrical nerve stimulation.

Early studies on mechanisms of action of TENS were performed in normal, uninjured animals. These studies provided valuable information regarding potential mechanisms of TENS. More recent studies have translated and extended these data by examining the mechanisms of TENS in animal models of pain. These studies have revealed pharmacological and anatomical pathways that mediate the reduction in pain produced by TENS [2,12,29,40,45,47,48,53,61,63,64,69,71,79,81–83,93,88]. The current data suggest that different frequencies of TENS produce analgesia through actions on different neurotransmitters and receptors.

Afferent Fibers Activated by TENS

Recordings from the median nerve in human subjects indicate that high-frequency stimulation at sensory intensity (100 Hz at three times the sensory threshold) activates only large-diameter Aβ fibers. Similarly, low-frequency (4-Hz) TENS, at a maximal tolerable intensity, activates only Aβ afferent fibers, whereas Aδ activation only occurs at intensities above maximal tolerable intensity [46]. Similarly, in animals, high- or low-frequency TENS at sensory intensity, or motor threshold, activates only large-diameter Aβ afferent fibers. Increasing the intensity to two times the motor threshold with both low- and high-frequency TENS will recruit Aδ fibers [64].

It is generally assumed that TENS reduces pain and hyperalgesia through activation of cutaneous afferent fibers because patients perceive the stimulus in the skin. However, one animal study provides evidence contradictory to this assertion. Specifically, in animals with knee joint inflammation, local anesthetic was applied to the skin under the electrodes or into the knee joint prior to TENS (either at low or high frequency at sensory intensities). TENS was still effective after cutaneous afferents were anesthetized with local anesthetic; however, it was ineffective when knee joint afferents were anesthetized with local anesthetic [64]. These findings support a role for deep-tissue afferents in the pain relief produced by TENS. Thus, it can be concluded that TENS must be applied at sufficient intensities to activate large-diameter deep-tissue afferent fibers to produce significant pain relief.

Electrode Placement

Few studies have addressed electrode placement. In one animal study, the effect of electrode placement was evaluated by placing electrodes within the receptive field for a spinothalamic tract neuron, outside the receptive field of the neuron but on the same limb, and at the mirror site [44]. The greatest degree of inhibition of spinothalamic tract cell activity occurred with electrodes placed within the receptive field for the neuron, and only minimal inhibition occurred when electrodes were placed on the same hindlimb but outside the receptive field. In animals with chronic muscle inflammation that resulted in bilateral hyperalgesia, electrode placement over either the inflamed or the contralateral non-inflamed muscle reduced secondary hyperalgesia [2]. Similarly, in animals with acute cutaneous inflammation, application of TENS to the contralateral hindpaw reduced primary hyperalgesia at the site of inflammation [71]. Together, these data suggest that TENS produces a widespread analgesic response; the greatest effect may occur if electrodes are placed at the site of injury, but application to the contralateral mirror side also may be effective in reducing hyperalgesia.

Neuronal Pathways Activated by TENS

Research over several years has discovered that TENS produces its analgesic effects through activation of pathways within the peripheral and central nervous systems. As stated above, large-diameter afferent fibers are activated by TENS. This input is sent through the central nervous system to activate the descending inhibitory systems to reduce hyperalgesia. Specifically, blockade of activity in the ventrolateral periaqueductal gray (PAG), rostral ventromedial medulla (RVM), and spinal cord inhibits the analgesic effects of TENS [22,40,81]. Further, receptors at the site of injury also play a role in the analgesia produced by TENS [42,71]. Thus, TENS activates a complex neuronal network to result in a reduction in pain. Details of the pathways, neurotransmitters, and receptors involved in the analgesia by low- and high-frequency TENS are presented below.

Effects of TENS in Animal Models of Pain

In animals without tissue injury, responses to noxious thermal stimuli increase after treatment with either high- or low-frequency TENS [94,95]. In parallel, dorsal horn neuron activity is reduced by both low- and high-frequency TENS in intact animals [26,27,27,44,76,77]. These data show that increasing frequency, pulse amplitude, or pulse duration results in a greater reduction in dorsal horn neuron activity and further reduces the response to peripherally applied noxious stimuli [27].

In animal models with tissue injury induced by inflammation of the skin, joint, or muscle, both primary and secondary hyperalgesia are reversed by either low-frequency (4-Hz) or high-frequency (100-Hz) TENS [2,29,67,79,88]. In a model of chronic muscle inflammation, hyperalgesia spreads to the contralateral hindlimb [62]. In this case, application of TENS to the inflamed or the contralateral non-inflamed muscle equally reduces the secondary hyperalgesia, which suggests widespread effects of TENS. Furthermore, sensitization of dorsal horn neurons to both noxious and innocuous stimuli after peripheral inflammation is also reduced by either high- or low-frequency TENS [47]. In animal models of neuropathic pain, either high- or low-frequency TENS reduces hyperalgesia as well as the sensitization of spinal neurons that normally occurs in these models [45,53,87]. Thus, TENS is analgesic in normal animals, reduces primary and secondary hyperalgesia in animals with tissue injury, and reduces central sensitization produced by tissue injury.

Analgesic Mechanisms of TENS

High-Frequency TENS

In animals that were spinalized to remove descending inhibitory pathways, inhibition of the tail flick by high-frequency TENS still occurred but was reduced by about 50% [95]. Thus, these studies suggest that both segmental spinal inhibition and descending inhibition are involved in the analgesia produced by high-frequency TENS. Later studies prevented the antihyperalgesia by blocking δ-opioid receptors in the RVM, or by blocking synaptic transmission in the ventrolateral PAG, further supporting a role for supraspinal pathways in TENS analgesia [40].

Opioid peptides mediate the effects of high-frequency TENS. High-frequency TENS increases the concentration of β-endorphins in the bloodstream and cerebrospinal fluid, and increases methionine-enkephalin in the cerebrospinal fluid, in human subjects [31,72]. In animals with knee joint inflammation, blockade of δ-opioid receptors in the spinal cord or the RVM reverses the antihyperalgesia produced by high-frequency TENS [40,81]. Repeated daily application of high-frequency, motor-intensity TENS produces analgesic tolerance to the antihyperalgesic effects of TENS by the fourth day (i.e., the effectiveness of TENS is reduced) [12]. High-frequency TENS also reduces release of the excitatory neurotransmitters glutamate and substance P in the spinal cord dorsal horn in animals with inflammation [69,84]. The reduction in glutamate is prevented by blockade of δ-opioid receptors. Thus, one consequence of activation of inhibitory pathways of TENS is to reduce excitation and consequent neuron sensitization in the spinal cord.

High-frequency TENS also enhances release of the inhibitory neurotransmitter γ-aminobutyric acid (GABA) in the spinal cord dorsal horn, and TENS-induced antihyperalgesia is reduced by blockade of $GABA_A$ receptors in the spinal cord [48]. Muscarinic receptors are also commonly implicated in analgesia at the level of the spinal cord, particularly with respect to opioid analgesia mechanisms. Indeed, the antihyperalgesia produced by high-frequency TENS is reduced by blockade of muscarinic receptors (M1, M3) in the spinal cord [63]. However, blockade of serotonergic or noradrenergic receptors in the spinal cord has no effect on the reversal of hyperalgesia produced by high-frequency TENS [61]. Thus, a complicated neural circuitry is activated in response to high-frequency TENS that engages descending opioid inhibitory pathways—including the PAG, RVM, and spinal cord—to reduce excitability of dorsal horn neurons by decreasing release of glutamate and increasing release of GABA, endogenous opioids, and acetylcholine to result in reduction of nociception and consequently pain.

Peripherally, the primary afferent neuropeptide substance P, which is normally increased in injured animals, is reduced in dorsal root ganglion neurons by high-frequency, sensory-intensity TENS in animals injected with the inflammatory irritant formalin [69]. In α_{2A}-adrenoreceptor knockout mice, antihyperalgesia is not elicited by high-frequency TENS [42]. Blockade of peripheral, but not of spinal or supraspinal, α_2 receptors prevents the antihyperalgesia produced by TENS [42], suggesting a role for peripheral α_{2A}-adrenoreceptors in analgesia produced by TENS. Further, high-frequency TENS effects autonomic function and blood flow. Blood flow changes with high-frequency TENS are minimal and transient, with intensities tested always within the sensory range [14,15,73]. Thus, current evidence suggests that some of the analgesic effects of TENS are mediated through actions on primary afferent fibers and through modulation of autonomic activity.

Low-Frequency TENS

The antihyperalgesia produced by low-frequency TENS ($\leq$10 Hz) is mediated by classic descending inhibitory pathways that include the PAG, RVM, and spinal cord [22,40,81]. Low-frequency TENS-induced antihyperalgesia is prevented by blockade of μ-opioid receptors in the spinal cord or the RVM [40,81]. Further, repeated daily application of TENS produces tolerance to the antihyperalgesic effects of treatment by the fourth day, with concomitant cross-tolerance to μ-opioid receptor agonists in the spinal cord [12], further supporting a role for μ-opioid receptors in TENS antihyperalgesia. The antihyperalgesia produced by low-frequency, sensory-intensity TENS is also reduced by blockade of $GABA_A$, serotonin 5-HT_{2A} and 5-HT_3, and muscarinic M1 and M3 receptors in the spinal cord [48,61,63]. Similarly, serotonin is released during low-frequency TENS in animals with joint inflammation [83]. Taken together, these studies suggest that opioid, GABA, serotonin, and muscarinic receptors in the spinal cord are activated by low-frequency TENS to reduce dorsal horn neuron activity, nociception, and the consequent pain.

Low-frequency TENS also has effects on the peripheral and autonomic nervous systems. Blockade of peripheral opioid receptors with naloxone at the site of application prevents the antihyperalgesic effects of low-frequency, but not high-frequency, TENS in an animal model of inflammatory pain [71], showing a role for peripheral opioid receptors in TENS analgesia. In another study, a reduction in cold allodynia by low-frequency TENS was reduced by administration of systemic phentolamine to block α-adrenergic receptors [53]. In parallel, the antihyperalgesia produced by low-frequency TENS in animals with joint inflammation was reduced in α_{2A}-noradrenergic receptor knockout mice, and it was prevented by peripheral blockade of α_{2A}-noradrenergic receptors (but not by spinal or supraspinal blockade) [42]. Results from studies assessing blood flow changes—a measure of autonomic activity—are mixed, with small, transient increases in blood flow in some cases with low-frequency TENS at intensities below or just above motor threshold. However, significant increases occur with stronger intensities that produce motor contractions with an intensity greater than 25% above motor threshold [14–16,73,75]. Thus, peripheral effects of TENS may involve changes in sympathetic activity mediated by local α_{2A}-noradrenergic receptors.

Translation of Mechanisms of TENS Analgesia to the Clinic

Clinically, TENS more than likely will not be the only treatment the patient is receiving. TENS is a complementary and adjunct treatment to control pain, allowing patients to engage in an active exercise program and return to their normal roles in society. Physical therapists who treat pain, particularly chronic pain, use a combination of exercise and functional training. They use electrotherapeutic modalities as an adjunct to modulate and reduce pain to allow the subject to participate in a more active program. The patient's medical treatment will probably include prescription medications such as nonsteroidal anti-inflammatory drugs (NSAIDs), opioids (e.g., fentanyl or oxycodone), α_{2A}-adrenergic agonists (e.g., clonidine), and/or muscle relaxants (e.g., cyclobenzaprine). Understanding the mechanisms of action for TENS will better assist the clinician in the appropriate choice of pain control treatments.

Use of TENS (in combination with other therapies) will allow patients to increase their activity level and improve their level of function. For inpatients, it can reduce the length of hospital stay. Treatment with TENS increases joint function in patients with arthritis [1,43,49,50,98]. In patients with chronic low back pain, TENS yields improvements on the physical and mental component summary of the SF-36 quality-of-life survey [28]. TENS treatment after thoracic surgery reduces recovery room stay, and it improves pulmonary function (as measured by postoperative PO_2, vital capacity, and functional residual capacity) when compared to sham-treated controls [3,65,93]. Thus, decreasing pain with TENS may increase function and allow the patient to tolerate other therapies and activities, resulting in an improved quality of life.

Every practitioner should be aware of the medications a patient is taking and know the effects they may have on the outcome of TENS. If a patient is taking opioids (currently the majority of those available target μ-opioid receptors), high-frequency TENS may be more appropriate. This recommendation is based on the fact that low-frequency, but not high-frequency, TENS is ineffective in animals tolerant to morphine [82]. Clinically, in patients who had taken enough opioids to become tolerant to morphine, TENS was ineffective in reducing postoperative pain [86]. Thus, low-frequency TENS is ineffective in patients with μ-opioid tolerance.

Combining pharmaceutical interventions with TENS could enhance the analgesic effects of treatment. Preclinical studies show that either high- or low-frequency TENS is more effective in reducing primary hyperalgesia if given in combination with acute administration of morphine [78] or clonidine [80] and should thus reduce the dosage necessary to reduce hyperalgesia and lessen the side effects of the drugs. Clinically, TENS allows patients to reduce their intake of opioids [28,70,85,86,92] and mitigates the nausea, dizziness, and pruritis associated with morphine intake [92]. Based on the known mechanisms of TENS presented above, one could hypothesize that selective serotonin reuptake inhibitors would prolong the effects of low-frequency TENS, that NSAIDs could enhance the effectiveness of TENS, or that patients taking acetylcholinesterase (ACE) inhibitors for cardiac disease might obtain reduced benefit with TENS.

Tolerance and TENS

Given that the effects of TENS are opioid mediated, it follows that repeated application of TENS would produce tolerance to its analgesic effects. In animals with joint inflammation, repeated daily application of either low- or high-frequency TENS was ineffective by the fourth day [12], and this finding was associated with a cross-tolerance at spinal opioid receptors. Pharmacological studies show that application of μ- and δ-opioid agonists simultaneously, blockade of N-methyl D-aspartate (NMDA) glutamate receptors, or blockade of cholecystokinin (CCK) receptors prevents the development of tolerance to exogenous opioid agonists, and thus similar strategies could be used to prevent tolerance to TENS. In animals with joint inflammation, simultaneous administration of low- and high-frequency TENS in the same session, or alternating administration of low- and high-frequency TENS in subsequent sessions, significantly delays the development of tolerance [20]. Pharmacological blockade of NMDA glutamate receptors or CCK receptors during application of TENS prevents the development of tolerance to either high- or low-frequency TENS [21,32].

Thus, prevention of tolerance to TENS is critical for full effectiveness of treatment. Physical therapists can easily modulate frequencies of TENS in the clinic to prevent or delay the development of tolerance. Pharmacological treatments aimed at blocking NMDA receptors (i.e., ketamine or dextromethorphan) or CCK receptors (i.e., proglumide) could enhance the efficacy of TENS by preventing tolerance (Fig. 5).

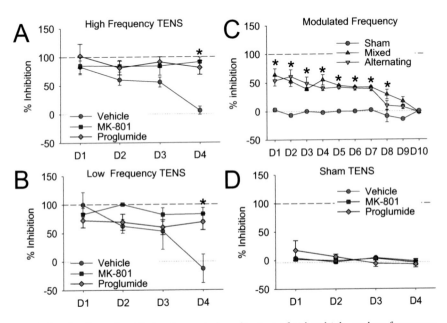

Fig. 5. Graphs show the effects of repeated application of either high- or low-frequency TENS in animals that received a vehicle control (A,B, red) compared to those that received the NMDA antagonist MK-801 (A,B, blue), the CCK antagonist proglumide (A,B, green), or a combined application of low- and high-frequency TENS in the same session (C, mixed, blue) or alternating sessions (C, alternating, green). Withdrawal thresholds of the paw were measured before and after daily application of TENS to the inflamed knee joint (induced with 3% kaolin and carrageenan). Those that received sham TENS showed no change in withdrawal thresholds before or after treatment throughout the testing period. Notice the development of tolerance by day 4 in animals that received either (A) high-frequency or (B) low-frequency TENS and a vehicle (red symbols). In animals treated with MK-801 or proglumide, tolerance to either high- or low-frequency TENS did not develop. In those treated with mixed or alternating TENS, development of tolerance was significantly delayed. Data are represented as a percentage change in hyperalgesia, induced by knee joint inflammation 24 hours earlier, before and after TENS on each day. Dotted lines represent no change in hyperalgesia, i.e., 0%. Hatched lines represent a complete reversal of hyperalgesia, i.e., 100%. Data are means ± SEM. Asterisks (*) denote a significant increase from sham TENS in animals treated with vehicle. Based on data from [21,32] and unpublished data (K.A. Sluka et al.).

Analgesic Mechanisms of IFT

The mechanisms of action for IFT remain speculative. A recent animal study showed that IFT delivered at 4,000 Hz carrier frequency, 140 Hz beat frequency, with a pulse duration of 125 µs and pulse amplitude of 5 mA for 1 hour reduced spontaneous activity produced by formalin inflammation and lessened primary mechanical hyperalgesia produced by carrageenan inflammation [38].

Clinical Efficacy of TENS and IFT

TENS

Although TENS is most commonly used for pain management, it has also been associated with other benefits such as anti-emetic effects [39] and the promotion of wound healing [8]. In an attempt to highlight the limitations of clinical research to date, Table II summarizes key systematic reviews and meta-analyses that have been published on TENS. It highlights the small number of eligible randomized controlled trials (RCTs) that meet the inclusion criteria for such reviews. In addition, lack of details on TENS application, poor methodological quality of trials, and heterogeneous study populations are all common problems specific to TENS research.

Several systematic reviews report negative or inconclusive findings for chronic pain conditions: general chronic pain [54], poststroke shoulder pain [59], chronic low back pain [41], and cancer pain [68]. In contrast, Osiri et al. [56] and Brosseau et al. [7] report more positive findings for knee osteoarthritis and rheumatoid arthritis of the hand, respectively. More recently, Johnson and Martinson [35] published a meta-analysis on the efficacy of electrical nerve stimulation (ENS) for chronic musculoskeletal pain. The types of stimulation assessed were both TENS and percutaneous electrical nerve stimulation (PENS), and the range of conditions included rheumatoid arthritis, low back pain, osteoarthritis, ankylosing spondylitis, and myofascial trigger points. They included 38 studies from 29 papers for a total of 335 subjects receiving placebo, 474 subjects receiving ENS, and 418 crossover subjects (receiving both placebo and at least one ENS treatment). Data analyses of these studies indicated a significant

Table II
Evidence for TENS efficacy

Disease/Pain Condition	Ref.	Type of Review	No. Studies	Results
Postoperative pain	[11]	Systematic review	17	Ineffective
Postoperative pain	[6]	Meta-analysis	21	Effective; adequate parameters necessary to get a positive effect
Labor pain	[10]	Systematic review	10	Ineffective
Knee osteoarthritis	[56]	Cochrane review	7	TENS and AL-TENS more effective than placebo
Poststroke shoulder pain	[59]	Cochrane review	4	Inconclusive
Primary dysmenorrhea	[60]	Cochrane review	9	High-frequency TENS more effective than placebo; low-frequency TENS similar to placebo
Rheumatoid arthritis of the hand	[7]	Cochrane review	3	AL-TENS improved pain intensity and muscle power scores over placebo; C-TENS had no clinical benefit on pain intensity compared to placebo; C-TENS showed more clinical benefit on patient assessment of changes in disease over AL-TENS
Dementia	[9]	Cochrane review	9	Inconclusive
Chronic musculoskeletal pain	[35]	Meta-analysis	38	Effective; concluded that prior studies had inadequate statistical power
Chronic low back pain	[41]	Cochrane review	4	Conflicting evidence
Chronic pain	[54]	Cochrane review	25	Inconclusive
Cancer pain	[68]	Cochrane review	2	Inconclusive

Abbreviations: AL = acupuncture-like; C = conventional; TENS = transcutaneous electrical nerve stimulation.

decrease in pain with ENS compared to placebo. The authors highlight that lack of statistical power was the main reason for disparity in their findings compared with other studies and meta-analyses in this area.

Although TENS is commonly used as an intervention for chronic pain, its efficacy for acute pain conditions has also been examined.

Systematic reviews have produced mixed results for postoperative pain [6,11], labor pain [10], and primary dysmenorrhea [60]. Bjordal et al.'s meta-analysis on postoperative pain highlights the importance of considering the inclusion criteria in a meta-analysis or systematic review when interpreting the results [6]. Bjordal et al. only included studies that used "optimal" stimulation parameters (i.e., appropriate dose), whereas Carroll's earlier systematic review [11] did not impose this inclusion criterion. Bjordal et al. concluded that TENS can significantly reduce analgesic consumption for postoperative pain, whereas Carroll et al. determined that the majority of studies they reviewed showed no benefit for TENS. Furthermore, there is no universally accepted scoring system in systematic reviews to assess the efficacy of an intervention. Caution is therefore warranted in areas such as the scoring of blinding in an RCT of TENS, because blinding is inherently problematic with electrophysical treatments.

As pain is multidimensional, assessment of other parameters may be equally important as measurement of pain intensity at rest on a visual analogue scale (VAS). Recently, deSantana and colleagues showed that TENS reduced both the affective and sensory dimensions of pain, as measured by the McGill Pain Questionnaire, in patients with inguinal hernia surgery and in patients undergoing sterilization procedures [23,24]. Further, pain with movement—which probably represents a form of hyperalgesia—is particularly problematic postoperatively. Rakel and Franz [65] showed that in patients recovering from abdominal surgery, pain with walking or with deep breathing was significantly reduced by high-frequency TENS. However, they showed no effect on pain at rest [65].

Lastly, recent evidence supports the notion of adequate dosing, in particular for stimulation pulse amplitude. In an experimental pain study, Rakel and colleagues [66] show that pressure pain threshold (PPT) increased in healthy volunteers with pulse amplitudes greater than 18 mA when compared to a placebo. Pulse amplitudes below 18 mA showed only a small increase in PPT. Similarly, Bjordal et al. [6] and Rakel and Franz [65] show that TENS was only effective if given at pulse amplitudes greater than 12 mA, or 9 mA, respectively, in people with postoperative pain. Together, these data indicate that TENS needs to be applied at a relatively high pulse amplitude to obtain significant reductions in pain.

The current literature supports the conclusion that further evidence is required on the efficacy, parameter-specific effects, and cost-effectiveness of TENS. Optimal stimulation parameters and treatment durations should be considered when interpreting the outcome of systematic reviews and meta-analyses on TENS.

Interferential Therapy

The main clinical indications for using IFT are pain management [17], reduction of swelling [34], and muscle strengthening [5,19]. Traditionally, IFT was applied in a physical therapy clinic, which limited its use for different pain conditions. However, small portable IFT units are now widely available (see Fig. 2), which allows IFT to be applied for similar pain conditions to TENS. In a postal survey of 416 physical therapists in the United Kingdom and Hong Kong on the use of TENS for pain management, Hong Kong physical therapists reported using TENS and IFT more frequently than their U.K. colleagues [91]. When asked to rate the perceived effectiveness of the two modalities for acute and chronic pain, both groups indicated that IFT was more effective for acute pain. However, Hong Kong physical therapists rated IFT as more effective for chronic pain, whereas their U.K. counterparts felt that TENS was more effective. Poitras et al. [58] highlighted the popularity of IFT in physical therapy clinics in Canada for low back pain, and a further two surveys have reported that IFT is the most widely used electrotherapeutic modality for this condition in the United Kingdom and Ireland [25,30].

Experimental pain models show no consistent effect of IFT for measures of cold pain, ischemic pain, delayed-onset muscle soreness, or PPT [4,36,37,52]. However, recent clinical data show that for acute back pain, IFT alone, manipulative therapy alone, or IFT and manipulative therapy combined produced long-term improvements (for up to 12 months) in functional disability, pain, quality of life, analgesic medication consumption, and exercise participation [33]. Although improvements were noted in all three treatment groups, there were no significant differences between groups. IFT was applied using two electrodes applied over the appropriate spinal nerve roots (3.85-kHz carrier frequency, 140-Hz beat frequency). However, no placebo control was used in this study.

Zambito et al. [97] compared the effects of IFT (200-Hz modulated beat frequency, dermatome application, for 10 minutes' duration, 5 times per week for 2 weeks), horizontal therapy (HT, a form of electrical stimulation), and sham HT in a sample of patients with multiple vertebral compression fractures or degenerative disk disease. In a more recent study on multiple vertebral compression fractures, Zambito et al. [96] again compared IFT (as described above, except that the duration of each session was 30 minutes) compared to HT or sham-HT groups. Results from the two studies showed a significant reduction in pain in both HT and IFT groups compared to the sham-HT group at weeks 6 and 14. Interestingly, in both of the above studies, subjects in all treatment groups performed flexion and extension stretching exercises during the 2 weeks of IFT/HT treatment, suggesting that stretching exercises alone were not sufficient to improve pain.

Cheing et al. 2008 [13] recently compared the effects of acupuncture and exercise, IFT and exercise, and no treatment in individuals with idiopathic frozen shoulder. The IFT group received 10 treatment sessions over 4 weeks. IFT was delivered to the affected shoulder at a beat frequency of 80–120 Hz for 20 minutes at an intensity just below the pain threshold. Participants in the two intervention groups were instructed to perform a standard set of shoulder mobilization exercises five times daily until the 6-month follow-up. Data analysis showed a significant reduction in pain intensity (on a VAS) and an increase in shoulder function (Constant Murley Assessment) in the two intervention groups (both $P < 0.001$); however, no significant difference was found between the two intervention groups. The observed improvement was well maintained in both intervention groups, at least until the 6-month follow-up session.

In people with knee osteoarthritis, Defrin et al. [17] demonstrated that IFT delivered with a carrier frequency of 4,000 Hz reduced pain and morning stiffness compared to sham-treated and no-treatment control groups. Interestingly, pain was reduced if the intensity was delivered at either a noxious intensity (30% above pain threshold) or an innocuous intensity (30% below pain threshold). This study also reported no significant differences in treatment outcomes if the patients routinely adjusted the stimulation intensity to prevent the sensation fading, as opposed to not adjusting the intensity even though the sensation was fading. This study was the first to clinically examine the concept of accommodation associated with the application of electrical currents. Thus, emerging evidence from placebo-controlled trials suggests that IFT is effective for reduction of pain associated with osteoarthritis, degenerative disk disease, or vertebral fractures. However, no systematic reviews on the efficacy of IFT have been published to date.

Summary

In summary, there is evidence from basic science, as well as clinical studies, that TENS is an effective treatment for pain control in both acute and chronic pain conditions. Evidence suggests that frequency of stimulation activates different endogenous analgesia systems, and that intensity of stimulation is critical to pain relief. For IFT, evidence is emerging from RCTs to support its use. However, the mechanisms by which IFT produces its analgesic effect are unknown.

References

[1]   Abelson K, Langley GB, Vlieg M, Wigley RD. Transcutaneous electrical nerve stimulation in rheumatoid arthritis. N Z Med J 1983;96:156–8.
[2]   Ainsworth L, Budelier K, Clinesmith M, Fiedler A, Landstrom R, Leeper BJ, Moeller L, Mutch S, O'Dell K, Ross J, et al. Transcutaneous electrical nerve stimulation (TENS) reduces chronic hyperalgesia induced by muscle inflammation. Pain 2006;120:182–7.
[3]   Ali J, Yaffe CS, Sessle BJ. The effect of transcutaneous electric nerve stimulation on postoperative pain and pulmonary function. Surgery 1981;89:507–12.
[4]   Alves-Guerreiro J, Noble JG, Lowe AS, Walsh DM. The effect of three electrotherapeutic modalities upon peripheral nerve conduction and mechanical pain threshold. Clin Physiol 2001;21:704–11.
[5]   Bircan C, Senocak O, Peker O, Kaya A, Tamci SA, Gulbahar S, Akalin E. Efficacy of two forms of electrical stimulation in increasing quadriceps strength: a randomized controlled trial. Clin Rehabil 2002;16:194–9.
[6]   Bjordal JM, Johnson MI, Ljunggreen AE. Transcutaneous electrical nerve stimulation (TENS) can reduce postoperative analgesic consumption. A meta-analysis with assessment of optimal treatment parameters for postoperative pain. Eur J Pain 2003;7:181–8.
[7]   Brosseau L, Judd MG, Marchand S, Robinson VA, Tugwell P, Wells G, Yonge K. Transcutaneous electrical nerve stimulation (TENS) for the treatment of rheumatoid arthritis in the hand. Cochrane Database Syst Rev 2003;CD004377.
[8]   Burssens P, Forsyth R, Steyaert A, Van OE, Praet M, Verdonk R. Influence of burst TENS stimulation on collagen formation after Achilles tendon suture in man. A histological evaluation with Movat's pentachrome stain. Acta Orthop Belg 2005;71:342–6.
[9]   Cameron M, Lonergan E, Lee H. Transcutaneous electrical nerve stimulation (TENS) for dementia. Cochrane Database Syst Rev 2003;CD004032.
[10] Carroll D, Moore RA, Tramer MR, McQuay H. Transcutaneous electrical nerve stimulation does not relieve labor pain: updated systematic review. Contemp Issues Obstet Gynecol 1997;September:195–205.

[11] Carroll D, Tramer M, McQuay H, Nye B, Moore A. Randomization is important in studies with pain outcomes: systematic review of transcutaneous electrical nerve stimulation in acute postoperative pain. Br J Anaesth 1996;77:798–803.

[12] Chandran P, Sluka KA. Development of opioid tolerance with repeated transcutaneous electrical nerve stimulation administration. Pain 2003;102:195–201.

[13] Cheing GL, So EM, Chao CY. Effectiveness of electroacupuncture and interferential electrotherapy in the management of frozen shoulder. J Rehabil Med 2008;40:166–70.

[14] Chen CC, Johnson MI, McDonough S, Cramp F. The effect of transcutaneous electrical nerve stimulation on local and distal cutaneous blood flow following a prolonged heat stimulus in healthy subjects. Clin Physiol Funct Imaging 2007;27:154–61.

[15] Cramp AF, Gilsenan C, Lowe AS, Walsh DM. The effect of high- and low-frequency transcutaneous electrical nerve stimulation upon cutaneous blood flow and skin temperature in healthy subjects. Clin Physiol 2000;20:150–7.

[16] Cramp FL, McCullough GR, Lowe AS, Walsh DM. Transcutaneous electric nerve stimulation: the effect of intensity on local and distal cutaneous blood flow and skin temperature in healthy subjects. Arch Phys Med Rehabil 2002;83:5–9.

[17] Defrin R, Ariel E, Peretz C. Segmental noxious versus innocuous electrical stimulation for chronic pain relief and the effect of fading sensation during treatment. Pain 2005;115:152–60.

[18] Delaney E, Cusack T. A postal questionnaire surveying the use of electrophysical agents in outpatient physiotherapy departments in Irish hospitals. Physiother Ireland 2008;29:61–7.

[19] Demirturk F, Akbayrak T, Karakaya IC, Yuksel I, Kirdi N, Demirturk F, Kaya S, Ergen A, Beksac S. Interferential current versus biofeedback results in urinary stress incontinence. Swiss Med Wkly 2008;138:317–21.

[20] deSantana JM, Santana-Filho VJ, Sluka KA. Modulation between high- and low-frequency transcutaneous electric nerve stimulation delays the development of analgesic tolerance in arthritic rats. Arch Phys Med Rehabil 2008;89:754–60.

[21] deSantana JM, Sluka KA. Blockade of CCK receptors, systemically and spinally prevents the development of tolerance to TENS. Abstract presented at: 12th World Congress on Pain, Glasgow, 2008.

[22] deSantana JM, Sluka KA. Blockade of the ventrolateral PAG prevents the effects of TENS. Neuroscience 2009; in press.

[23] deSantana JM, Sluka KA. Hypoalgesic effect of the transcutaneous electrical nerve stimulation following inguinal herniorrhaphy: a randomized controlled trial. J Pain 2008;9:623–9.

[24] deSantana JM, Sluka KA, Lauretti GR. High and low frequency TENS reduce postoperative pain intensity after laparoscopic sterilization for tubal ligation: a randomized controlled trial. Clin J Pain 2009;25:12–9.

[25] Foster NE, Thompson KA, Baxter GD, Allen JM. Management of nonspecific low back pain by physiotherapists in Britain and Ireland. A descriptive questionnaire of current clinical practice. Spine 1999;24:1332–42.

[26] Garrison DW, Foreman RD. Decreased activity of spontaneous and noxiously evoked dorsal horn cells during transcutaneous electrical nerve stimulation (TENS). Pain 1994;58:309–15.

[27] Garrison DW, Foreman RD. Effects of prolonged transcutaneous electrical nerve stimulation (TENS) and variation of stimulation variables on dorsal horn cell activity. Eur J Phys Med Rehabil 1997;6:87–94.

[28] Ghoname EA, Craig WF, White PF, Ahmed HE, Hamza MA, Gajraj NM, Vakharia AS, Nohr D. The effect of stimulus frequency on the analgesic response to percutaneous electrical nerve stimulation in patients with chronic low back pain. Anesth Analg 1999;88:841–6.

[29] Gopalkrishnan P, Sluka KA. Effect of varying frequency, intensity and pulse duration of TENS on primary hyperalgesia in inflamed rats. Arch Phys Med Rehabil 2000;81:984–90.

[30] Gracey JH, McDonough SM, Baxter GD. Physiotherapy management of low back pain: a survey of current practice in northern Ireland. Spine 2002;27:406–11.

[31] Han JS, Chen XH, Sun SL, Xu XJ, Yuan Y, Yan SC, Hao JX, Terenius L. Effect of low and high frequency TENS on met-enkephalin-arg-phe and dynorphin A immunoreactivity in human lumbar CSF. Pain 1991;47:295–8.

[32] Hingne PM, Sluka KA. Blockade of NMDA receptors prevents analgesic tolerance to repeated transcutaneous electrical nerve stimulation (TENS) in rats. J Pain 2008;9:217–25.

[33] Hurley DA, McDonough SM, Dempster M, Moore AP, Baxter GD. A randomized clinical trial of manipulative therapy and interferential therapy for acute low back pain. Spine 2004;29:2207–16.

[34] Jarit GJ, Mohr KJ, Waller R, Glousman RE. The effects of home interferential therapy on post-operative pain, edema, and range of motion of the knee. Clin J Sport Med 2003;13:16–20.

[35] Johnson M, Martinson M. Efficacy of electrical nerve stimulation for chronic musculoskeletal pain: a meta-analysis of randomized controlled trials. Pain 2007;130:157–65.

[36] Johnson MI, Tabasam G. An investigation into the analgesic effects of different frequencies of the amplitude-modulated wave of interferential current therapy on cold-induced pain in normal subjects. Arch Phys Med Rehabil 2003;84:1387–94.

[37] Johnson MI, Tabasam G. An investigation into the analgesic effects of interferential currents and transcutaneous electrical nerve stimulation on experimentally induced ischemic pain in otherwise pain-free volunteers. Phys Ther 2003;83:208–23.

[38] Jorge S, Parada CA, Ferreira SH, Tambeli CH. Interferential therapy produces antinociception during application in various models of inflammatory pain. Phys Ther 2006;86:800–8.

[39] Kabalak AA, Akcay M, Akcay F, Gogus N. Transcutaneous electrical acupoint stimulation versus ondansetron in the prevention of postoperative vomiting following pediatric tonsillectomy. J Altern Complement Med 2005;11:407–13.

[40] Kalra A, Urban MO, Sluka KA. Blockade of opioid receptors in rostral ventral medulla prevents antihyperalgesia produced by transcutaneous electrical nerve stimulation (TENS). J Pharmacol Exp Ther 2001;298:257–63.

[41] Khadilkar A, Odebiyi DO, Brosseau L, Wells GA. Transcutaneous electrical nerve stimulation (TENS) versus placebo for chronic low-back pain. Cochrane Database Syst Rev 2008;CD003008.

[42] King EW, Audette K, Athman GA, Nguyen HOX, Sluka KA, Fairbanks CA. Transcutaneous electrical nerve stimulation activates peripherally located alpha-2A adrenergic receptors. Pain 2005;115:364–73.

[43] Kumar VN, Redford JB. Transcutaneous nerve stimulation in rheumatoid arthritis. Arch Phys Med Rehabil 1982;63:595–6.

[44] Lee KH, Chung JM, Willis WD. Inhibition of primate spinothalamic tract cells by TENS. J Neurosurg 1985;62:276–87.

[45] Leem JW, Park ES, Paik KS. Electrophysiological evidence for the antinociceptive effect of transcutaneous electrical nerve stimulation on mechanically evoked responsiveness of dorsal horn neurons in neuropathic rats. Neurosci Lett 1995;192:197–200.

[46] Levin MF, Hui-Chan CW. Conventional and acupuncture-like transcutaneous electrical nerve stimulation excite similar afferent fibers. Arch Phys Med Rehabil 1993;74:54–60.

[47] Ma YT, Sluka KA. Reduction in inflammation-induced sensitization of dorsal horn neurons by transcutaneous electrical nerve stimulation in anesthetized rats. Exp Brain Res 2001;137:94–102.

[48] Maeda Y, Lisi TL, Vance CG, Sluka KA. Release of GABA and activation of GABAA receptors in the spinal cord mediates the effects of TENS in rats. Brain Res 2007;1136:43–50.

[49] Mannheimer C, Carlsson C-A. The analgesic effect of transcutaneous electrical nerve stimulation (TNS) in patients with rheumatoid arthritis. A comparative study of different pulse patterns. Pain 1979;6:329–34.

[50] Mannheimer C, Lund S, Carlsson C-A. The effect of transcutaneous electrical nerve stimulation (TNS) on joint pain in patients with rheumatoid arthritis. Scand J Rheumatol 1978;7:13–6.

[51] Melzack R, Wall PD. Pain mechanisms: a new theory. Science 1965;150:971–8.

[52] Minder PM, Noble JG, Alves-Guerreiro J, Hill ID, Lowe AS, Walsh DM, Baxter GD. Interferential therapy: lack of effect upon experimentally induced delayed onset muscle soreness. Clin Physiol Funct Imaging 2002;22:339–47.

[53] Nam TS, Choi Y, Yeon DS, Leem JW, Paik KS. Differential antinociceptive effect of transcutaneous electrical stimulation on pain behavior sensitive or insensitive to phentolamine in neuropathic rats. Neurosci Lett 2001;301:17–20.

[54] Nnoaham KE, Kumbang J. Transcutaneous electrical nerve stimulation (TENS) for chronic pain. Cochrane Database Syst Rev 2008;CD003222.

[55] Noble JG, Henderson G, Cramp AF, Walsh DM, Lowe AS. The effect of interferential therapy upon cutaneous blood flow in humans. Clin Physiol 2000;20:2–7.

[56] Osiri M, Welch V, Brosseau L, Shea B, McGowan J, Tugwell P, Wells G. Transcutaneous electrical nerve stimulation for knee osteoarthritis. Cochrane Database Syst Rev 2000;CD002823.

[57] Ozcan J, Ward AR, Robertson VJ. A comparison of true and premodulated interferential currents. Arch Phys Med Rehabil 2004;85:409–15.

[58] Poitras S, Blais R, Swaine B, Rossignol M. Management of work-related low back pain: a population-based survey of physical therapists. Phys Ther 2005;85:1168–81.

[59] Price CI, Pandyan AD. Electrical stimulation for preventing and treating post-stroke shoulder pain. Cochrane Database Syst Rev 2000;CD001698.

[60] Proctor ML, Smith CA, Farquhar CM, Stones RW. Transcutaneous electrical nerve stimulation and acupuncture for primary dysmenorrhoea. Cochrane Database Syst Rev 2002;CD002123.

[61] Radhakrishnan R, King EW, Dickman J, Richtsmeier C, Schardt N, Spurgin M, Sluka KA. Blockade of spinal 5-HT receptor subtypes prevents low, but not high, frequency TENS-induced antihyperalgesia in rats. Pain 2003;105:205–13.

[62] Radhakrishnan R, Moore SA, Sluka KA. Unilateral carrageenan injection into muscle or joint induces chronic bilateral hyperalgesia in rats. Pain 2003;104:567–77.

[63] Radhakrishnan R, Sluka KA. Spinal muscarinic receptors are activated during low or high frequency TENS-induced antihyperalgesia in rats. Neuropharmacology 2003;45:1111–9.

[64] Radhakrishnan R, Sluka KA. Deep tissue afferents, but not cutaneous afferents, mediate TENS-induced antihyperalgesia. J Pain 2005;6:673–80.

[65] Rakel B, Frantz R. Effectiveness of transcutaneous electrical nerve stimulation on postoperative pain with movement. J Pain 2003;4:455–64.

[66] Rakel BA, Adams HJ, Cooper NA, Dannen DR, Granquist MJ, Messer BR, Miller CA, Mitchelson AC, Ruggle RC, Vance CG, et al. Increasing TENS intensity produces greater analgesia when compared to a new placebo that allows true investigator blinding. Abstract presented at: 12th World Congress on Pain, Glasgow, 2008.

[67] Resende MA, Sabino GG, Candido CRM, Pereira LSM, Francischi JN. Transcutaneous electrical stimulation (TENS) effects in experimental inflammatory edema and pain. Eur J Pharmacol 2004;504:217–22.

[68] Robb K, Oxberry SG, Bennett MI, Johnson MI, Simpson KH, Searle RD. A Cochrane systematic review of transcutaneous electrical nerve stimulation for cancer pain. J Pain Symptom Manage 2009;37:746–53.

[69] Rokugo T, Takeuchi T, Ito H. A histochemical study of substance P in the rat spinal cord: effect of transcutaneous electrical nerve stimulation. J Nippon Med Sch 2002;69:428–33.

[70] Rosenberg M, Curtis L, Bourke DL. Transcutaneous electrical nerve stimulation for the relief of postoperative pain. Pain 1978;5:129–33.

[71] Sabino GS, Santos CM, Francischi JN, de Resende MA. Release of endogenous opioids following transcutaneous electric nerve stimulation in an experimental model of acute inflammatory pain. J Pain 2008;9:157–63.

[72] Salar G, Job I, Mingrino S, Bosio A, Trabucchi M. Effect of transcutaneous electrotherapy on CSF beta-endorphin content in patients without pain problems. Pain 1981;10:169–72.

[73] Sandberg ML, Sandberg MK, Dahl J. Blood flow changes in the trapezius muscle and overlying skin following transcutaneous electrical nerve stimulation. Phys Ther 2007;87:1047–55.

[74] Shealy CN. Transcutaneous electrical stimulation for control of pain. Clin Neurosurg 1974;21:269–77.

[75] Sherry JE, Oehrlein KM, Hegge KS, Morgan BJ. Effect of burst-mode transcutaneous electrical nerve stimulation on peripheral vascular resistance. Phys Ther 2001;81:1183–91.

[76] Sjolund BH. Peripheral nerve stimulation suppression of C-fiber evoked flexion reflex in rats. Part 1: parameters of continuous stimulation. J Neurosurg 1985;63:612–6.

[77] Sjolund BH. Peripheral nerve stimulation suppression of C-fiber evoked flexion reflex in rats. Part 2: parameters of low rat train stimulation of skin and muscle afferent nerves. J Neurosurg 1988;68:279–83.

[78] Sluka KA. Systemic morphine in combination with TENS produces an increased analgesia in rats with acute inflammation. J Pain 2000;1:204–11.

[79] Sluka KA, Bailey K, Bogush J, Olson R, Ricketts A. Treatment with either high or low frequency TENS reduces the secondary hyperalgesia observed after injection of kaolin and carrageenan into the knee joint. Pain 1998;77:97–102.

[80] Sluka KA, Chandran P. Enhanced reduction in hyperalgesia by combined administration of clonidine and TENS. Pain 2002;100:183–90.

[81] Sluka KA, Deacon M, Stibal A, Strissel S, Terpstra A. Spinal blockade of opioid receptors prevents the analgesia produced by TENS in arthritic rats. J Pharmacol Exp Ther 1999;289:840–6.

[82] Sluka KA, Judge MA, McColley MM, Reveiz PM, Taylor BM. Low frequency TENS is less effective than high frequency TENS at reducing inflammation-induced hyperalgesia in morphine-tolerant rats. Eur J Pain 2000;4:185–93.

[83] Sluka KA, Lisi TL, Westlund KN. Increased release of serotonin in the spinal cord during low, but not high, frequency TENS in rats with joint inflammation. Arch Phys Med Rehabil 2006;87:1137–40.
[84] Sluka KA, Vance CGT, Lisi TL. High-frequency, but not low-frequency, transcutaneous electrical nerve stimulation reduces aspartate and glutamate release in the spinal cord dorsal horn. J Neurochem 2005;95:1794–801.
[85] Smith CR, Lewith GT, Machin D. TNS and osteoarthritis: preliminary study to establish a controlled method of assessing transcutaneous electrical nerve stimulation as a treatment for pain caused by osteoarthritis. Physiotherapy 1983;69:266–8.
[86] Solomon RA, Viernstein MC, Long DM. Reduction of postoperative pain and narcotic use by transcutaneous electrical nerve stimulation. Surgery 1980;87:142–6.
[87] Somers DL, Clemente FR. High-frequency transcutaneous electrical nerve stimulation alters thermal but not mechanical allodynia following chronic constriction injury of the rat sciatic nerve. Arch Phys Med Rehabil 1998;79:1370–6.
[88] Vance CG, Radhakrishnan R, Skyba DA, Sluka KA. Transcutaneous electrical nerve stimulation at both high and low frequencies reduces primary hyperalgesia in rats with joint inflammation in a time-dependent manner. Phys Ther 2007;87:44–51.
[89] Wall PD, Sweet WH. Temporary abolition of pain in man. Science 1967;155:108–9.
[90] Walsh DM. TENS: clinical applications and related theory. Edinburgh: Churchill Livingstone; 1997.
[91] Walsh DM, Scudds RA, Baxter GD, McDonough SM, Scudds RJ. Transcutaneous electrical nerve stimulation for the treatment of pain in physiotherapy practice. Abstract presented at: 12th World Congress on Pain, Glasgow, 2008.
[92] Wang B, Tang J, White PF, Naruse R, Sloninsky A, Kariger R, Gold J, Wender RH. Effect of the intensity of transcutaneous acupoint electrical stimulation on the postoperative analgesic requirement. Anesth Analg 1997;85:406–13.
[93] Warfield CA, Skein JM, Frank HA. The effect of transcutaneous electrical nerve stimulation on pain after thoracotomy. Ann Thorac Surg 1985;39:462–5.
[94] Woolf CJ, Barrett GD, Mitchell D, Myers RA. Naloxone-reversible peripheral electroanalgesia in intact and spinal rats. Eur J Pharmacol 1977;45:311–4.
[95] Woolf CJ, Mitchell D, Barrett GD. Antinociceptive effect of peripheral segmental electrical stimulation in the rat. Pain 1980;8:237–52.
[96] Zambito A, Bianchini D, Gatti D, Rossini M, Adami S, Viapiana O. Interferential and horizontal therapies in chronic low back pain due to multiple vertebral fractures: a randomized, double blind, clinical study. Osteoporos Int 2007;18:1541–9.
[97] Zambito A, Bianchini D, Gatti D, Viapiana O, Rossini M, Adami S. Interferential and horizontal therapies in chronic low back pain: a randomized, double blind, clinical study. Clin Exp Rheumatol 2006;24:534–9.
[98] Zizic TM, Hoffman KC, Holt PA, Hungerford DS, Odell JR, Jacobs MA, Lewis CG, Deal CL, Caldwell JR, Cholewcznski JG, et al. The treatment of osteoarthritis of the knee with pulsed electrical stimulation. J Rheumatol 1995;22:1757–61.

Correspondence to: Prof. Kathleen A. Sluka, PT, PhD, Graduate Program in Physical Therapy and Rehabilitation Science, The University of Iowa, 1-252 Medical Education Building, Iowa City, IA 52242-1190, USA. Tel: 1-319-335-9791; fax: 1-319-335-9707; email: kathleen-sluka@uiowa.edu.

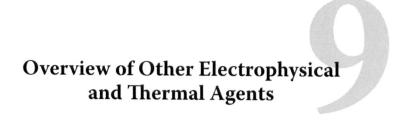

Overview of Other Electrophysical and Thermal Agents

G. David Baxter[a] and Jeffery R. Basford[b]

[a]School of Physiotherapy, University of Otago, Dunedin, New Zealand; [b]Department of Physical Medicine and Rehabilitation, Mayo Clinic, Rochester, Minnesota, USA

The roles of transcutaneous electrical nerve stimulation (TENS) and interferential therapy (IFT) were reviewed in Chapter 8. The focus of this chapter is on the analgesic capabilities of other commonly used electrophysical agents, whether they be purely thermal (e.g., hot and cold packs), sound-based (ultrasound), or electromagnetic (shortwave diathermy and low-intensity laser therapy). The chapter will focus on relevant mechanisms of action and current evidence of clinical effectiveness for each agent. A detailed examination of the principles of application for each of these modalities is beyond the scope of the current chapter; the reader is directed to some of the specialist texts that are available [2,4,46,69]. In particular, in using thermal modalities, a thorough understanding of the contraindications and precautions is essential, given the risk of burns or scalds; further details on these precautions are presented elsewhere [6].

Thermotherapy

The analgesic capabilities of the thermal agents (heat and cold) have been known since antiquity and are widely accepted. All rely on one of three processes: conduction (hot and cold packs), convection (whirlpool baths), and conversion of another form of energy to heat (ultrasound and short-wave diathermy). The latter are the only modalities capable of heating deeper structures and lesions. Although a wide variety of agents are available, this chapter will concentrate on hot packs, shortwave diathermy, ice therapy, and ultrasound, which represent the most popular forms of thermotherapy.

Hot Packs

Hot packs are a popular choice for the relief of pain because of their cost-effectiveness and ease of use [2]. Hot packs used in physical therapy are usually kept suspended in hot water baths at temperatures of up to 80°C and are drained and wrapped in toweling prior to application. Application time is typically up to 20 minutes, limited by patient tolerance and cooling of the pack. Packs for patient self-use are widely marketed and are typically designed to be heated in a microwave oven prior to use; alternative forms of conductive heating are also available, including electrical heating pads and hot water bottles.

Shortwave Diathermy

Shortwave diathermy machines are transmitters that produce electromagnetic radiation within the radiofrequency range (regulated to operate at a frequency of 27.12 MHz). Operation can be continuous (where the aim is to cause tissue heating) or pulsed, usually with the aim of producing non-thermal effects (also called *pulsed electromagnetic energy*). Treatments are based on tuning the circuit (comprising the patient and the machine) in a similar fashion to a radio set; tuning occurs automatically on contemporary units. Once tuning is completed, treatments usually last for up to 20–30 minutes, during which time patient feedback is used to monitor treatment. Contemporary units consist of a base unit, along with applicators that may comprise pairs of electrodes (for capacitive treatments) or pads or arm-mounted drums (for inductive applications). Rubber-coated cables as applicators (coiled over or around a body part), although once popular, are now rarely used due to concerns about an increased risk of overheating and prolonged setup time.

Tissue heating with continuous shortwave diathermy can be significant (6–15°C depending upon depth and type of tissue). Heat is produced by electrical "eddy" currents (when inductive application is used) or by electrical fields (capacitive application) within the tissue [23,49]. The inductive technique predominantly causes heating of muscle tissue (through the tissues' resistance to the current), while capacitive application produces more heat in structures such as ligaments, tendons, and joint capsules (through continuously reversing field polarity) [23,49]. This difference is an important consideration in targeting the treatment to a particular anatomical site of pain (e.g., tendinopathy versus myogenic pain).

Cold Therapy (Cryotherapy)

A variety of means are used to provide cold therapy or cryotherapy, including relatively simple ice packs (bags filled with crushed ice from an ice machine), ice massage, or packs of frozen peas, as well as the more sophisticated (and more expensive) gel-filled packs. Apart from ice massage, which is typically applied directly to the skin in paper or Styrofoam cups in which water has been frozen and the top peeled away to expose the ice, a wet towel is usually used as a barrier between the pack and the skin to prevent ice burn. In some cases, oil may also be lightly applied to the skin to reduce such risk.

A range of alternative cooling media are also available. Examples include vapocoolant sprays and chemical "break and apply" packs; however, for routine use these agents do not seem to offer any additional benefit over ice application, and some may indeed be less efficient in cooling treated tissues [15,45,59].

Although cryotherapy is by its nature a superficial thermal modality, its physiological and thus clinical effects can be significant and systemic. Cryotherapy produces a rapid vasoconstriction in superficial tissues (after 5 minutes of cooling), which becomes evident in deeper tissues (including periarticular structures, muscles, and bones) after 20 minutes of application [1,42,59]. While treatments may last for up to 20–25 minutes, when ice is applied directly over the site of pain, cryotherapy can produce localized analgesia within a much shorter period (reported by the patient as "numbness" after 10 minutes or less). Apart from significant changes in skin temperature during treatment (up to 20°C in some cases), temperature changes in deeper structures can also be profound. For example, ice treatment in osteoarthritic knee joints was found to reduce intraarticular temperatures by 6°C [45,59].

Mechanisms of Pain Relief with Thermal Modalities

Thermal therapies achieve their clinical effects by changing tissue temperature, which in turn produces alterations in cellular and physiological function. Both heat and cold packs increase pain thresholds in healthy controls [53,61]. The effects of thermal modalities for pain reduction are aimed at reducing activation of nociceptors in the periphery. Thus, these modalities are used to treat peripheral sites of injury. Although changes in temperature produced during treatment may in some circumstances be relatively modest (around 5°C or less), the effects upon cellular and physiological functions such as nerve conduction or blood flow can be significant. In addition to causing local changes in blood flow, thermal modalities can alter blood flow in distal parts of the body [1,20,47,48]. Altered nerve conduction and changes in blood flow are considered to be particularly important in terms of the pain-relieving effects of heat and cold [1,47,48]. Changes in blood flow may improve tissue healing, remove inflammatory irritants, and consequently decrease the activity of nociceptive afferents to ultimately alleviate pain. Ice clearly decreases the conduction velocity of primary afferent fibers and simultaneously increases pain threshold and pain tolerance [1]. In fact, if the temperature of the primary afferent fibers is lowered to 4°C, conduction of afferent fibers is stopped, which would prevent afferent input from reaching the spinal cord. Decreasing the conduction velocity of afferent fibers thus would produce analgesia by decreasing the firing of afferent fibers and consequently reducing input to the central nervous system.

Heat has been long employed by physical therapists to help mobilize tissues and joints by increasing tissue extensibility and reducing muscle spasm. Heat would be expected to remove mechanical irritants from nociceptors and decrease input to the central nervous system. Heat-induced alterations in muscle spindle activity and in firing of Golgi tendon organs are thought to be responsible for the observed reductions in muscle tone [56]. Group II spindle afferent fibers show reduced activity after heating, whereas Group I spindle afferent fibers show increased activity. As Group II spindle afferents monitor muscle length, decreased activity should result in decreased activity of the alpha-motor neuron to decrease muscle spasm. A concomitant increase in Golgi tendon organ firing would also decrease alpha-motor neuron firing through an interneuron circuit in the spinal cord. Joint stiffness as a feature of inflammatory arthritis (and some other forms of arthritic pain and joint irritability) can be reduced with heating [73]. While cooling can have similar effects to heating in terms of reducing muscle tone or spasticity [1,35,57], it can also increase stiffness, at least in the small joints of the hand [43,73].

Effectiveness of Heat and Cold Therapy

The evidence base to support the use of thermal modalities in the alleviation of pain is limited by the quality of a number of relatively dated investigations. Most of the studies to date have been completed on musculoskeletal pain, including low back and arthritic pain; recent Cochrane reviews in these areas have indicated potential benefits of superficial heat and cold [13,16,30,63]. In the management of rheumatoid arthritis, no differences were found between the effectiveness of (or patient preference for) most types of thermotherapy; superficial heat and cryotherapy were recommended for use as palliative therapy, and wax or paraffin baths with exercises for short-term effects for arthritic hands [63]. In osteoarthritis, ice packs may provide benefits in terms of swelling and range of movement but appear ineffective in terms of pain [13]. For low back pain, a recent review of the effectiveness of superficial heat found moderate evidence of short-term reductions in pain in cases of acute or subacute low back pain; there was insufficient evidence to assess the effectiveness of cryotherapy [30].

Ice has long been recognized—by clinicians and the public alike—as an important component of the RICE management of musculoskeletal injuries in the acute stage (rest, ice, compression, and elevation). However, a review of the evidence on the effectiveness of ice and compression in acute soft-tissue injuries found only limited evidence to support effectiveness or to recommend any particular regimen of treatment [11]. A recent review of superficial cooling for postpartum perineal pain found limited evidence for reduction in pain in the short term following local cooling treatments (i.e., ice packs, cold gel pads, or cold/iced baths) [28].

Despite an extensive history of clinical use of shortwave diathermy for alleviation of musculoskeletal pain, the evidence base for such use is limited and contradictory. One recent controlled trial of continuous shortwave diathermy in knee osteoarthritis found significant reductions in pain [44], whereas another reported no additional benefit for back pain (however, this study used pulsed treatment) [27].

Ultrasound

Ultrasound has been used for treatment of pain for decades [2]. Contemporary machines combine a base or controller unit, which allows the operator to select treatment parameters (typically treatment time, continuous wave or pulsed operation, and intensity), with treatment applicators operating at fixed pulsing frequencies. Increasingly sophisticated units have become more popular in recent years, providing basic clinical decision-making support and parameter selection systems. Patient treatment involves moving the ultrasound applicator over the painful area or lesion, using a circular or back-and-forth motion, with a water-based gel applied as a coupling medium. For areas that are more difficult to treat (such as the small joints of the hands), the applicator and the limb to be treated may both be immersed in a water bath filled with degassed water. Treatment times are typically 5–10 minutes.

Ultrasound is a form of mechanical energy, comprising alternating compressions and rarefactions of the medium, at frequencies above the human audible range (which is approximately 20 kHz). Typical ultrasound frequencies range from 0.8 to 3 MHz. Ultrasound shares common physical properties with sound energy. Depending upon the parameters used, ultrasound may produce thermal or nonthermal effects; higher power intensities and continuous wave operation are more commonly used in North America (compared to the United Kingdom) to provide thermal effects, including increased blood flow and soft-tissue extensibility, as well as for pain relief, possibly linked to reported effects on peripheral nerve function [19]. A variety of other effects predominate at nonthermal intensities (typically <0.5 W/cm^2) and using pulsed mode, including cavitation, acoustic streaming, and deformation of the insonated tissue. The primary goal of treatment at nonthermal intensities is promotion of tissue repair, through enhanced cellular function and other metabolic processes [24,25,26,58].

While intensity (specified in watts per square centimeter) is important in determining the amount of heating produced, the frequency of the ultrasound determines its depth of penetration and is thus an important parameter in targeting treatment to particular anatomical structures. Higher frequencies (e.g., 3.0 MHz) are used to treat more superficial tissues (up to 2 cm deep, such as the superficial paraspinal musculature), while lower frequencies (<1.0 MHz) are employed for more deeply seated structures or lesions [34]. Tissue type and orientation also determine penetration, with ultrasound penetrating fat and muscle more readily than bone [33,50,51].

Temperature changes resulting from ultrasound treatment can be significant (5–10°C) and may be most pronounced at interfaces between tissues with different transmission characteristics (e.g., bone and muscle) [50,52]. Thus, although the depth and uneven aspects of ultrasound heating are a concern, the safety concerns related to ultrasound are primarily those associated with other forms of heating. However, even at nonthermal intensities, mechanical effects of ultrasound (e.g., cavitation) can be potentially damaging, and thus treatment over sensitive structures such as the eyes must be avoided as well as treatment over the pregnant uterus, heart, brain, and cervical ganglia. Caution should also be used with treatment of the back, and high intensities should not be used over the spine. Direct treatment over laminectomy or surgical sites with metal implants has long been recognized as a prudent contraindication [32]. While ultrasound has found popular application in the treatment of arthritic pain, as with other forms of heating, its use at thermal intensities should be avoided in younger people with immature growth plates as well as in acute exacerbations of inflammatory disease or over inflamed joints, because it may exacerbate the inflammatory process [52,72].

Effectiveness of Ultrasound

Despite long-standing and widespread use in musculoskeletal physical therapy, research findings to support the use of ultrasound for the treatment of pain are limited and inconclusive [14,18,41,63]. In particular, the Philadelphia Panel's evidence-based guidelines for musculoskeletal rehabilitation reported that although there was evidence of benefit in ultrasound for some shoulder disorders (calcific tendonitis) [29], there was no convincing evidence of benefit in the treatment of musculoskeletal pain of other etiologies [41]. Review of current research findings for different interventions in the treatment of heel pain found no convincing evidence of benefit of therapeutic ultrasound [18]. A randomized controlled trial in lateral epicondylalgia found that continuous wave ultrasound offered better pain relief than rest, but was no more effective than sham treatment [54]; a subsequent study using pulsed ultrasound reported similar results [40]. Recent work, as part of two small-scale controlled studies on myofascial trigger points, found low-intensity ultrasound to be effective in desensitizing trapezius and infraspinatus trigger points [65,66].

A Cochrane review of thermal therapies found no significant clinical benefit of therapeutic ultrasound in the treatment of rheumatoid arthritis [63]. However, a more focused review of ultrasound treatment reported a range of benefits (including reduced early-morning stiffness and increased range of motion) in the treatment of rheumatoid hands [14], and these findings are supported by the recommendations of the Ottawa Panel on electrophysical agents for treatment of rheumatoid arthritis [60]. A recent review has highlighted a range of potential benefits in osteoarthritis, including pain relief [64].

Neurogenic pain, particularly postherpetic neuralgia, has been treated with therapeutic ultrasound, apparently with some success [31,68]; however, published studies are rather dated, poorly controlled, and contradictory.

Low-Intensity Laser Therapy

Since initial reports first appeared in the late 1960s and early 1970s, low-power laser devices have found a range of treatment applications in physical therapy, primarily to accelerate tissue healing in conditions ranging from chronic ulcers to soft-tissue injuries [4]. Such devices have also been used in the management of pain of various etiologies, although such use, as is true of use in wound healing, remains contentious [21]. Since the 1980s, most devices used in physiotherapy have been diode-based systems (rather than the former helium-neon gas-based systems), comprising either single (laser/diode) source treatment applicators, or—increasingly—multidiode arrays comprising up to several hundred diodes (including both laser and superluminous monochromatic diodes) [4]. Device outputs can vary from less than 10 mW to several hundred milliwatts; recent times have seen higher outputs as the norm (>30 mW). Most systems produce radiation at single wavelengths between the visible red to near-infrared part of the spectrum (around 630–904 nm), although for pain relief and musculoskeletal (i.e., non-wound-healing) applications, use of infrared wavelengths is the norm. Dosages used for treatment of musculoskeletal pain have been variable. Suggested irradiation parameters for a range of tendinopathies and arthritic conditions are available from the World Association for Laser Therapy (www.walt.nu). Treatments usually consist of the treatment of localized areas of tenderness and pain in a grid or sweeping pattern, as well as the irradiation of acupuncture or trigger points.

Mechanisms of Laser Therapy

The mechanisms underpinning the observed pain-relieving effects of laser therapy are unclear. Studies of direct neurophysiological effects of laser irradiation at various parameters have reported variable results in terms of nerve conduction latencies and action potentials [3,7,39]. In contrast, investigations in animal models of pain have typically reported significant antinociceptive effects of laser irradiation, which are dependent upon the dosage [71] and the pulse repetition rate used [62]. Such effects are apparently based on a variety of neuropharmacological mechanisms, which may [70], or may not [62], be opioid mediated.

Unlike the modalities considered above, laser therapy is essentially athermic (nonheating), and thus the safety considerations are less onerous. In particular, laser therapy can be used in many cases to treat acute pain or injury without the risk of exacerbating the inflammatory process. Other safety considerations and contraindications are a minor risk to the unprotected eye and avoidance in cases of active or suspected carcinoma [6].

Effectiveness of Laser Therapy

The effectiveness of laser therapy for alleviation of pain has been a matter of ongoing debate, in part because of dispute over the putative mechanism of action [5,21]. Systematic reviews of clinical effectiveness have found laser therapy to provide clinically significant benefits in chronic joint pain [8], in osteoarthritis of the knee [9], and for short-term alleviation of pain and morning stiffness in rheumatoid arthritis [12]. Additionally, a review of physical therapies for temporomandibular joint pain found that laser therapy was effective, and more effective than other electrophysical agents [55]. In other conditions, the evidence is less clear: contradictory findings have been reported in two reviews in mechanical neck pain (although the later, more focused review found evidence of some benefit with infrared wavelengths) [17,37]. For shoulder pain, adhesive capsulitis is the only condition for which laser therapy has shown benefit [36]. While previous reviews have reported no convincing evidence of benefit of laser therapy in lateral epicondylitis [10], a more recent review and meta-analysis found short-term pain relief with laser treatment at some wavelengths (principally 904 nm) [67]. The most recent review of laser therapy in treatment of low back pain reported that there was insufficient evidence to draw any conclusions on potential benefits [74].

Clinical trials in other conditions have reported potential benefits of laser therapy in the treatment of fibromyalgia [38] and as an adjunctive treatment when combined with exercise in the management of chronic low back pain [22].

In the United States, since the relaxation of registration requirements, the Food and Drug Administration has approved more than 25 different laser therapy devices for the treatment of pain since 2002 [2].

Summary

The electrophysical agents described in this chapter, in addition to the use of TENS and IFT as discussed in Chapter 8, are important options in the clinical treatment of pain. Nevertheless, a number of caveats are in order. First, the evidence base for their effectiveness, particularly for anything more than short-term pain relief, is discouragingly limited (see Table I). Second, with the exception of the tissue-penetrating capabilities of agents such as ultrasound and the diathermies, there is little evidence that the newer modalities are any more effective than the old standbys of heat and cold. Third, as emphasized in Chapter 6, electrophysical agents are almost always most beneficial as adjuncts to a program focused on exercise, strengthening, mobilization, and education. And, fourth, treatment choice depends on the etiology of the pain, treatment goals, pain

Table I
Evidence for heat, cold, ultrasound, and laser therapy

Disease/Pain Condition	Ref.	Type of Review	No. Studies	Results
Low back pain	[16]	American Pain Society guidelines	Based on systematic reviews	Superficial heat effective for acute low back pain
Low back pain	[30]	Systematic review	9	Heat wrap therapy (superficial heat) effective for acute and subacute low back pain; insufficient evidence to evaluate cold therapy
Rheumatoid arthritis	[63]	Cochrane review	7	No effect of superficial heat or cold; can be used as palliative care
Rheumatoid arthritis	[14]	Cochrane review	2	Ultrasound applied to the hand improved grip strength, range of motion, number of swollen joints, number of painful joints; no difference between ultrasound with exercises compared with paraffin baths and exercises
Rheumatoid arthritis	[60]	Ottawa Panel guidelines	5 laser, 1 ultrasound, 2 thermal	Recommends low-level laser therapy, ultrasound, and thermotherapy
Osteoarthritis	[13]	Cochrane review	3	Cold therapy improved range of motion, function, and knee strength and reduced edema, but had no effect on pain; superficial heat had no effect on edema
Acute soft tissue injury	[11]	Systematic review	22	Ice plus exercise is effective
Plantar heel pain	[18]	Cochrane review	1 laser, 1 ultrasound	No evidence for ultrasound or laser therapy for chronic heel pain
Musculoskeletal pain	[41]	Philadelphia Panel guidelines	Unclear	Recommends ultrasound for calcific tendonitis of the shoulder

duration (e.g., ice for acute musculoskeletal injury), the area to be covered (ultrasound for limited areas, hot packs for wider areas), pain intensity (ice massage versus cool packs), and the depth of the painful tissue (ultrasound versus hot packs).

References

[1] Algafly AA, George KP. The effect of cryotherapy on nerve conduction velocity, pain threshold and pain tolerance. Br J Sports Med 2007;41:365–9.

[2] Basford JR, Baxter GD. Therapeutic physical agents. In: Physical medicine and rehabilitation: principles and practice, 5th ed. Philadelphia: Lippincott Williams & Wilkins; 2009. In press.

[3] Basford J, Daube J, Hallman H, Millard T, Moyer S. Does low-intensity helium-neon laser irradiation alter sensory nerve active potentials or distal latencies. Lasers Surg Med 1990;10:35–9.

[4] Baxter GD. Therapeutic lasers: theory and practice. Edinburgh: Churchill Livingstone; 1994. p. 259.

[5] Baxter GD, Basford JR. Laser therapy: state of the art? Focus Alternative Complement Ther 2008;13:11–13.

[6] Baxter GD, Bazin S, Diffy B, et al. Guidance for the clinical use of electrophysical agents. London: Chartered Society of Physiotherapy; 2006.

[7] Baxter GD, Walsh DM, Allen JM, Lowe AS, Bell AJ. Effects of low intensity infrared laser irradiation upon conduction in the human median nerve in vivo. Exp Physiol 1994;79:227–34.

[8] Bjordal JM, Couppe C, Chow RT, Tuner J, Ljunggren EA. A systematic review of low level laser therapy with location-specific doses for pain from chronic joint disorders. Aust J Physiother 2003;49:107–16.

[9] Bjordal JM, Johnson MI, Lopes-Martins RA, Bogen B, Chow R, Ljunggren AE. Short-term efficacy of physical interventions in osteoarthritic knee pain. A systematic review and meta-analysis of randomised placebo-controlled trials. BMC Musculoskelet Disord 2007;8:51.

[10] Bjordal JM, Lopes-Martins RA, Joensen J, et al. A systematic review with procedural assessments and meta-analysis of low level laser therapy in lateral elbow tendinopathy (tennis elbow). BMC Musculoskelet Disord 2008;9:75.

[11] Bleakley C, McDonough S, MacAuley D. The use of ice in the treatment of acute soft-tissue injury: a systematic review of randomized controlled trials. Am J Sports Med 2004;32:251–61.

[12] Brosseau L, Wells G, Marchand S et al. Randomized controlled trial on low level laser therapy (LLLT) in the treatment of osteoarthritis (OA) of the hand. Lasers Surg Med 2005;36:210–9.

[13] Brosseau L, Yonge KA, Robinson V, Marchand S, Judd M, Wells G, Tugwell P. Thermotherapy for treatment of osteoarthritis. Cochrane Database Syst Rev 2003;CD004522.

[14] Casimiro L, Brosseau L, Robinson V, Milne S, Judd M, Wells G, Tugwell P, Shea B. Therapeutic ultrasound for the treatment of rheumatoid arthritis. Cochrane Database Syst Rev 2002;CD003787.

[15] Chesterton LS, Foster NE, Ross L. Skin temperature response to cryotherapy. Arch Phys Med Rehabil 2002; 83:543–9.

[16] Chou R, Huffman LH. Nonpharmacologic therapies for acute and chronic low back pain: a review of the evidence for an American Pain Society/American College of Physicians clinical practice guideline. Ann Intern Med 2007;147:492–504.

[17] Chow RT, Barnsley L. Systematic review of the literature of low-level laser therapy (LLLT) in the management of neck pain. Lasers Surg Med 2005;37:46–52.

[18] Crawford F, Thomson C. Interventions for treating plantar heel pain. Cochrane Database Syst Rev 2003;CD000416.

[19] Currier DP, Greathouse D, Swift T. Sensory nerve conduction: effect of ultrasound. Arch Phys Med Rehabil 1978;59:181–5.

[20] Denys EH. AAEM minimonograph #14: The influence of temperature in clinical neurophysiology. Muscle Nerve 1991;14:795–811.

[21] Devor M. What's in a laser beam for pain therapy? Pain 1990;43:139.

[22] Djavid GE, Mehrdad R, Ghasemi M, Hasan-Zadeh H, Sotoodeh-Manesh A, Pouryaghoub G. In chronic low back pain, low level laser therapy combined with exercise is more beneficial than exercise alone in the long term: a randomised trial. Aust J Physiother 2007;53:155–60.

[23] Draper DO, Knight K, Fujiwara T, Castel JC. Temperature change in human muscle during and after pulsed short-wave diathermy. J Orthop Sports Phys Ther 1999;29:13–8.

[24] Dyson M. Non-thermal cellular effects of ultrasound. Br J Cancer Suppl 1982;5:165–71.

[25] Dyson M, Brookes M. Stimulation of bone repair by ultrasound. Ultrasound Med Biol 1983;61–6.

[26] Dyson M, Suckling J. Stimulation of tissue repair by ultrasound: a survey of the mechanisms involved. Physiotherapy 1978;64:105–8.

[27] Dziedzic K, Hill J, Lewis M, Sim J, Daniels J, Hay EM. Effectiveness of manual therapy or pulsed shortwave diathermy in addition to advice and exercise for neck disorders: a pragmatic randomized controlled trial in physical therapy clinics. Arthritis Rheum 2005;53:214–22.

[28] East CE, Begg L, Henshall NE, Marchant P, Wallace K. Local cooling for relieving pain from perineal trauma sustained during childbirth. Cochrane Database Syst Rev 2007;CD006304.

[29] Ebenbichler GR, Erdogmus CB, Resch KL, Funovics MA, Kainberger F, Barisani G, Aringer M, Nicolakis P, Wiesinger GF, Baghestanian M, et al. Ultrasound therapy for calcific tendinitis of the shoulder. N Engl J Med 1999;340:1533–8.

[30] French SD, Cameron M, Walker BF, Reggars JW, Esterman AJ. A Cochrane review of superficial heat or cold for low back pain. Spine 2006;31:998–1006.

[31] Garrett AS, Garrett M. Ultrasound therapy for herpes zoster pain. J R Coll Gen Pract 1982;32:709, 711.

[32] Gersten JW. Effect of metallic objects on temperature rises produced in tissue by ultrasound. Am J Phys Med 1958;37:75–82.

[33] Gersten JW. Relation of ultrasound effects to the orientation of tendon in the ultrasound field. Arch Phys Med Rehabil 1956;37:201–9.

[34] Gersten JW. Temperature rise of various tissues in the dog on exposure to ultrasound at different frequencies. Arch Phys Med Rehabil 1959;40:187–92.

[35] Gracies JM. Physical modalities other than stretch in spastic hypertonia. Phys Med Rehabil Clin N Am 2001;12:769–92.

[36] Green S, Buchbinder R, Hetrick S. Physiotherapy interventions for shoulder pain. Cochrane Database Syst Rev 2003;CD004258.

[37] Gross AR, Goldsmith C, Hoving JL, Haines T, Peloso P, Aker P, Santaguida P, Myers C. Conservative management of mechanical neck disorders: a systematic review. J Rheumatol 2007;34:1083–102.

[38] Gur A. Physical therapy modalities in management of fibromyalgia. Curr Pharm Des 2006;12:29–35.

[39] Hadian M, Moghagdam B. The effects of low power laser on electrophysiological parameters of sural nerve in normal subjects: a comparison between 670 and 780 nm wavelengths. Acta Med Iranica 2003;41:138–42.

[40] Haker E, Lundeberg T. Pulsed ultrasound treatment in lateral epicondylalgia. Scand J Rehabil Med 1991;23:115–8.

[41] Harris GR, Susman JL. Managing musculoskeletal complaints with rehabilitation therapy: summary of the Philadelphia Panel evidence-based clinical practice guidelines on musculoskeletal rehabilitation interventions. J Fam Pract 2002;51:1042–6.

[42] Ho SS, Illgen RL, Meyer RW, Torok PJ, Cooper MD, Reider B. Comparison of various icing times in decreasing bone metabolism and blood flow in the knee. Am J Sports Med 1995;23:74–6.

[43] Hunter J, Kerr EH, Whillans MG. The relation between joint stiffness upon exposure to cold and the characteristics of synovial fluid. Can J Med Sci 1952;30:367–77.

[44] Jan MH, Chai HM, Wang CL, Lin YF, Tsai LY. Effects of repetitive shortwave diathermy for reducing synovitis in patients with knee osteoarthritis: an ultrasonographic study. Phys Ther 2006;86:236–44.

[45] Kanlayanaphotporn R, Janwantanakul P. Comparison of skin surface temperature during the application of various cryotherapy modalities. Arch Phys Med Rehabil 2005;86:1411–5.

[46] Lehmann JF. Therapeutic heat and cold, 4th ed. Baltimore: Williams & Wilkins; 1990. p. 725.

[47] Lehmann JF, DeLateur BJ. Therapeutic heat. In: Lehmann JF, editor. Therapeutic heat and cold, 4th ed. Baltimore: Williams & Wilkins; 1990. p. 417–581.

[48] Lehmann JF, DeLateur BJ. Cryotherapy. In: Lehmann JF, editor. Therapeutic heat and cold, 4th ed. Baltimore: Williams & Wilkins; 1990. p. 590–632.

[49] Lehmann JF, DeLateur BJ, Stonebridge JB. Selective muscle heating by shortwave diathermy with a helical coil. Arch Phys Med Rehabil 1969;50:117–23.

[50] Lehmann JF, DeLateur BJ, Stonebridge JB, Warren CG. Therapeutic temperature distribution produced by ultrasound as modified by dosage and volume of tissue exposed. Arch Phys Med Rehabil 1967;48:662–6.

[51] Lehmann JF, DeLateur BJ, Warren CG, Stonebridge JS. Heating produced by ultrasound in bone and soft tissue. Arch Phys Med Rehabil 1967;48:397–401.

[52] Lehmann JF, DeLateur BJ, Warren CG, Stonebridge JB. Heating of joint structures by ultrasound. Arch Phys Med Rehabil 1968;49:28–30.

[53] Lerman Y, Jacubovich R, Green MS. Pregnancy outcome following exposure to shortwaves among female physiotherapists in Israel. Am J Ind Med 2001;39:499–504.

[54] Lundeberg T, Abrahamsson P, Haker E. A comparative study of continuous ultrasound, placebo ultrasound and rest in epicondylalgia. Scand J Rehabil Med 1988;20:99–101.

[55] Medlicott MS, Harris SR. A systematic review of the effectiveness of exercise, manual therapy, electrotherapy, relaxation training, and biofeedback in the management of temporomandibular disorder. Phys Ther 2006;86:955–73.

[56] Mense S. Effects of temperature on the discharges of muscle spindles and tendon organs. Pflugers Arch 1978;374:159–66.

[57] Miglietta O. Action of cold on spasticity. Am J Phys Med 1973;52:198–205.

[58] Nyborg WL. Biological effects of ultrasound: development of safety guidelines. Part II: general review. Ultrasound Med Biol 2001;27:301–33.

[59] Oosterveld FG, Rasker JJ, Jacobs JW, Overmars HJ. The effect of local heat and cold therapy on the intraarticular and skin surface temperature of the knee. Arthritis Rheum 1992;35:146–51.

[60] Ottawa Panel. Evidence-based clinical practice guidelines for electrotherapy and thermotherapy interventions in the management of rheumatoid arthritis in adults. Phys Ther 2004;84:1016–43.

[61] Ouellet-Hellstrom R, Stewart WF. Miscarriages among female physical therapists who report using radio- and microwave-frequency electromagnetic radiation. Am J Epidemiol 1993;138:775–86.

[62] Ponnudurai RN, Zbuzek VK, Wu W. Hypoalgesic effect of laser photobiostimulation shown by rat tail flick test. Int J Acupuncture Electrother Res 1987;12:93–100.

[63] Robinson V, Brosseau L, Casimiro L, Judd M, Shea B, Wells G, Tugwell P. Thermotherapy for treating rheumatoid arthritis. Cochrane Database Syst Rev 2002;CD002826.

[64] Srbely JZ. Ultrasound in the management of osteoarthritis: part I: a review of the current literature. JCCA J Can Chiropr Assoc 2008;52:30–7.

[65] Srbely JZ, Dickey JP. Randomized controlled study of the antinociceptive effect of ultrasound on trigger point sensitivity: novel applications in myofascial therapy? Clin Rehabil 2007;21:411–7.

[66] Srbely JZ, Dickey JP, Lowerison M, Edwards AM, Nolet PS, Wong LL. Stimulation of myofascial trigger points with ultrasound induces segmental antinociceptive effects: a randomized controlled study. Pain 2008;139:260–6.

[67] Trudel D, Duley J, Zastrow I, Kerr EW, Davidson R, MacDermid JC. Rehabilitation for patients with lateral epicondylitis: a systematic review. J Hand Ther 2004;17:243–66.

[68] Walker E. Ultrasound therapy for herpes zoster pain. J R Coll Gen Pract 1984;34:627–8.

[69] Watson T, editor. Electrotherapy: evidence-based practice, 12th ed. Edinburgh: Elsevier; 2008. p. 400.

[70] Wedlock PM, Shephard RA. Cranial irradiation with GaA1As laser leads to naloxone reversible analgesia in rats. Psychol Rep 1996;78:727–31.

[71] Wedlock P, Shephard RA, Little C, McBurney F. Analgesic effects of cranial laser treatment in two rat nociception models. Physiol Behav 1996;59:445–8.

[72] Weinberger A, Fadilah R, Lev A, Levi A, Pinkhas J. Deep heat in the treatment of inflammatory joint disease. Med Hypotheses 1988;25:231–3.

[73] Wright V, Johns RJ. Quantitative and qualitative analysis of joint stiffness in normal subjects and in patients with connective tissue diseases. Ann Rheum Dis 1961;20:36–46.

[74] Yousefi-Nooraie R, Schonstein E, Heidari K, Rashidian A, Pennick V, Akbari-Kamrani M, Irani S, Shakiba B, Mortaz Hejri SA, Mortaz Hejri SO, Jonaidi A. Low level laser therapy for nonspecific low-back pain. Cochrane Database Syst Rev 2008;CD005107.

Correspondence to: Prof. David Baxter, TD, PT, MBA, DPhil, School of Physiotherapy, University of Otago, P.O. Box 56, Dunedin 9054, New Zealand. Tel: 011-643479-7411, fax: 011-643479-7184; email: david.baxter@otago.ac.nz.

Manual Therapy

Kathleen A. Sluka[a] and Stephan Milosavljevic[b]

[a]Graduate Program in Physical Therapy and Rehabilitation Science, The University of Iowa, Iowa City, Iowa, USA; [b]Centre for Physiotherapy Research, School of Physiotherapy, University of Otago, Dunedin, New Zealand

Manual Therapy Techniques

Depending on the nature of the presenting clinical disorder, contemporary manual therapists will use the detailed information derived from subjective and physical examinations to plan and offer various clinical interventions. Manual therapy techniques may include traditional massage, soft-tissue mobilization, joint mobilizations and manipulations, nerve or "neural" mobilization procedures, joint stabilization exercises, and self-mobilization exercises. Importantly, treatment should include advising patients on appropriate self-management strategies as well as devising strategies for reducing the risk of injury recurrence.

Traditional massage includes techniques such as effleurage and petrissage that are delivered to the body part affected. Massage is typically applied to relieve muscle and soft-tissue tightness and to reduce pain. Soft-tissue mobilization techniques involve sustained stretching of the muscle or connective tissue and are similarly used to reduce soft-tissue tightness and pain. These techniques include trigger point therapy, myofascial therapy, and deep-tissue massage. Neural mobilization uses techniques designed to restore the ability of the nerve and surrounding structures to shift in relation to the surrounding structures, either by putting the nerve and its surrounding tissue in a stretched position, or by using mobilization techniques designed to facilitate movement at this interface. Joint mobilizations are performed either by holding sustained positions or by applying oscillatory repetitive movements within the normal physiological range. Mobilizations have been graded from I to IV, with grade I described as an oscillation at the beginning of the range, II within the mid-range, III up to the end of the range, and IV within the end of the range for the joint. Manipulations are generally high-velocity, low-amplitude movements of a joint, sometimes termed type V manipulation/mobilization. This chapter will explain the basic science mechanisms underlying these types of treatments and review the clinical evidence to support their use for common pain conditions.

Basic Science Mechanisms

Massage

The literature on basic science mechanisms underlying the effects of massage includes evidence aimed at deciphering central pathways activated by massage. In addition, several theories are used to support the use of massage. In an animal model used to investigate the mechanisms of massage, 10 minutes of massage to the abdomen increased pain thresholds, and cumulative effects on pain thresholds occurred with daily treatments [21]. In this model, the neuropeptide oxytocin increased in the plasma and in the periaqueductal gray (PAG) in the midbrain in response to the massage treatment when compared to a control treatment [21]. Conversely, blockade of oxytocin receptors, either systemically or in the PAG, will reduce the analgesic effect of massage [1]. Studies in human subjects also show that massage decreases pain intensity and simultaneously decreases cortisol in the blood in patients with juvenile rheumatoid arthritis [13] or burn injury [20]. An increase in plasma serotonin has also been observed in response to massage in people with either burn injury or migraine [12]. Thus, massage may activate descending inhibitory pathways that include the PAG, using oxytocin and possibly serotonergic systems to produce analgesia.

Theoretically, massage could also produce its pain-relieving effects indirectly by helping to restore normal movement patterns, reduce muscle spasms, and improve healing by increasing blood flow to the area. These effects would be likely to reduce mechanical or chemical irritants that activate nociceptors and thus lessen input to the central nervous system and consequently diminish pain.

Joint Mobilization and Manipulation

Joint manipulation and mobilization produce effects both peripherally and centrally. Peripherally, high-thrust manipulations and mobilizations increase pain thresholds and decrease motor neuron excitability, as measured by the H-reflex, in human subjects [3,5,7,16]. This reduction in motor neuron excitability lasts only approximately 10–20 seconds in healthy controls. However, in people with low back pain, spinal manipulation increases the activity of the oblique abdominal muscle for several minutes, but has no effect in normal healthy controls [10], suggesting longer-term and greater effects on motor neuron excitability in people with chronic pain. In an animal model, at the time of a lumbar spinal thrust there is a reduction in the activity of muscle spindle afferent fibers that lasts for several seconds [29]. This reduction in muscle spindle activity is accompanied by a decrease in electromyographic activity in the paraspinal muscles that lasts for at least the duration of the recording period, approximately 6 minutes [25]. Sympathetic excitation also increases in response to mobilization of the cervical spine, as measured by an increase in heart rate, respiratory rate, and blood pressure and changes in skin conductance in human subjects [30], suggesting widespread activation of the autonomic nervous system. Thus, peripherally, spinal manipulation can decrease muscle spindle activity, reduce motor neuron excitability, and reduce electromyographic activity of the paraspinal muscles and would therefore be expected to decrease spasm of the paraspinal musculature. Decreasing muscle spasm would be expected to decrease muscle ischemia and thus reduce nociceptor sensitization and lessen central input to the spinal dorsal horn.

In healthy controls, there is a decrease in temporal summation—a measure of central nervous system excitability—following spinal manipulation, suggesting that central mechanisms may play a role [3,16]. Further support for central mechanisms, in both human and animal studies, comes from the observation that application of joint mobilization to an uninjured joint reduces pain and hyperalgesia in an injured joint. For example, in people with lateral epicondylalgia, joint mobilization of the cervical spine (grade III lateral glide of C5/6) increases pressure pain thresholds, pain-free range of motion on the upper-limb tension test, and pain-free grip force [31]. Similarly, in animal models of inflammatory pain, grade III mobilizations of the knee joint reduce the hyperalgesia associated with inflammation of the knee or the ankle [22,27,28]. In people with knee osteoarthritis, application of joint mobilization to the knee increases pressure pain thresholds at the knee (primary hyperalgesia) and the heel (secondary hyperalgesia), suggesting that central mechanisms, in addition to peripheral mechanisms, play a role in pain reduction [22].

Pharmacological studies in humans and animals have begun to decipher potential mechanisms in the central nervous system underlying the analgesia produced by joint manipulation. The analgesia produced by joint manipulation and mobilization is not reversed by the opioid antagonist naloxone, either in human subjects [24,32,33] or in an animal model of mobilization-induced analgesia [27]. The analgesia produced using grade III mobilization of the knee joint, in an animal model of ankle inflammation, is prevented by spinal blockade of serotonin $5-HT_{1A}$ and α_2-noradrenergic receptors [27]. However, blockade of γ-aminobutyric acid (GABA) or opioid receptors spinally has no effect on the analgesia produced by mobilization [27]. These data suggest that joint mobilizations reduce pain through effects in the central nervous system by activating non-opioidergic descending inhibitory pathways from the rostral ventromedial medulla and dorsolateral pontine tegmentum.

It could be hypothesized that joint mobilizations and manipulations, similar to massage, also produce their effects by improving normal joint range of motion and helping to restore normal movement and muscle recruitment patterns. These effects would reduce mechanical irritation to peripheral nociceptors, reducing input to the central nervous system and thus lessening pain.

Table I
Evidence for manual therapy

Disease/Pain Condition	Ref.	Type of Study	No. Studies	Results
Low back pain	[15]	Cochrane review	13	Effective for subacute and chronic low back pain when combined with exercise and education; acupuncture massage more effective than traditional massage; similar to exercise, superior to joint mobilization and self-care
Mechanical neck disorders	[19]	Cochrane review	19	Inconclusive effects for massage therapy
Mechanical neck disorders	[18]	Cochrane review	33	Manipulation or mobilization with exercise more effective than no treatment
Tension-type headache	[9]	Systematic review	6	Ineffective for spinal manipulation; limited evidence for soft-tissue massage
Low back pain	[2]	Cochrane review	39	Spinal mobilization/manipulation effective when compared to sham therapy but not other therapies
Low back pain	[6]	American Pain Society guidelines	Primary source was published systematic reviews	Spinal mobilization/manipulation effective for acute and chronic low back pain
Lateral epicondylalgia	[4]	Systematic review	3	Cervical mobilization reduced pain and increased pressure pain thresholds; wrist mobilization similar to other treatments
Musculoskeletal pain	[8]	Systematic review	11	Limited evidence that neural mobilization reduces pain

Clinical Evidence

Several systematic reviews have examined the use of manipulation and mobilization for the neck and back (Table I). These reviews generally used the same literature base to produce their conclusions. This chapter presents evidence from Cochrane systematic reviews as the primary source for effectiveness, supplemented by subsequent systematic reviews that have highlighted the effectiveness of mobilization and manipulation. For the use of massage and peripheral mobilizations, the literature is minimal, and we have included randomized controlled trials (RCTs) to highlight their effectiveness. One difficulty with RCTs for manual therapy is devising an appropriate placebo treatment. Most studies have investigated effectiveness compared to no treatment or to another treatment that might be equally effective; however, a few studies have attempted to provide a placebo for mobilization.

Massage Therapy and Soft-Tissue Mobilization

There is limited evidence for the use of massage therapy for treatment of painful conditions. Nevertheless, massage is commonly used to treat musculoskeletal pain conditions. In an experimental muscle pain model (delayed-onset muscle soreness) in human subjects, both superficial cutaneous massage (used as a placebo) and deep-tissue massage reduced muscle pain, as measured by pressure pain thresholds and ratings of stretch-induced pain [14], supporting a role for massage in deep-tissue muscle pain. In an RCT comparing massage to mind-body therapy or standard therapy in patients with chronic musculoskeletal pain, 1 hour of weekly massage reduced the unpleasantness of pain after 8 weeks. However, there were no long-term effects for massage [26], supporting only a short-term effect for this intervention at reducing pain. The massage in this study was delivered by a licensed massage therapist with techniques applied at the discretion of the therapist that included Swedish, deep-tissue, neuromuscular, and pressure-point techniques. In a Cochrane systematic review, the effects of massage therapy for low back pain were evaluated compared to either an inert treatment or other therapies [15]. The review concluded that massage was effective for subacute and chronic low back pain when combined with exercises and education. The authors further concluded, based on one study, that acupressure massage was more effective than traditional massage. Lastly, the authors found that the effects of massage were similar to those of exercise and superior to those of joint mobilization and self-care. Similar results were found for the effectiveness of massage for mechanical neck pain [19]. For tension-type headache, soft-tissue mobilization and massage techniques have limited evidence for reduction in pain intensity and frequency [9]. Thus, there is moderate evidence to support the use of massage therapy (traditional or soft-tissue) for the control of musculoskeletal pain conditions.

Cervical Manipulation/Mobilization

For cervical pain, manipulation and mobilization procedures are commonly used to reduce pain. A Cochrane review of the literature examined the effects of manipulation and mobilization for mechanical neck pain [18]. For the 33 trials selected, there was a reduction in pain and an improved ability to perform activities of daily living for people who received exercises in combination with mobilization or manipulation compared to those who received no treatment. However, there was no improvement in those who received manipulation or mobilization alone. A more recent systematic review, by the same group of authors, continued to support the use of mobilization or manipulation in combination with exercises for treatment of mechanical neck disorders [17].

      For lateral epicondylalgia, one systematic review showed that cervical mobilization decreases subjective pain scores and increases pressure pain thresholds [4]. These effects were only studied over the short term, but the findings support the use of cervical mobilization for upper-limb pain conditions.

Lumbar Manipulation and Mobilization

Manipulation and mobilization are common treatments for back pain. Several reviews and evidence-based guidelines have been published, including a Cochrane systematic review that identified 39 RCTs. For patients with acute or chronic low back pain, spinal manipulative therapy was more effective than a sham procedure in reducing subjective pain ratings.

However, spinal manipulative therapy was not significantly more effective when compared to other therapies including general practitioner care, analgesics, other physical therapy modalities, exercises, or back school [2]. Despite these somewhat equivocal findings, current evidence-based guidelines developed by the American Pain Society for low back pain recommend manipulation and mobilization for both acute and chronic low back pain [6]. Interestingly, an RCT of 240 patients with nonspecific low back pain comparing spinal manipulative therapy, general exercise therapy (strengthening and aerobic exercise), and specific motor control exercises (designed to retrain trunk muscles) showed improved short-term effects of spinal manipulation and motor control exercises compared to general exercise therapy, but similar long-term outcomes [11].

Peripheral Joint Mobilization or Manipulation

Most studies have examined the effects of spinal mobilizations on pain reduction, but some have investigated the effects of mobilization of peripheral joints. In people with osteoarthritis, a grade III accessory glide of the tibia increases pressure pain threshold of the knee and the heel, and also increases function as measured by the timed up-and-go test (TUG), when compared to a placebo treatment or a no-treatment control [22]. For people with lateral epicondylalgia, application of Mulligan's mobilization with movement (a manual therapy technique in which a passive accessory movement is combined with an active physiological movement) increased pain-free grip strength and pressure pain thresholds in the treatment group but not in a placebo group or in a no-treatment control group [23]. Thus, peripheral mobilization appears to reduce both local and referred pain and hyperalgesia.

Neural Mobilization

One systematic review examined the efficacy of neural mobilization for treatment of a variety of musculoskeletal conditions. Of the 11 studies examined, the authors concluded that there was limited evidence (Level 3) for the effectiveness of neural mobilization techniques, which included pain reduction [8]. It should be noted, however, that all 11 studies utilized different techniques, were single-blinded or unblinded, and were rated as being of moderate to low quality.

Conclusion

There is moderate evidence to support the effectiveness of manipulation and mobilization techniques for acute and chronic neck or back pain and lateral epicondylalgia. There is limited evidence to support the use of massage therapy, soft-tissue mobilization, neural mobilization, and peripheral mobilization and manipulation for treatment of various musculoskeletal pain conditions. The use of peripheral mobilization and soft-tissue massage techniques, while common practice for physical therapists, at present has limited to no evidence to support its use. Most studies show that the effects of manual therapy, even when it is applied repetitively, are short-term. As with electrothermal modalities, the use of manual therapy techniques should be used as an adjunct to a program of exercise and education. Clearly, future studies need to use appropriate placebo controls and examine a greater proportion of pain conditions.

References

[1]   Agren G, Lundeberg T, Uvnas-Moberg K, Sato A. The oxytocin antagonist 1-deamino-2-D-Tyr-(Oet)-4-Thr-8-Orn-oxytocin reverses the increase in the withdrawal response latency to thermal, but not mechanical nociceptive stimuli following oxytocin administration or massage-like stroking in rats. Neurosci Lett 1995;187:49–52.
[2]   Assendelft WJ, Morton SC, Yu EI, Suttorp MJ, Shekelle PG. Spinal manipulative therapy for low back pain. Cochrane Database Syst Rev 2004;CD000447.
[3]   Bialosky JE, Bishop MD, Robinson ME, Barabas JA, George SZ. The influence of expectation on spinal manipulation induced hypoalgesia: an experimental study in normal subjects. BMC Musculoskelet Disord 2008;9:19.
[4]   Bisset L, Paungmali A, Vicenzino B, Beller E. A systematic review and meta-analysis of clinical trials on physical interventions for lateral epicondylalgia. Br J Sports Med 2005;39:411–22.
[5]   Bulbulian R, Burke J, Dishman JD. Spinal reflex excitability changes after lumbar spine passive flexion mobilization. J Manipulative Physiol Ther 2002;25:526–32.
[6]   Chou R, Huffman LH. Nonpharmacologic therapies for acute and chronic low back pain: a review of the evidence for an American Pain Society/American College of Physicians clinical practice guideline. Ann Intern Med 2007;147:492–504.
[7]   Dishman JD, Bulbulian R. Spinal reflex attenuation associated with spinal manipulation. Spine 2000;25:2519–24.
[8]   Ellis RF, Hing WA. Neural mobilization: a systematic review of randomized controlled trials with an analysis of therapeutic efficacy. J Man Manipulative Ther 2008;16:8–22.
[9]   Fernandez-de-las-Penas C, onso-Blanco C, Cuadrado ML, Miangolarra JC, Barriga FJ, Pareja JA. Are manual therapies effective in reducing pain from tension-type headache? A systematic review. Clin J Pain 2006;22:278–85.
[10] Ferreira ML, Ferreira PH, Hodges PW. Changes in postural activity of the trunk muscles following spinal manipulative therapy. Man Ther 2007;12:240–8.
[11] Ferreira ML, Ferreira PH, Latimer J, Herbert RD, Hodges PW, Jennings MD, Maher CG, Refshauge KM. Comparison of general exercise, motor control exercise and spinal manipulative therapy for chronic low back pain: a randomized trial. Pain 2007;131:31–7.
[12] Field T, Hernandez-Reif M, Diego M, Schanberg S, Kuhn C. Cortisol decreases and serotonin and dopamine increase following massage therapy. Int J Neurosci 2005;115:1397–413.

[13] Field T, Hernandez-Reif M, Seligman S, Krasnegor J, Sunshine W, Rivas-Chacon R, Schanberg S, Kuhn C. Juvenile rheumatoid arthritis: benefits from massage therapy. J Pediatr Psychol 1997;22:607–17.

[14] Frey Law LA, Evans S, Knudtson J, Nus S, Scholl K, Sluka KA. Massage reduces pain perception and hyperalgesia in experimental muscle pain: a randomized, controlled trial. J Pain 2008;9:714–21.

[15] Furlan AD, Imamura M, Dryden T, Irvin E. Massage for low back pain. Cochrane Database Syst Rev 2008:CD001929.

[16] George SZ, Bishop MD, Bialosky JE, Zeppieri G Jr, Robinson ME. Immediate effects of spinal manipulation on thermal pain sensitivity: an experimental study. BMC Musculoskelet Disord 2006;7:68.

[17] Gross AR, Goldsmith C, Hoving JL, Haines T, Peloso P, Aker P, Santaguida P, Myers C. Conservative management of mechanical neck disorders: a systematic review. J Rheumatol 2007;34:1083–102.

[18] Gross AR, Hoving JL, Haines TA, Goldsmith CH, Kay T, Aker P, Bronfort G. Manipulation and mobilisation for mechanical neck disorders. Cochrane Database Syst Rev 2004;CD004249.

[19] Haraldsson BG, Gross AR, Myers CD, Ezzo JM, Morien A, Goldsmith C, Peloso PM, Bronfort G. Massage for mechanical neck disorders. Cochrane Database Syst Rev 2006:CD004871.

[20] Hernandez-Reif M, Field T, Largie S, Hart S, Redzepi M, Nierenberg B, Peck TM. Children's distress during burn treatment is reduced by massage therapy. J Burn Care Rehabil 2001;22:191-5.

[21] Lund I, Ge Y, Yu LC, Uvnas-Moberg K, Wang J, Yu C, Kurosawa M, Agren G, Rosen A, Lekman M, Lundeberg T. Repeated massage-like stimulation induces long-term effects on nociception: contribution of oxytocinergic mechanisms. Eur J Neurosci 2002;16:330–8.

[22] Moss P, Sluka KA, Wright A. The initial effects of knee joint mobilisation on osteoarthritic hyperalgesia. Man Ther 2007;12:109–18.

[23] Paungmali A, O'Leary S, Souvlis T, Vicenzino B. Hypoalgesic and sympathoexcitatory effects of mobilization with movement for lateral epicondylalgia. Phys Ther 2003;83:374–83.

[24] Paungmali A, O'Leary S, Souvlis T, Vicenzino B. Naloxone fails to antagonize initial hypoalgesic effect of a manual therapy treatment for lateral epicondylalgia. J Manipulative Physiol Ther 2004;27:180–5.

[25] Pickar JG. Neurophysiological effects of spinal manipulation. Spine J 2002;2:357–71.

[26] Plews-Ogan M, Owens JE, Goodman M, Wolfe P, Schorling J. A pilot study evaluating mindfulness-based stress reduction and massage for the management of chronic pain. J Gen Intern Med 2005;20:1136–8.

[27] Skyba DA, Radhakrishnan R, Rohlwing JJ, Wright A, Sluka KA. Joint manipulation reduces hyperalgesia by activation of monoamine receptors but not opioid or GABA receptors in the spinal cord. Pain 2003;106:159–68.

[28] Sluka KA, Wright A. Knee joint mobilization reduces secondary mechanical hyperalgesia induced by capsaicin injection into the ankle joint. Eur J Pain 2001;5:81–7.

[29] Sung PS, Kang YM, Pickar JG. Effect of spinal manipulation duration on low threshold mechanoreceptors in lumbar paraspinal muscles: a preliminary report. Spine 2005;30:115–22.

[30] Vicenzino B, Collins D, Benson H, Wright A. An investigation of the interrelationship between manipulative therapy-induced hypoalgesia and sympathoexcitation. J Manipulative Physiol Ther 1998;21:448–53.

[31] Vicenzino B, Gutschlag F, Collins D, Wright A. An investigation of the effects of spinal manual therapy on forequarter pressure and thermal pain thresholds and sympathetic nervous system activity in asymptomatic subjects: a preliminary report. In: Shacklock M, editor. Moving in on pain. Adelaide: Butterworth-Heinemann; 1995. p. 185–93.

[32] Vicenzino B, O'Callahan J, Kermode F, Wright A. No influence of naloxone on the initial hypoalgesic effect of spinal manual therapy. In: Devor M, Rowbotham MC, Wiesenfeld-Hallin Z, editors. Proceedings of the 9th World Congress on Pain. Seattle: IASP Press; 2000. p. 1039–44.

[33] Zusman M, Edwards BC, Donaghy A. Investigation of a proposed mechanism for the relief of spinal pain with passive joint movement. J Manual Med 1989;4:58–61.

Correspondence to: Stephan Milosavljevic, PhD, Centre for Physiotherapy Research, School of Physiotherapy, University of Otago, P.O. Box 56, Dunedin, New Zealand. Tel: +1-64-3-479-7193; fax: +1-64-3-479-8414; email: stephan. milosavljevic@otago.ac.nz.

Section III

Interdisciplinary Pain Management

Interdisciplinary Pain Management

Harriët Wittink

*Lifestyle and Health Research Group, Faculty of Health Care,
University of Applied Sciences, Utrecht, The Netherlands*

Chronic pain has been defined as a function of a complex interaction among demographic, physical, psychological, social, and economic factors, including age, sex, education, medical status, pain severity, alcohol and substance abuse, beliefs about pain, increased use of medications and health care services, and a generalized adoption of the sick role [18].

Because chronic pain is multifactorial, the use of any one treatment modality is bound to fail. John Bonica saw the idea of interdisciplinary collaboration as the key to the understanding of pain and was the first to establish a multidisciplinary pain clinic, which he founded at the University of Washington in 1960. Many multidisciplinary pain clinics have been developed since then that offer a variety of therapeutic approaches to effective pain management. In 2003, more than 3,500 programs, clinics, centers, and solo practices in the United States provided care for 9 million persons with pain [12]. Some of these clinics or practices are modality specific (providing, for example, nerve blocks, acupuncture, or biofeedback), some are diagnosis specific (specializing in facial pain or pelvic pain, for example), and some are specialized pain centers in which clinicians with

Mechanisms and Management of Pain for the Physical Therapist
edited by Kathleen A. Sluka
IASP Press, Seattle, © 2009

expertise in various pain-related disciplines (including physicians, physical therapists, and psychologists) work as a team to provide comprehensive pain care.

The Joint Commission on Accreditation of Healthcare Organizations (JCAHO) developed standards [3] that address the assessment and management of pain in hospitals and other health care settings. The standards acknowledge that patients have a right to effective pain management and require that the presence of pain be routinely assessed for all patients. These standards, which have been endorsed by the American Pain Society [5], underscore the importance of effective pain management and establish it as an essential component of quality patient care. The standards apply to ambulatory care facilities, behavioral health care facilities, health care networks, home care, hospitals, long-term care organizations, long-term care pharmacies, and managed behavioral health care organizations. The Commission on Accreditation of Rehabilitation Facilities (CARF) [6] also incorporates principles of the interdisciplinary approach to pain treatment in its pain program accreditation standards. CARF surveys and accredits rehabilitation facilities, including those involved in chronic pain management. Table I summarizes the most important JCAHO and CARF standards for pain management.

The International Association for the Study of Pain (IASP) believes that patients throughout the world would benefit from the establishment of a set of recommendations for pain treatment services and has defined three different types of pain programs [10], described as follows (the IASP task force recommendations are given in full at www.iasp-pain.org).

Multidisciplinary pain centers are distinguished by the broad range of their clinical staff, patient care services, pain conditions treated, and educational and research activities. They should be part of or affiliated with a higher education and/or research institution. In general the staff should include clinicians from a variety of medical and other health care disciplines; all clinicians should have expertise in pain management. The clinicians who assess and treat patients in the pain center should include physicians, nurses, mental health professionals (e.g., clinical psychologists or psychiatrists), and physical therapists. The center should be able to treat any type of pain problem; thus, there must be a system for obtaining consultation as needed from physicians from disciplines not included on the staff.

A multidisciplinary pain *clinic* differs from a multidisciplinary pain center only in that research and academic teaching activities are not necessarily included in its regular programs.

A single provider may have a *pain practice* if he or she is licensed in his or her specialty, has completed specialty pain medicine training or the equivalent, and is certified in pain management by the appropriate local or national credentialing organization. This provider must be knowledgeable about the contributions of biological, psychological, and social/environmental factors to pain problems. There must be a system for obtaining consultation as needed from health care providers from other specialties. In addition, the provider should refer patients to a multidisciplinary pain clinic or center whenever there are diagnostic or therapeutic issues that exceed the provider's capabilities.

Although the IASP task force has recommendations for pain treatment services, it does not differentiate between multidisciplinary and interdisciplinary care. There is a difference, however. Multidisciplinary care is treatment in which multiple providers from different disciplines contribute to care. Interdisciplinary care is treatment provided by multiple providers from different disciplines that integrate care as a team, through frequent communication and common goals. As can be seen in the recommendations, the IASP supports a team-oriented approach to pain management in multidisciplinary pain treatment centers and clinics. This chapter will discuss interdisciplinary pain management and the evidence for its efficacy.

Interdisciplinary Pain Management

The biopsychosocial approach to pain and disability is widely accepted as the most heuristic perspective to the understanding and treatment of chronic pain disorders and has replaced the outdated, reductionistic biomedical approach. The biopsychosocial approach views pain and disability as a complex and dynamic interaction among physiological, psychological, and social factors that perpetuates—and may even worsen—the clinical presentation [9]. Psychosocial factors such as abuse, mood disorder, employment disability, poor coping skills, and other psychosocial problems are commonly found in patients with chronic pain referred to clinics [17].

Table I

Joint Commission on Accreditation of Healthcare Organizations (JCAHO) and Commission on Accreditation of Rehabilitation Facilities (CARF) standards for pain management

JCAHO Standards	CARF Standards
Recognize the right of patients to appropriate assessment and management of pain	Leadership standards and excellence Pain services are recognized and supported by the facility's executive leaders Leaders at all levels serve as advocates for people with "activity limitations" There is a strategic plan for pain services, and this plan is reviewed and modified regularly
Screen for the existence of pain and assess its nature and intensity in all patients	Rehabilitation process standards* Admission criteria Comprehensive pain assessments are completed at admission and include measures of participant characteristics and physical, psychological, social, financial, and vocational status in addition to pain At admission, predicted outcomes are established, as well as a discharge plan Intake information should allow for internal comparisons (at the same program over time) and external comparisons (with other facilities)
Record the results of the assessment in a way that facilitates regular reassessment and follow-up	Information and outcomes management standards Comprehensive, appropriate, and useful outcomes data must be gathered at admission, discharge, and follow-up using reliable and valid instruments tapping all major outcome domains (e.g., pain, activity, psychosocial factors, work) Data must be analyzed regularly and clearly linked to performance improvement activities Programs must compare their actual performance to their expected level of performance; they must contrast changes in outcomes measures between admission and discharge, and between discharge and follow-up Outcomes must be communicated to stakeholders and to all staff Interdisciplinary pain rehabilitation standards Programs use outcomes to identify areas for improvement, develop a plan for improvement, implement change, and measure the effects of the change

Determine and ensure staff competency in pain assessment and management, and address pain assessment and management in the orientation of all new staff	Staff competencies, team functioning Involvement of the consumer in the decision-making process Interdisciplinary pain rehabilitation standards Team composition and function; scope and intensity of treatment; program director, medical director, psychologist, and physician qualifications and responsibilities; staff training Leadership standards Staff are competent in the area of pain services or receive training and supervision in the area according to policies and standards Staffing levels match pain program outcomes objectives
Establish policies and procedures that support the appropriate prescription or ordering of effective pain medications	Rehabilitation process standards Interdisciplinary pain rehabilitation standards
Educate patients and their families about effective pain management	Interdisciplinary pain rehabilitation standards Consumer education, family services
Address patient needs for symptom management in the discharge planning process	Rehabilitation process standards Discharge criteria Comprehensive pain assessments are completed at discharge and include measures of physical, psychological, social, and financial factors; work capability; satisfaction with services; type, duration, and intensity of services provided; and characteristics of the home/transition environment
Maintain a pain control performance improvement plan	Rehabilitation process standards At some point after discharge, follow-up measures of physical, psychological, social, and financial factors; work capability; satisfaction with services; and home environment are conducted from a representative sample of participants The time frame chosen for follow-up should allow for measurement of the durability of the rehabilitation outcomes attained

* Rights of the persons served at the level of the organization, program, and treatment team.

Chronic pain affects multiple domains of life, and patients with chronic pain therefore require multidimensional assessment and treatment, which is best done by an interdisciplinary team.

CARF has defined interdisciplinary pain rehabilitation programs as "outcomes-focused, coordinated, goal-oriented interdisciplinary team services" [11]. Such programs can benefit those "who have impairments associated with pain that impact their activity and participation." They are designed to measure and improve the function of individuals with pain and encourage them to use health care systems and services appropriately.

Interdisciplinary pain management in comprehensive pain programs (CPPs) involves health care providers from several disciplines, each of whom specializes in different features of the pain experience. Fordyce [8] wrote: "In a multidisciplinary exercise, two or more professions may make their respective contributions, but each contribution stands on its own and could emerge without the input of the other. In an interdisciplinary effort, life is not so simple. The end product requires that there be an interactive and symbiotic interplay of the contributions from different disciplines. Without that interaction, the outcome will fall short of the need. … The essence of the matter is that each of the participating professions needs the others to accomplish what, collectively, they have agreed are their objectives."

In the interdisciplinary management of chronic pain, the core team typically comprises a pain management physician, a psychologist, a nurse specialist, a physical and occupational therapist, a vocational counselor, and a pharmacist, although owing to poor reimbursement issues, many interdisciplinary teams have had to scale back in personnel. CARF [6] requires that all accredited programs have a board-certified medical director and a psychologist on staff. The various disciples have different roles within the team (Table II). These roles may overlap, predominantly regarding behavioral approaches offered to the patient by the psychologist and occupational and physical therapists. It helps to reinforce the message to the patient when the same message is given by the various care providers.

The initial screening of the patient by a member of the core team determines which members of the team will be needed for a complete assessment of the patient. The assessment should include all major outcome domains—pain and physical, psychological, social, and vocational

Table II
Roles of the members of the interdisciplinary pain management team

Team Member	Role in Team
Physician	Comprehensive assessment of patient and review of prior records and previous treatments. Consideration of medical, nerve block, or implantation interventions.
Psychologist	Comprehensive psychological assessment, with a focus on coping mechanisms and the presence of psychological and/or psychiatric comorbidities, and substance abuse potential. Development of psychological interventions, including education on the use of self-management techniques, education on the pathophysiology of pain, pain coping skills, and cognitive-behavioral therapy.
Nurse	Coordination of care, education, and medical therapy.
Physical therapist	Comprehensive assessment of strength, flexibility, and physical endurance, with emphasis on the musculoskeletal system. Assessment of functional activities and behavior. Education on pain pathophysiology and active physical coping skills. Management of the physical rehabilitation process.
Occupational therapist	Assessment of the worksite and home. Assessment of the need for adaptive equipment. Setting of functional goals. Education on active coping skills, assertiveness training, and relaxation and distraction techniques.
Vocational rehabilitation specialist	Assessment of vocational skills and identification of opportunities and strategies to return to work.
Pharmacist	Comprehensive review of past and current pharmacological interventions, including the use of herbal and homeopathic substances, education of patient with regard to appropriate use of pharmacological interventions.
Psychiatrist	Diagnosis and treatment of psychiatric comorbidities. Medication management of psychiatric problems.

Source: Adapted from Ashburn and Staats [2].

functioning—using reliable and valid instruments that preferably are sensitive to change.

After this evaluation, the entire core team discusses the case, and a comprehensive treatment plan is developed. The care team tailors the care plan according to the individual needs of the patient, with a focus on achieving measurable treatment goals that are established with the patient. Therapeutic goals for CPPs are generally multifaceted. Some of the most common goals are to (1) reduce pain, (2) improve function, (3) permit return to work, (4) resolve medication issues, and (5) reduce health care utilization [15].

The plan must fit the patient's abilities and expectations. For some individuals, education and medical management suffice, whereas others may need an inpatient pain program that requires them to remain at a treatment center 24 hours a day, 7 days a week, for 3–4 weeks, or an outpatient pain rehabilitation program that can vary according to the facility from 8 hours a day, 5 days a week for 2–4 weeks, to 2 hours per day, 3 days a week for 6–8 weeks. Negotiating the overall treatment plan is the collective responsibility of the team and the patient.

Contingencies for possible outcomes should also be agreed on by the team and patient. Agreements should be clear and are best put in writing. Contracts are a simple and effective means of avoiding future confusion about the plan. Written contracts offer the patient the opportunity to review and consider the information over time.

Team unity is critical to managing any patient, but especially the difficult patient. Unity is largely a function of communication and understanding and respecting the expertise of the other team members. Frequent team meetings connect key representatives of the treatment team. Patient progress should be discussed during the meetings. If patients are not meeting their goals, are inconsistent with their attendance, or do not follow through with recommendations, the team should make recommendations for continuation of therapy or discharge. Because it might be impossible for the entire team to meet, there should be a mechanism for disseminating the plan among clinicians. Preferentially, the plan is put in writing, which both documents the interdisciplinary effort of the team and provides a sequence of events during the treatment of a patient. Frequent reassessment can help determine if the patient is progressing according to plan and whether he or she can be discharged with all goals met. At discharge a follow-up plan should be made with the patient, and comprehensive pain assessments should be completed that include measures of physical, psychological, social, financial, and work capability; satisfaction with services; the type, duration, and intensity of services provided; and characteristics of the home/transition environment.

The percentage of pain programs that claimed they could document outcomes data declined from 67% in 2001 to 59% in 2003. Although 87% of true multidisciplinary pain programs could document outcomes in 2003, only 40% of anesthesia-based modality-oriented programs could.

These figures represent a decline from 1999, when fully 77% of all pain programs surveyed reported that they could document outcomes data [12]. The authors of the analysis stated that the main reason for the decline may be due to the increase in the number of solo anesthesiologists practicing pain management.

Evidence for Interdisciplinary Treatment

In a survey of the most commonly used techniques for the treatment of chronic pain [12], a worrying trend was noted: the use of nerve blocks increased from 79% of pain practices surveyed in 2001 to 82% in 2003, while physical therapy use dropped from 85% in 2001 to 71% of programs in 2003. The multidisciplinary approach also declined in use from 81% of programs in 2001 to 77% in 2003. This change seems most likely to be due to reimbursement issues, because there is considerable evidence that interdisciplinary pain programs are effective [7,9,14,21], especially for patients with long-standing nonspecific chronic pain.

A meta-analysis of studies evaluating chronic pain treatment programs found that, in comparison to no treatment and single-modality methods, patients participating in interdisciplinary programs demonstrated greater long-term improvement [7]. Chronic pain patients in this type of treatment functioned better than 75% of control patients. They had significant improvements regarding activity level, pain intensity, pain behaviors, and use of medication and health services compared with the no-treatment group. In addition, 68% of the patients returned to work, versus 36% of the untreated patients.

Pain rehabilitation programs provide comparable reduction in pain to alternative pain treatment modalities, but with significantly better outcomes for medication use, health care utilization, functional activities, return to work, and closure of disability claims and with substantially fewer iatrogenic consequences and adverse events. Surgery, spinal cord stimulators, and implantable drug devices appear to have substantial benefits on some outcome criteria for carefully selected patients, but these options are expensive. Pain rehabilitation programs are significantly more cost-effective than implantation of spinal cord stimulators or implantable drug devices, conservative care, and surgery, even for selected patients [19].

In a systematic review of studies comparing participants in comprehensive chronic pain programs (CPPs) to unimodal treatment or no-treatment control patients, which involved a total of 3,089 participants, McCracken and Turk [13] reported the following outcomes comparisons: return to work, 68% of CPP patients versus 32% patients in unimodal programs or receiving no treatment; pain reduction, 37% versus 4%; medication reduction, 63% versus 21%; and increases in activity, 53% versus 13%, respectively. Gatchel and Okifuji [9] conducted a comprehensive review of all studies in the scientific literature reporting treatment outcomes for patients with chronic pain. They found that CPPs result in varying degrees of pain reduction, ranging from 14% to 60% with an average of 20% to 30%. These figures are comparable to the most conventional medical management of chronic pain with opioids, which yields an average pain reduction of 30%.

Approximately a 65% increase in physical activity is observed following CPP treatments. In contrast, only a 35% increase is reported in patients receiving conventional medical care. Return-to-work rates following CPP treatment range from 29% to 86%, with a mean of 66%, whereas conventional medical treatments consistently yield lower rates, from 0% to 42%, with a mean rate of 27%. Health care utilization data from CPP trials generally yield favorable results, with reduced seeking of additional therapy for pain within 1 year of treatment, along with reductions in subsequent hospitalization, surgical intervention, and medication use.

Robbins et al. [16] showed that patients who completed interdisciplinary pain management demonstrated significant improvements on the majority of outcome measures and maintained these gains at 1-year follow-up, relative to treatment dropouts. This was true for measures of both physical and psychosocial functioning, suggesting that the treatment program had a significant effect on all aspects of the experience of chronic pain. Treatment completers showed significant positive changes in work status from pretreatment to after treatment, with only 14.6% not working because of the original injury. These gains were maintained at 1-year follow-up, again revealing that interdisciplinary pain management has a lasting positive effect on vocational status.

Interestingly, patients who did not have physical therapy (due to reimbursement issues) exhibited significantly worse functioning relative to those who did [16]. In terms of vocational status, the percentage of subjects who were not working because of their original injury decreased in patients who had physical therapy, and these gains were maintained at a 1-year follow-up.

Conversely, patients who did not receive physical therapy did not show significant changes in vocational status, either immediately after treatment or at a 1-year follow-up. These findings suggest that patients who did not receive physical therapy did not experience the same benefits of interdisciplinary pain management as those who received all of their treatment in the same clinic.

As a group, in comparison to clinical trials in other areas of therapy, randomized controlled trials related to pain tend to be of low quality due to several factors—the small numbers of patients enrolled; flaws in patient randomization, assignment, and retention; scanty descriptions of the patients enrolled; and heterogeneity in the methods and timing of assessment of pain and other outcomes [22]. Many interventions in randomized controlled trials of pain control are sparse and too disparate to consolidate [1]. Thus, for much of clinical practice there is no "best evidence." The studies cited above seem to indicate that interdisciplinary pain management helps patients with chronic pain. Patients with chronic pain are not a homogeneous group, and different interventions may be indicated for different subgroups of patients [20]. Matching treatment to patient characteristics has been shown to improve outcomes of clinical care [4]. We still have a long way to go in determining which patients benefit from which treatments, but we need to solve this issue in interdisciplinary teams.

What to Do When You Cannot "Go Interdisciplinary"

Most physical therapy interventions for patients with chronic pain are unidisciplinary, meaning that care is not integrated with other health care providers. It is helpful to form (un)official alliances with the patient's various care providers. Although time-consuming, such cooperation is necessary, as it prevents misunderstandings between care providers and prevents the patient from getting conflicting information from different providers. Physical therapists must work with pain psychologists for optimal treatment of patients. Patients with chronic pain have high rates of concurrent anxiety and depression, and some may have suicidal ideation. Many have diagnosed (and some have undiagnosed) psychiatric illnesses or personality disorders, or both. For a physical therapist to address psychological problems is not only far beyond the scope of physical therapy practice—it is also irresponsible. Referral to psychologists specialized in the treatment of patients with chronic pain is discussed in Chapter 13.

References

[1] Abram SE, Hopwood M. Can meta-analysis rescue knowledge from a sea of unintelligible data? Reg Anesth 1996;21:514–6.
[2] Ashburn MA, Staats PS. Management of chronic pain. Lancet 1999;353:1865–9.
[3] Berry PH, Dahl JL. The new JCAHO pain standards: implications for pain management nurses. Pain Manag Nurs 2000;1:3–12.
[4] Brennan GP, Fritz JM, Hunter SJ, Thackeray A, Delitto A, Erhard RE. Identifying subgroups of patients with acute/subacute "nonspecific" low back pain: results of a randomized clinical trial. Spine 2006;31:623–31.
[5] Chapman R. New JCAHO standards for pain management: carpe diem! APS Bull 2000;10.
[6] Commission on Accreditation of Rehabilitation Facilities. Medical rehabilitation: standards manual. Tucson: Commission on Accreditation of Rehabilitation Facilities;2003.
[7] Flor H, Fydrich T, Turk DC. Efficacy of multidisciplinary pain treatment centers: a meta-analytic review. Pain 1992;49:221–30.
[8] Fordyce WE, Fowler RS Jr, Lehmann JF, Delateur BJ, Sand PL, Trieschmann RB. Operant conditioning in the treatment of chronic pain. Arch Phys Med Rehabil 1973;54:399–408.
[9] Gatchel RJ, Okifuji A. Evidence-based scientific data documenting the treatment and cost-effectiveness of comprehensive pain programs for chronic nonmalignant pain. J Pain 2006;7:779–93.
[10] International Association for the Study of Pain. Desirable characteristics for pain treatment facilities. 2009. Available at: www.iasp-pain.org.
[11] .MacDonell CM, Ervin E. Interdisciplinary pain rehabilitation programs: an update from CARF. APS Bull 2003;13(2).
[12] Marketdata Enterprises. Chronic pain management clinics: a market analysis. 2003. Available at: http://www.marketresearch.com.
[13] McCracken LM, Turk DC. Behavioral and cognitive-behavioral treatment for chronic pain: outcome, predictors of outcome, and treatment process. Spine 2002;27:2564–73.
[14] Okifuji AA, Turk DC, Kalauokalani D. Clinical outcomes and economic evaluation of the multidisciplinary pain centers. In: Block A, Kremer EE, Fernandez E, editors. Handbook of pain syndromes. Mahwah, NJ: Lawrence Erlbaum; 1999. p. 77–97.
[15] Okifuji A. Interdisciplinary pain management with pain patients: evidence for its effectiveness. Semin Pain Med 2003;1:110–9.
[16] Robbins H, Gatchel RJ, Noe C, Gajraj N, Polatin P, Deschner M, Vakharia A, Adams L. A prospective one-year outcome study of interdisciplinary chronic pain management: compromising its efficacy by managed care policies. Anesth Analg 2003;97:156–62.
[17] Tunks ER, Weir R, Crook J. Epidemiologic perspective on chronic pain treatment. Can J Psychiatry 2008;53:235–42.
[18] Turk DC. Biopsychosocial perspective on chronic pain. In: Gatchel R, Turk DC, editors. Psychological approaches to pain management. New York: Guilford Press; 1996. p. 3–32.
[19] Turk DC. Clinical effectiveness and cost-effectiveness of treatments for patients with chronic pain. Clin J Pain 2002;18:355–65.
[20] Turk DC. The potential of treatment matching for subgroups of patients with chronic pain: lumping versus splitting. Clin J Pain 2005;21:44-55.

[21] Turk DC, Okifuji A. Efficacy of multidisciplinary pain centres: an antidote to anecdotes. Baillieres Clin Anaesthesiol 1998;103–19.

[22] Zucker DR, Schmid CH, McIntosh MW, D'Agostino RB, Selker HP, Lau J. Combining single patient [N-of-1] trials to estimate population treatment effects and to evaluate individual patient responses to treatment. J Clin Epidemiol 1997;50:401–10.

Correspondence to: Prof. Harriët Wittink, PT, MS, PhD, Lifestyle and Health Research Group, Faculty of Health Care, University of Applied Sciences Utrecht, Bolognalaan 101, 3584CJ Utrecht, The Netherlands. Tel: +1-030-2585156; fax: +1-030-2540608; email: harriet.wittink@hu.nl.

Medical Management of Pain

Eva Kosek

*Department of Clinical Neuroscience, Karolinska Institute
and Stockholm Spine Center, Stockholm, Sweden*

Pain can be conceptualized as a primarily motivational state to induce a behavioral drive with the purpose of restoring homeostasis. Acute pain can be regarded as an important warning signal, which is supported by the severe tissue injuries sustained by people with an inherited inability to feel pain. The intensity of acute pain is normally proportional to the extent of injury (i.e., nociceptive input), but that is not necessarily true for chronic pain. On the contrary, the intensity of chronic pain often correlates poorly with the degree of peripheral pathology, as in osteoarthritis [72] and rheumatoid arthritis [89]. Pain can even persist without any identifiable organic pathology, as in fibromyalgia [23]. The perception of pain can be described in terms of sensory-discriminative, affective, and cognitive dimensions [70].

The multidimensionality of the pain experience is supported by studies using functional magnetic resonance imaging (fMRI) to assess cerebral activation during stimulus-evoked pain in human subjects. These studies have documented activation of brain areas traditionally associated with the perception of sensory features, as well as regions associated with emotional and motivational aspects of pain [24]. In a recent fMRI study of patients with chronic low back pain, activation of the somatosensory cortex was seen only during brief periods of spontaneously increasing pain intensity. During periods of ongoing low back pain, only brain regions of importance for emotional and cognitive aspects of pain (the prefrontal and cingulate cortices) were activated [12]. These results are in accordance with two recent positron emission tomography (PET) studies of joint pain, showing increased activation of brain areas implicated in emotional/evaluative aspects of pain during the experience of clinical pain compared to the experience of stimulus-evoked heat pain in patients with osteoarthritis [58] and rheumatoid arthritis [79]. These studies indicate a greater emotional salience of clinical pain compared to experimental pain and stress the importance of coping strategies influencing the perception of chronic pain. Chronic pain should therefore be regarded not solely as a symptom, but as a medical problem in itself.

Clinical Assessment of the Pain Patient

The medical assessment of a pain patient always includes a careful history and physical examination. Depending on the results, the physician must decide whether additional laboratory tests or radiological or neurophysiological examinations are needed in order to define the diagnosis and to exclude potentially dangerous and treatable medical conditions. The physician must always consider whether the cause of pain can be treated. For example, surgery may be appropriate in patients with severe pain due to osteoarthritis, or disease-modifying treatments may be helpful in patients with rheumatoid arthritis. Unfortunately, causal treatment is not always possible.

The next step is to consider treatments that can relieve the pain (i.e., symptomatic treatment), such as physiotherapy or pharmacotherapy. Despite these interventions, many patients are still left with chronic pain that affects their function and quality of life in a negative way. Chronic pain can severely affect psychological well-being, cognitive functions, and physical activity. In order to make a complete assessment of a chronic pain patient, all dimensions of pain (sensory, affective, cognitive, and motor) must be analyzed in addition to the social context (the patient's ability to function as a spouse, parent, or employee). Interventions to help patients to cope better with their pain and to reduce the negative effects of pain on daily life should be considered. Cognitive-behavioral therapy (see Chapter 13) and multiprofessional team-based rehabilitation programs (see Chapter 11) have proven effective in this regard.

History

A careful history in combination with a pain drawing is usually sufficient to give a good working hypothesis as to the nature of the pain problem and provide guidance for further investigations. The history should include heredity of interest, past and present disease, previous investigations, and previous treatments and their results. The patient should be asked to fill in a pain drawing, mapping the location of pain and other symptoms such as numbness and paresthesias. Ratings of the present, minimal, and maximal pain intensity should be gathered. The duration of pain, diurnal variation in pain intensity, as well as pain-aggravating factors (such as movements or stress) and pain-relieving factors need to be assessed. The history should also include psychosocial factors of relevance (especially in chronic pain patients), such as depression, anxiety, anger, coping strategies, cognitive difficulties, sleep disturbance, and the patient's perception of stress, problems with relationships, and function (including work capacity).

Physical Examination

All patients should be examined with the goal of identifying the cause of pain. In nonsevere acute pain conditions, the examination can usually be restricted to the painful part of the body, whereas patients with long-term or severe pain need a more extensive examination. Neurological evaluation (including sensitivity testing, reflexes, and exclusion of paresis and fasciculation), relevant examination of the musculoskeletal system (examination of joints and muscles, including functional measures), and a psychological assessment (assessment of depression and anxiety) usually form part of the examination. Additional investigations that may be required for certain patients include laboratory tests, radiological examinations, neurophysiological examinations—quantitative sensory testing (QST), electroneurography, and electromyography—and/or referral to other specialists for further investigation and treatment. Given that the diagnosis of neuropathic pain relies heavily on the presence of sensory dysfunction, the examination of sensitivity is of great importance. A complete bedside examination includes assessment of different modalities, such as vibration (tuning fork; Aβ fibers), light touch (brush; Aβ fibers), pinprick (needle; Aδ/C fibers), cold (metal; Aδ fibers), and warmth (heated metal; C fibers). The examination should be guided by the suspected diagnosis. In certain cases, complementary examinations using more sophisticated methods such as QST can be required [44]. Dysfunction of small fibers (Aδ and C fibers) cannot be detected by electroneurography, and thus electroneurography can never replace bedside sensory testing (or QST).

The clinical assessment should result in the definition of the type or types of pain (i.e., nociceptive pain, neuropathic pain, pain of unknown origin, or psychogenic pain) and a pain diagnosis according to the ICD-10 classification criteria [100]. It is important to acknowledge that one diagnostic entity can give rise to several different pain types, which can be illustrated by lumbar disk herniations, which commonly cause nociceptive pain in the back and neuropathic pain in the leg. The dominant type of pain in a patient with lumbar disk herniation will guide the physician to choose the correct treatment. Accordingly, the same type of pain can occur across various diagnostic entities; for example, nociceptive pain is seen in patients with acute fractures, osteoarthritis, rheumatoid arthritis, and ischemic ulcers—conditions that clearly demand different medical treatments.

Multidimensional Pain Analysis

In the complex, subjective experience of pain, the sensory, emotional, cognitive, and motor dimensions are constantly interacting. In patients presenting with severe or long-term pain, the role of a multidimensional pain analysis is to assess all of these dimensions in order to obtain a specific profile, which is used to guide the choice of further treatment (see Fig. 1). It is well known that depression [1,33], pain-related anxiety or fear [9,13], kinesiophobia or movement avoidance [8,96], and catastrophizing [88] are strong negative predictors for good treatment outcomes in chronic pain patients. On the other hand, acceptance has been identified as a predictor for good treatment outcomes [66,67,68]. The beneficial effects of cognitive-behavioral therapy in chronic pain patients are most likely explained by the reduction of negative psychological factors in combination with increased acceptance and self-efficacy [93] (see Chapter 13).

A multidimensional pain analysis is best performed as a multi-professional, team-based assessment, resting on the biopsychosocial pain model. In addition to the sensory aspects (the intensity, localization, and type of pain), emotional and cognitive aspects must be examined (see Chapter 11). Anxiety, depression, pain-related anger, coping strategies, fear-avoidance, and degree of acceptance can be assessed during an interview with the patient. Self-administered, standardized questionnaires can be used as a complement to the interview and are also valuable for the assessment of treatment outcome.

Pain can also have negative effects on physical function. Inactivity due to movement-related pain is common in chronic pain patients and leads to decreased muscle strength, reduced endurance, and decreased aerobic capacity. An adequate training regimen can often improve physical

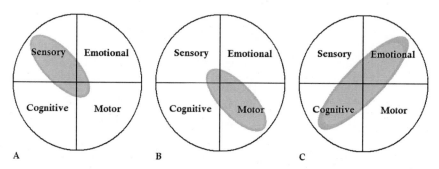

Fig. 1. Multidimensional pain analysis of chronic pain patients and its implication for treatment. (A) The pain profile of a 67-year-old female patient with nociceptive pain due to osteoarthritis of the hip. She has no psychological symptoms, has good coping strategies, and has remained physically active. This patient was helped by transdermal buprenorphine (5 μg/hour), which reduced her pain at rest, lessened her sleep disturbance, and improved her quality of life. (B) The pain profile of a 46-year-old male after surgery for lumbar disk herniation. He was totally relieved of his radicular pain, and his lumbar pain was tolerable. He had no psychological or cognitive complications. However, he was hesitant to resume normal physical activity and had a low functional capacity. This patient improved his function following physical therapy (a graded training regimen). (C) The pain profile of a 52-year-old female patient 2 years after a whiplash trauma. She had developed depression and pain-related anxiety. Her coping strategies were dominated by catastrophizing and avoidance. She was convinced that because physical activity increased her pain it was harmful to her neck. This patient participated in a multimodal, team-based rehabilitation program including cognitive-behavioral therapy, social counseling, and physical therapy. Despite residual pain, she improved her function and returned to work half-time.

capacity and even reduce pain. Nonfunctional body postures, selectively increased muscle tension, problems with coordination, and coactivation of antagonists can develop as a consequence of pain and can be treated by a physical therapist. Fear of movement constitutes a special problem leading to avoidance of certain physical activities. In analogy to treatment of phobias, treatment consists of a gradual exposure to the physical activity that the patient fears and avoids [96]. Patients with a complex pain profile, involving severe pain along with depression or anxiety, inadequate coping strategies and/or fear-avoidance, should be considered for multiprofessional team-based pain treatment and rehabilitation programs.

When Should a Physical Therapist Refer to a Pain Specialist?

The physical therapist should refer a patient to a pain physician if one or more of the following situations is present: (1) lack of a pain diagnosis, or symptoms that are not in accordance with the analysis made; (2) lack of a positive treatment effect of physical therapy despite adequate compliance and duration of treatment; (3) worsening of pain or presentation of new symptoms requiring investigation; (4) inadequate pain treatment (i.e., the need for pharmacotherapy or other forms of pain relief that cannot be provided by the physical therapist); (5) "red flags" such as weight loss, severe fatigue, initial pain onset at 55 years or older, recent trauma, pain that worsens at night, a history of cancer, steroid consumption, very poor general health or disability, a severe sleep disorder, any sign of systemic disease such as infection, an inflammatory disorder, a neurological disorder (unless accounted for and adequately treated), or any suspicion of a previously unrecognized medical condition; (6) suspicion of overconsumption of analgesics, drug abuse, or alcohol abuse; (7) psychological symptoms that need additional treatment (depression, anxiety, or catastrophizing); (8) a complex pain profile indicating that the patient is likely to need treatment by a multiprofessional team.

Different Types of Pain

According to the IASP terminology, four types of pain are currently acknowledged: nociceptive pain, pain of unknown origin (including dysfunctional pain), neuropathic pain, and psychogenic pain [71]. The correct identification of the type of pain is clinically important because each type of pain requires a different treatment strategy.

Nociceptive Pain

Nociceptive pain is induced by tissue injury (which can be caused by lacerations, infection, inflammation, and/or ischemia) and is mediated by a healthy nervous system. The intensity of acute nociceptive pain is usually proportional to the degree of injury or tissue pathology and responds well to antinociceptive pharmacotherapy. In cases of long-term nociceptive pain, changes in the function of endogenous pain modulatory mechanisms (i.e., central sensitization and disinhibition) are commonly seen. There are currently no acknowledged diagnostic criteria to detect central hyperexcitability, but increased pain intensity, spread of pain to previously unaffected parts of the body, and increased sensitivity to stimulus-evoked pain in the absence of corresponding aggravation of the peripheral pathology are considered characteristic. The distinction between nociceptive pain with profound central hyperexcitability and dysfunctional pain (where the central hyperexcitability is believed to be the dominating pain generator) is difficult, and there are currently no acknowledged guidelines for the clinician to use. However, this distinction can be important for the correct choice of pharmacotherapy.

Another diagnostic difficulty is to differentiate between nociceptive and neuropathic pain. Sensory aberrations can be found in patients with nociceptive pain [53,54]. Furthermore, referred pain, especially if combined with sensory abnormalities in the areas of referred pain, can mimic neuropathic pain (i.e., radiculopathies).

Referred pain, characterized as perception of pain in an area distant from the site of nociceptive input (the primary pain focus), is a normal physiological phenomenon that is often reported by patients with musculoskeletal pain. Referred pain is most likely a consequence of a misinterpretation of the origin of input from the area of nociceptive stimulation. When nociceptive input becomes strong enough, neurons with projected fields in the area of referred pain become excited somewhere along the neuroaxis, giving rise to the perception of pain [56]. Results from fMRI studies show activation of the primary somatosensory cortex corresponding to the focal pain area only during perception of localized pain, whereas subjects experiencing localized and referred pain have activation of the somatosensory cortex corresponding to the central representation of the local and referred pain areas [62]. Several characteristics can be used to recognize referred pain (and to differentiate between referred pain and neuropathic pain).

First, referred pain typically has a distribution distal to the primary pain focus (with the exception of cervicogenic headache) [91] (see Fig. 2). Second, the intensity and distribution of referred pain are directly proportional to the pain intensity in the primary pain focus [41,42]. This phenomenon can be illustrated by a patient with lumbar pain reporting no pain in the legs when the lumbar pain is of low intensity, pain in the dorsal part of the thighs when the lumbar pain is moderate, and pain in the dorsal part of the thighs and also in the dorsal part of the calves when the lumbar pain is intense. Previous studies have shown larger areas of referred pain, including proximal referral of pain, in patients with whiplash-associated disorder [49], fibromyalgia [81], and osteoarthritis [11], compared to healthy controls following the same painful stimulation (i.e., pain intensities were higher in the patient groups). However, a larger distribution of referred pain, including proximal pain referral, was recently documented following the same subjectively painful stimuli, indicating a truly different pattern of pain referral in the patient group (see Fig. 3) [57].

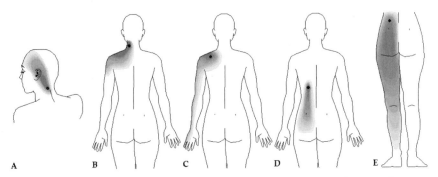

Fig. 2. The typical distribution of referred pain. (A) A primary pain focus in the upper cervical structures typically gives rise to referred pain in the form of occipital headache, spreading toward the forehead. (B) Pain originating in the lower cervical structures is typically referred to the ipsilateral shoulder/arm/hand and the thoracic spine. (C) Pain originating in the shoulders is typically referred to the ipsilateral arm/hand. (D) Thoracic pain is typically referred distally to the lumbar spine. (E) When the primary pain focus is localized at the lumbar spine, pain is typically referred to the buttocks, thighs, calves, and ankles.

Third, referred pain is usually perceived as diffuse and variable [55]. Sensory abnormalities can be present in the primary pain focus as well as in the area of referred pain. The sensory aberrations are diffuse and are influenced by pain intensity, thus differing in distribution, character, and severity over time [55]. So far, no pathognomonic profile has been identified for the sensory abnormalities seen in areas of referred pain [55].

In conclusion, several characteristics differ between referred and neuropathic pain. The distribution of neuropathic pain is less variable than that of referred pain, and the sensory abnormalities in neuropathic pain states typically have a clear neuroanatomical correlate and are more consistent over time [55]. Diagnostic blocks can be used to recognize referred pain, because the sensory abnormalities normalize when the input from the primary pain focus is blocked [60,94].

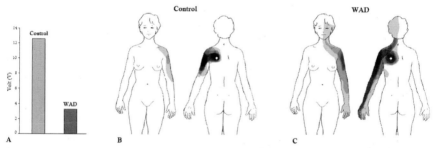

Fig. 3. Increased pain sensitivity and abnormal distribution of referred pain in patients with whiplash-associated disorder (WAD) (adapted from [57]). (A) The intensity (in volts) of intramuscular (i.m.) electrical stimuli at the infraspinatus muscle that gave rise to pain ratings corresponding to 4/10 on a Borg category-ratio scale [17] in 12 WAD patients and 12 age- and sex-matched healthy controls. The WAD patients had increased sensitivity to i.m. electrical stimulation compared to controls ($P < 0.01$). The i.m. electrical stimulus gave rise to referred pain in all subjects. (B) The pattern of referred pain during i.m. electrical stimulation at the infraspinatus muscle in healthy controls. (C) The pattern of referred pain during i.m. electrical stimulation at the infraspinatus muscle in WAD patients. Compared to controls, WAD patients had larger areas of referred pain ($P < 0.003$), and they also had proximal pain referral, which was never seen in healthy controls.

Neuropathic Pain

Definition

According to the most recent classification, neuropathic pain is defined as "pain arising as a direct consequence of a lesion or disease affecting the somatosensory system" [92]. This definition is proposed to replace the current definition of neuropathic pain as "pain initiated or caused by a primary lesion or dysfunction in the nervous system" because the older definition did not clearly distinguish between neuropathic and dysfunctional pain (i.e., nociceptive/idiopathic pain with central hyperexcitability). Central neuropathic pain (pathology within the central nervous system) is distinguished from peripheral neuropathic pain (pathology within the peripheral nervous system). Because of the lack of a specific diagnostic tool for neuropathic pain, a grading system has been proposed for clinical and research purposes [92].

Grading System

Neuropathic pain is graded according to the following conditions:

1) Pain with a distinct neuroanatomically plausible distribution. (A region corresponding to a peripheral innervation territory or to the topographic representation of a body part in the central nervous system.)

2) A history suggestive of a relevant lesion or disease affecting the peripheral or central nervous system. (The suspected lesion or disease is reported to be associated with pain, including a temporal relationship typical for the condition.)

3) Demonstration of a distinct neuroanatomically plausible distribution by at least one confirmatory test. (As part of the neurological examination, these tests confirm the presence of negative or positive neurological signs concordant with the distribution of pain. Clinical sensory examination may be supplemented by laboratory and objective tests to uncover subclinical abnormalities.)

4) Demonstration of a relevant lesion or disease by at least one confirmatory test. (As part of the neurological examination, these tests confirm the diagnosis of the suspected lesion or disease. These confirmatory tests depend on which lesion or disease is causing neuropathic pain.)

Definite neuropathic pain is diagnosed when all conditions (1–4) are fulfilled. A diagnosis of probable neuropathic pain requires conditions 1 and 2, plus either condition 3 or 4. A diagnosis of possible neuropathic pain requires conditions 1 and 2, without confirmatory evidence from conditions 3 or 4.

Pain of Unknown Origin

Frequently, the cause of pain cannot be identified, which is especially common in patients with chronic pain localized in the musculoskeletal system. The pain is then classified as pain of unknown origin (idiopathic pain). Often, a nociceptive pain focus was initially present, but it can no longer account for the intensity and distribution of pain. In many of these patients, various signs of central hyperexcitability can be found, and in these cases the term "dysfunctional pain" is often used. Pain syndromes such as fibromyalgia have traditionally been classified as "pain of unknown origin." However, the extensive documentation of central hyperexcitability (pain amplification) in fibromyalgia and the fact that centrally acting drugs have been shown to have pain-relieving effects in patients make the term "pain of unknown origin" problematic. Until a new, more appropriate term is found for the pain in patients with central hyperexcitability, the term "dysfunctional pain" may be used (as will be the case in this chapter).

A problem with dysfunctional pain is a lack of consensus as to how to identify individual patients with central hyperexcitability (central sensitization, disinhibition, and/or facilitation). Based on clinical experience, certain symptom constellations are considered to indicate dysfunctional pain, although not all are specific for this kind of pain. The characteristics of dysfunctional pain are: (1) increased intensity and distribution of spontaneous ongoing pain in combination with increased sensitivity to stimulus-evoked pain, without a corresponding worsening of the underlying (peripheral) pathology; (2) aftersensations such as increased pain following palpation; (3) increased pain intensity following physical activity; and (4) increased pain during sitting or standing so that the patient reports a constant urge to change position. Central hyperexcitability, suggesting dysfunctional pain, has been found in many different pain syndromes such as whiplash-associated disorder [29,30,57,80], temporomandibular disorder [63], trapezius myalgia [61], chronic low back pain [38], and fibromyalgia [51]. Studies have found that central hyperexcitability is a major negative prognostic factor in patients with whiplash-associated disorder [48,85,86,87]. The best-studied disorder with regard to central hyperexcitability is fibromyalgia, which is associated with multimodal allodynia/hyperalgesia [51], increased temporal summation [82,83], dysfunction of endogenous pain inhibitory mechanisms [52,59], and increased transmission/processing of nociceptive input [40].

Psychogenic Pain

Psychogenic pain is defined as pain caused by psychiatric disorders such as major depression or schizophrenia. This phenomenon, in which pain is a hallucination, is extremely rare. Given the fact that pain is a subjective experience, psychological mechanisms, both affective and evaluative, form an integral part of all types of pain. However, this aspect of the pain experience should not be confounded with psychogenic pain.

Pharmacotherapy

Pharmacological Agents Used for Pain Relief

NSAIDS, Coxibs, and Acetaminophen (Paracetamol)

Nonsteroidal anti-inflammatory drugs (NSAIDs) and coxibs have anti-inflammatory, analgesic, and antipyretic effects through inhibition of the enzyme cyclooxygenase (COX), which is involved in the transformation of arachidonic acid to prostaglandins. Prostaglandins are involved in the induction of peripheral sensitization and also have pronociceptive effects in the central nervous system. There are two main kinds of COX, COX-1 and COX-2, the latter mainly present during inflammation. The traditional NSAIDs have a nonselective inhibitory effect on COX-1 and COX-2, while the coxibs are selective inhibitors of COX-2. The analgesic effects of NSAIDs and coxibs are equal. The difference is that the coxibs lack the anticoagulation effects and have fewer gastrointestinal side effects compared to traditional NSAIDs, but they do not have a lower risk for cardiovascular side effects or renal failure. In fact, several coxibs have been withdrawn from the market due to elevated cardiovascular risks. Acetaminophen (paracetamol) is an analgesic and an antipyretic, but it lacks anti-inflammatory effects. Its mechanisms of action are not completely understood, but it is considered to have a weak, possibly indirect, COX-inhibitory effect, most likely in the central nervous system [19]. NSAIDs, coxibs, and acetaminophen can also potentiate the analgesic effect of opioids.

Opioids

Seventy percent of the μ-opioid receptors in the dorsal horn of the spinal cord are located on presynaptic Aδ and C fibers [16], while Aβ fibers lack opioid receptors. The remaining 30% are located postsynaptically on interneurons and projecting neurons [16], including the wide-dynamic-range neurons [31]. The activation of μ-opioid receptors has inhibitory effects, consisting of presynaptic inhibition of primary nociceptive afferents and postsynaptic inhibition of projecting neurons. The opioid receptors are synthesized in the dorsal root ganglia (in the cell bodies of Aδ and C fibers) and are transported centrally and peripherally. Nerve damage has been reported to reduce the number of opioid receptors, most likely because of impaired axonal transport [15], whereas opioid receptors increase in the periphery during inflammation [84].

Opioids are traditionally divided into two arbitrary categories—weak and strong opioids [99]. However, it is important to remember that a high dose of weak opioids can be equivalent to treatment with the so-called strong opioids, and vice versa. Codeine, dextropropoxyphene, and tramadol are generally considered to be weak opioids. Codeine itself lacks analgesic effects, but it is metabolized to morphine in the liver (except in approximately 9% of the population) [20]. Tramadol is a weak μ-opioid receptor agonist and a weak reuptake inhibitor of serotonin and norepinephrine. Buprenorphine, a strong opioid, is equipotent to the weak opioids when administered transdermally (as a slow-release patch). Slow-release products (e.g., transdermal buprenorphine and oral slow-release tramadol) are believed to have a lower risk of tolerance development and abuse [46]. They provide a stable analgesic effect, including during the night, and are suited for treatment of patients with long-term pain.

There are several strong opioids, including morphine, methadone, fentanyl, hydromorphone, meperidine/pethidine, oxycodone, and buprenorphine. Treatment with a fixed dose of a long-acting, extended-release opioid is recommended for patients with chronic noncancer pain because it provides a more consistent analgesic effect, with less risk of end-of-dose breakthrough pain and better nighttime pain control [74].

Severe acute pain and cancer pain are often successfully treated by a combination of NSAIDS or coxibs and strong opioids. Patients with chronic nonmalignant pain constitute a more problematic group due to the risk of serious side effects and addiction or abuse. Treatment of pain with strong opioids in patients with chronic nonmalignant pain should be initiated by an experienced pain specialist. During the titration phase, frequent treatment evaluations are necessary. Many authorities consider that a positive treatment effect of opioids in long-term nonmalignant pain includes improvements in function and quality of life in addition to pain relief [78]. A history of psychiatric disease or ongoing/previous addiction is a risk factor for psychological addiction and abuse. The patient must be informed about the risk of side effects (constipation, sedation, nausea, vomiting, and dizziness) and also told of the risk of addiction. Furthermore, the patient must be willing to discontinue medication in the case of inadequate analgesic effects or uncontrolled dose escalation.

At the initial stage of opioid therapy, a distinction needs to be made between a true analgesic effect and an affective effect (an anxiolytic and/or euphoric effect). It is likely that a patient has a true analgesic effect if (a) a clear reduction of pain intensity is reported, (b) the duration of analgesia corresponds to the pharmacological drug effect, (c) the dose-response relationship is positive (i.e., increased analgesia with increased dose), (d) the reduced pain intensity leads to increased activity (mental and physical), and (e) the treatment leads to increased function and better quality of life. Characteristic for affective pain relief is that the patient reports that the pain intensity per se is not much different, but that he or she is no longer so bothered by the pain. Typically this phenomenon is described as "it is easier to relax," "I do not care as much about the pain, even though it is still there," or "I feel a bit groggy, so I do not care as much." Tolerance development is more pronounced for the affective than for the sensory, pain-reducing effect of opioids. Therefore, patients with an affective analgesic effect are at increased risk of psychological dependence and iatrogenic drug addiction and abuse [39,50,77]. For this reason, patients who mainly report an affective analgesic effect should be withdrawn from opioid medication.

Opioid tolerance refers to a shorter duration and reduced intensity of opioid effects with repeated use. In experimental settings, tolerance to respiratory suppression develops rapidly [76]. Tolerance for sedation, cognitive side effects, and nausea/vomiting take a longer time to develop; tolerance does not develop for opioid-induced meiosis and constipation

[76]. In correctly administered opioid treatment in patients with chronic, opioid-sensitive pain states, development of tolerance to the analgesic effect of the opioid is rare, and the opioid dose is basically only increased if the medical condition progresses [39,77]. However, there are exceptions in which tolerance to the analgesic effect of opioids occurs despite correct treatment. In these cases there is also a cross-tolerance to other opioids, but the cross-tolerance is incomplete [25]. This phenomenon has led to the tradition of opioid rotation, in which, when an insufficient treatment effect develops over time with one opioid, the patient is switched to another opioid [18,90]. Long-term opioid treatment always leads to the development of physical dependence, which should not be mistaken for abuse. The meaning of physical dependence is that a quick withdrawal from opioids will lead to opioid withdrawal symptoms. Therefore, a gradual withdrawal from opioids is always necessary following long-term use [76,77].

Opioid-induced hyperalgesia is a recently reported phenomenon and refers to the increased pain sensitivity reported in former drug addicts [64] and possibly also in pain patients following high doses of opioid therapy [22]. Former opioid addicts are reported to have an increased sensitivity to stimulus-induced pain that can remain after successful withdrawal from opioid abuse [75]. Increased pain sensitivity has also been reported in former opioid addicts on current substitution therapy with methadone or buprenorphine [26,27,35]. These patients are considered to have a long-term (perhaps permanent) change in the balance between opioid (antinociceptive) and cholecystokinin (pronociceptive) pain regulatory mechanisms [45]. This phenomenon must be considered when former addicts are treated for acute pain following trauma or surgery, because on average they need higher doses of opioids compared to individuals who have no history of addiction in order to achieve adequate analgesia [2,34].

Serotonin and Norepinephrine Reuptake Inhibitors

The pharmacological agents in this group were originally developed for the treatment of depression and are therefore known as antidepressants (which is inappropriate from the perspective of pain treatment). Drugs with a combined reuptake inhibitory effect on serotonin and norepinephrine—tricyclic antidepressants and serotonin-norepinephrine reuptake inhibitors (SNRIs)—have been reported to have analgesic effects in neuropathic pain states [10] and fibromyalgia [5]. There is also limited evidence for a beneficial effect in certain nociceptive pain states—osteoarthritis, rheumatoid arthritis, and acute low back pain [98]. The likely mechanism of action is that increased levels of serotonin and norepinephrine, two transmitter substances implicated in descending pain inhibitory pathways, increase the efficacy of endogenous pain inhibition. The analgesic effect is independent of the antidepressant effect [65]. Selective serotonin reuptake inhibitors (SSRIs) lack analgesic effects and should not be used for treatment of pain [65]. The tricyclic antidepressants have many side effects that limit their usefulness, especially in older patients. The most common side effects are dryness of the mouth, constipation, sweating, dizziness, fatigue, palpitations, orthostatic hypotension, sedation, and urine retention. The SNRIs are generally better tolerated, the main side effects being nausea, vomiting, constipation, somnolence, dry mouth, sweating, loss of appetite, and sexual dysfunction.

Anticonvulsive Medications (Gabapentin and Pregabalin)

Gabapentin and pregabalin bind to the $\alpha_2\delta$ subunit of the voltage-dependent calcium channels and thus presynaptically reduce the release of glutamate and substance P, which in turn leads to reduced activation of postsynaptic nociceptive neurons [36]. In animal models of neuropathic pain, upregulation of $\alpha_2\delta$ subunits has been documented that corresponds to the degree of allodynia as well as to the analgesic effect of gabapentin [36]. Both drugs have the same mechanism of action, but pregabalin has a linear relationship between dose and plasma concentration, which makes titration to the proper dose easier. The drugs have a documented pain-relieving effect in neuropathic pain [10,37] and fibromyalgia [4,3,69]. The analgesic effects are not related to the anxiolytic effects of the drugs [3]. The main side effects of the anticonvulsants are dizziness, somnolence, and peripheral edema.

Practical Aspects of Pharmacotherapy

As mentioned earlier, the treatment of patients with long-term pain should always rely on the biopsychosocial pain model, which takes the complexity of pain into account [97]. The possibility of treating the cause of pain (with surgery or disease-modifying pharmacological treatments) must always be considered before entering the path of symptomatic pharmacological pain relief. Patients must be informed that the treatment is symptomatic so that they do not continue to take medication in the belief that it will somehow beneficially affect the medical condition. They should be encouraged to discontinue medication when the pain is no longer present, or if the drug has lost its analgesic effects. Other treatment options such as physical therapy, cognitive-behavioral therapy, and multiprofessional team rehabilitation should be considered as an alternative to, or in addition to, pharmacological treatment. It is important to realize that not all forms of chronic pain can be successfully treated with pharmacotherapy. One of the most difficult tasks of the pain physician is to withdraw ineffective pain medications even in the absence of other options for pharmacological pain relief. The choice of drugs relies on the intensity and type of pain to be treated, as well as on the effects of the pharmacological treatment.

Pharmacotherapy for Nociceptive Pain

The choice of pharmacological treatment of nociceptive pain relies mainly on pain intensity, although NSAIDS/coxibs are preferred over acetaminophen in inflammatory pain states. Acetaminophen, NSAIDs, and coxibs are used for low and moderate pain intensities, and if the analgesia they provide is insufficient, the weak opioids are added (due to the synergistic effects of these drugs). The pharmacological treatment of severe acute pain and severe cancer pain (and in certain circumstances severe nonmalignant chronic pain) relies on the combination of acetaminophen/NSAIDS/coxibs and strong opioids. The general principle is to use the weakest possible category of drugs that give adequate pain relief.

In treatment of acute pain, the choice of drugs relies on the expected pain intensity following an injury, an acute illness, or a medical procedure. Patients should be provided with a sufficient amount of pain medication for the expected duration of pain and should be carefully instructed when and how to discontinue treatment and whom to contact in case of problems.

The rationale for treating long-term nociceptive pain is to start with acetaminophen, or (for pain with inflammatory components) with NSAIDs or coxibs, taken at regular intervals. If analgesia is insufficient, a weak opioid is added. In cases when long-term treatment is likely, slow-release preparations of an opioid should be considered due to the lower risk of tolerance development and abuse potential. In patients with disturbed sleep due to nocturnal pain, slow-release preparations are preferred due to their longer effect duration (reducing the need for further analgesic intake at night). Patients on weak opioids who experience insufficient pain relief, yet have an analgesic effect with a clear dose-response relationship, can be considered for strong opioids (see the previous section). These patients are encouraged to continue with acetaminophen (or NSAIDs/coxibs) but to discontinue the weak opioid. Generally, the dose of the strong opioid is titrated to the lowest effective dose, and a slow-release preparation is preferred. In patients with long-term nonmalignant pain who are taking long-acting opioids, the use of short-acting opioids as rescue medications during pain exacerbation should be avoided (to reduce the risk of opioid tolerance and abuse).

The treatment of long-term nonmalignant pain with strong opioids increases the demands on the physician to monitor treatment effects. Treatment effects should be evaluated not only for reductions in pain, but also for improvements in function and quality of life [78]. It is the responsibility of the physician not only to inform the patient about potential side effects and risk of addiction, but also to have an understanding with the patient regarding the estimated duration of treatment and under which circumstances the treatment with strong opioids will be discontinued.

Pharmacotherapy for Dysfunctional Pain and Pain of Unknown Origin

Pain of unknown origin is difficult to treat because the pathophysiological mechanisms are unknown. Naturally, no drugs have the indication of treatment of pain of unknown origin, although tricyclic antidepressants such as amitryptiline are commonly used. Pharmacotherapy of dysfunctional pain, i.e., pain in patients with documented central hyperexcitability such as in fibromyalgia, has been studied in several randomized, double-blind, placebo-controlled trials. The recommended drugs are similar to those used for treatment of neuropathic pain, described below. A special difficulty arises when treating patients who initially had nociceptive pain (and responded to antinociceptive treatment) but who in time developed signs of central hyperexcitability (i.e., they probably developed dysfunctional pain). In these patients, the initially effective medication usually loses its pain-relieving effects, which is in accordance with animal studies showing a decreased effect of opioids in animals with central hyperexcitability [32]. The patients should be encouraged to discontinue the ineffective medication. Theoretically, such patients would be likely to respond to similar pharmacotherapeutic strategies to those used to treat the dysfunctional pain of fibromyalgia; however, randomized controlled trials are necessary before any treatment recommendations can be given.

Patients with fibromyalgia have dysfunctional pain, or according to the official classification of IASP, pain of unknown origin. As mentioned, a great number of randomized controlled trials have been completed in fibromyalgia patients, and treatment guidelines, including pharmacotherapy, have recently been published [21]. Tricyclic antidepressants, such as amitryptiline, have been shown to have a beneficial effect on pain, sleep, fatigue, stiffness, and tenderness [5] in fibromyalgia patients. Several double-blind, placebo-controlled studies have reported that SNRIs such as duloxetine [6,7] and milnacipran [43,95] reduce pain, tenderness, and stiffness and improve function and quality of life in fibromyalgia patients. These effects were independent of the baseline levels of anxiety or depression and did not relate to the improvement of these psychological symptoms [6,7]. The SSRIs lack convincing pain-relieving effects in fibromyalgia [73]. The anticonvulsants pregabalin [3,28,69] and gabapentin [4] have beneficial effects on pain, sleep, and fatigue in fibromyalgia patients. Currently pregabalin, duloxetine, and milnacipran are the only drugs approved for the indication of fibromyalgia. Combination treatments have not been evaluated in fibromyalgia, but in clinical practice the combination of SNRIs and anticonvulsants has shown promising potential, with good treatment effects and reduced side effects (due to lower doses).

Tramadol (used alone or in combination with acetaminophen) has been documented to relieve pain and improve function in fibromyalgia patients [14]. There are no data assessing the effects of acetaminophen (monotherapy), codeine, dextropropoxyphene, buprenorphine, or strong opioids in dysfunctional pain syndromes. The use of strong opioids to treat the pain in fibromyalgia is generally not recommended [21], although there are cultural differences in treatment traditions.

Pharmacotherapy for Neuropathic Pain

Treatment recommendations regarding peripheral neuropathic pain [10] mainly rely on studies of patients with painful diabetic polyneuropathy and herpes zoster, under the assumption that the same treatments will also be effective for other peripheral neuropathic pain states (with the exception of trigeminal neuralgia).

The first line of recommended treatments is tricyclic antidepressants or anticonvulsive medications (pregabalin or gabapentin). The second line of treatments is the SNRIs, topical lidocaine (for patients with small areas of mechanical allodynia), or tramadol. Strong opioids are the last choice. No differences in the treatment effects of tricyclic antidepressants and SNRIs have been found. SNRIs and anticonvulsive medications have positive effects on sleep and quality of life, in addition to their pain-relieving effects. The pain-relieving effects of the antidepressants are not dependent on the antidepressant (mood) effects of the drugs, nor do SSRIs have positive pain-relieving effects [65]. Most studies indicate a lower efficacy of opioids in neuropathic compared to nociceptive pain. Long-term follow-ups have indicated that only a minority of patients continue with strong opioids after 1 year, generally because of intolerable side effects [47]. The relative inefficacy of opioids for the treatment of neuropathic pain, compared to nociceptive pain, has been discussed. The reduction of spinal opioid receptors due to nerve damage, the presence of Aβ-fiber-mediated pain (which is not responsive to opioids), and increased cholecystokinin- and/or NMDA-dependent activity (i.e., central sensitization) have all been proposed as possible explanations.

Summary

Medical management of pain requires a careful examination of the pain problem to classify pain as nociceptive, neuropathic, or dysfunctional (or of unknown origin). Understanding the cause of the pain is essential to adequate treatment. A biopsychosocial approach is likely to be necessary with chronic pain conditions, particularly when they are complex and difficult to treat. The choice of pharmacological treatments depends on the intensity and type of pain treated, and the best approach is to use the weakest possible category of drugs that give adequate pain relief.

References

[1]   Affleck G, Tennen H, Urrows S, Higgins P. Individual differences in the day-to-day experi-
       ence of chronic pain: a prospective daily study of rheumatoid arthritis patients. Health Psychol
       1991;10:419–26.
[2]   Alford DP, Compton P, Samet JH. Acute pain management for patients receiving maintenance
       methadone or buprenorphine therapy. Ann Intern Med 2006;144:127–34.
[3]   Arnold L, Crofford L, Martin S, Young J, Sharma U. The effect of anxiety and depression on im-
       provements in pain in a randomized, controlled trial of pregabalin for treatment of fibromyalgia.
       Pain Med 2007;8:633–8.
[4]   Arnold LM, Goldenberg DL, Stanford SB, Lalonde JK, Sandhu HS, Keck PE, Welge JA, Bishop F,
       Stanford KE, Hess EV, et al. Gabapentin in the treatment of fibromyalgia. A randomized, double-
       blind, placebo-controlled, multicenter trial. Arthritis Rheum 2007;56:1336–44.
[5]   Arnold LM, Keck PE, Welge JA. Antidepressant treatment of fibromyalgia. Psychosomatics
       2000;41:104–13.
[6]   Arnold LM, Lu Y, Crofford LJ, Wohlreich M, Detke MJ, Iyengar S, Goldstein DJ; Duloxetine
       Fibromyalgia Trial Group. A double-blind, multicenter trial comparing duloxetine with placebo
       in the treatment of fibromyalgia patients with or without major depressive disorder. Arthritis
       Rheum 2004;50:2974–84.
[7]   Arnold LM, Rosen A, Pritchett YL, D'Souza DN, Goldstein DJ, Iyengar S, Wernicke JF. A ran-
       domized, double-blind, placebo-controlled trial of duloxetine in the treatment of women with
       fibromyalgia with or without major depressive disorder. Pain 2005;119:5–15.
[8]   Asmundson G, Norton GR, Allerdings MD. Fear and avoidance in dysfunctional chronic back
       pain patients. Pain 1997;69:231–6.
[9]   Asmundson G, Vlaeyen J, Crombez G. Understanding and treating fear of pain. Oxford: Oxford
       University Press; 2004.
[10]   Attal N, Cruccu G, Haanpää M, Hansson P, Jensen TS, Nurmikko T, Sampaio C, Sindrup S,
       Wiffen P. EFNS guidelines on pharmacological treatment of neuropathic pain. Eur J Neurol
       2006;13:1153–69.
[11]   Bajaj P, Bajaj P, Graven-Nielsen T, Arendt-Nielsen L. Osteoarthritis and its association with mus-
       cle hyperalgesia: an experimental controlled study. Pain 2001;93:107–14.
[12]   Baliki MN, Chialvo DR, Geha PY, Levy RM, Harden RN, Parrish TB, Apkarian AV. Chronic
       pain and the emotional brain: specific brain activity associated with spontaneous fluctuations of
       intensity of chronic back pain. J Neurosci 2006;26:12165–73.
[13]   Benedetti F, Amanzio M, Vighetti S, Asteggiano G. The biochemical and neuroendocrine bases
       of the hyperalgesic nocebo effect. J Neurosci 2006;26:12014–22.
[14]   Bennett R, Schein J, Kosinski M, Hewitt D, Jordan D, Rosenthal N. Impact of fibromyalgia pain
       on health-related quality of life before and after treatment with tramadol/acetaminophen. Ar-
       thritis Rheum 2005;15:519–27.
[15]   Besse D, Lombard MC, Perrot S, Besson JM. Regulation of opioid binding sites in the superficial
       dorsal horn of the rat spinal cord following loose ligation of the sciatic nerve: comparisons with
       sciatic nerve section and lumbar dorsal rhizotomy. Neuroscience 1992;50:921–33.
[16]   Besse D, Lombard MC, Zajac JM, Roques BP, Besson JM. Pre- and postsynaptic distribution of
       mu, delta and kappa opioid receptors in the superficial layers of the cervical dorsal horn of the
       rat spinal cord. Brain Res 1990;521:15–22.
[17]   Borg G. Psychophysical bases of perceived exertion. Med Sci Sports Exerc 1982;14:377–81.
[18]   Bruera E, Pereira J, Watanabe S, Belzile M, Kuehn N, Hanson J. Opioid rotation in patients with
       cancer pain. A retrospective comparison of dose ratios between methadone, hydromorphone,
       and morphine. Cancer 1996;78:852–7.
[19]   Brune K, Zeilhofer HU. Antipyretic analgesics: basic aspects. In: McMahon SB, Koltzenburg M,
       editors. Textbook of pain. Amsterdam: Elsevier; 2006. p. 459–69.
[20]   Caraco Y, Sheller J, Wood A. Pharmacogenetic determination of the effects of codeine and pre-
       diction of drug interactions. J Pharmacol Exp Ther 1996;278:1165–74.
[21]   Carville SF, Arendt-Nielsen L, Bliddal H, Blotman F, Branco JC, Buskila D, DaSilva JAP, Dan-
       neskiøld-Samsøe B, Dincer F, Henriksson C, et al. EULAR evidence based recommendations for
       the management of fibromyalgia syndrome. Ann Rheum Dis 2008;67:536–41.

[22] Chu LF, Clark DJ, Angst MS. Opioid tolerance and hyperalgesia in chronic pain patients after one month of oral opioid therapy: a preliminary prospective study. J Pain 2006;7:43–8.

[23] Clauw D. Fibromyalgia: update on mechanisms and management. J Clin Rheumatol 2007;13:102–9.

[24] Coghill RC, Sang CN, Maisog JM, Iadarda MJ. Pain intensity processing within the human brain: a bilateral, distributed mechanism. J Neurophysiol 1999;82:1934–43.

[25] Collett B. Opioid tolerance: the clinical perspective. Br J Anesth 1998;81:58–68.

[26] Compton P, Charuvastra VC, Kintaudi K, Ling W. Pain responses in methadone-maintained opioid abusers. J Pain Symptom Manage 2000;20:237–45.

[27] Compton P, Charuvastra VC, Ling W. Pain intolerance in opioid-maintained former opiate addicts: effect of long-acting maintenance agent. Drug Alcohol Depend 2001;63:139–46.

[28] Crofford LJ, Rowbotham MC, Mease PJ, Russell IJ, Dworkin RH, Corbin AE, Young JP, LaMoreaux LK, Martin SA, Sharmaand U; Pregabalin 1008-105 Study Group Pregabalin for the treatment of fibromyalgia syndrome. Arthritis Rheum 2005;52:1264–73.

[29] Curatolo M, Arendt-Nielsen L, Petersen-Felix S. Evidence, mechanisms, and clinical implications of central hypersensitivity in chronic pain after whiplash injury. Clin J Pain 2004;20:469–76.

[30] Curatolo M, Petersen-Felix S, Arendt-Nielsen L, Giani C, Zbinden AM, Radanov BP. Central hypersensitivity in chronic pain after whiplash injury. Clin J Pain 2001;17:306–15.

[31] Dickenson A. Where and how do opioids act? In: Gebhart G, Hammond D, Jensen T, editors. Proceedings of the 7th World Congress on Pain. Progress in pain research and management. Seattle: IASP Press; 1994. p. 525–52.

[32] Dickenson AH. Spinal cord pharmacology of pain. Br J Anaesth 1995;75:193–200.

[33] Doan BD, Wadden NP. Relationship between depressive symptoms and descriptions of chronic pain. Pain 1989;36:329–38.

[34] Doverty M, Somogyi AA, White JM, Blochner F, Beare CH, Menelaou A, Ling W. Methadone maintenance patients are cross-tolerant to the antinociceptive effects of morphine. Pain 2001;93:155–63.

[35] Doverty M, White JM, Somogyi AA, Bochner F, Ali R, Ling W. Hyperalgesic responses in methadone maintenance patients. Pain 2001;90:91–6.

[36] Field MJ, Cox PJ, Stott E, Melrose H, Offord J, Su T-Z, Bramwell S, Corradini L, England S, Winks J, et al. Identification of the alpha2-delta-1 subunit of voltage-dependant calcium channels as a molecular target for pain mediating the analgesic actions of pregabalin. Proc Natl Acad Sci USA 2006;103:17537–42.

[37] Freynhagen R, Strojek K, Griesing T, Whalen E, Balkenohl M. Efficacy of pregabalin in neuropathic pain evaluated in a 12-week, randomised, double-blind, multicenter, placebo-controlled trial of flexible- and fixed-dose regimens. Pain 2005;115:254–63.

[38] Giesecke T, Gracely RH, Grant MAB, Nachemson A, Petzke F, Williams DA, Clauw DJ. Evidence of augmented central pain processing in idiopathic chronic low back pain. Arthritis Rheum 2004;50:613–23.

[39] Glynn C, Mather L. Clinical pharmacokinetics applied to patients with intractable pain: studies with pethidine. Pain 1982;13:237–46.

[40] Gracely R, Petzke F, Wolf J, Clauw D. Functional magnetic imaging evidence of augmented pain processing in fibromyalgia. Arthritis Rheum 2002;6:1333–43.

[41] Graven-Nielsen T, Arendt-Nielsen L, Svensson P, Jensen TS. Experimental muscle pain: a quantitative study of local and referred pain in humans following injection of hypertonic saline. J Musculoskel Pain 1997;5:49–69.

[42] Graven-Nielsen T, Arendt-Nielsen L, Svensson P, Jensen TS. Quantification of local and referred muscle pain in humans after sequential i.m. injections of hypertonic saline. Pain 1997;69:111–7.

[43] Grendreau RM, Thorn MD, Grendreau JF, Kranzler JD, Ribeiro S, Gracely RH, Williams DA, Mease PJ, McLean SA, Clauw DJ. Efficacy of milnacipran in patients with fibromyalgia. J Rheumatol 2005;32:1975–85.

[44] Hansson P, Backonja M, Bouhassira D. Usefulness and limitations of quantitative sensory testing: clinical and research application in neuropathic pain states. Pain 2007;129:256–9.

[45] Hebb ALO, Poulin J-F, Roach SP, Zacharko RM, Drolet G. Cholecystokinin and endogenous opioid peptides: interactive influence on pain, cognition, and emotion. Prog Neuropsychopharmacol Biol Psychiatry 2005;29:1225–38.

[46] Johnson RE, Fudala PJ, Payne R. Buprenorphine: considerations for pain management. J Pain Symptom Manage 2005;29:297–326.

[47] Kalso E, Edwards J, Moore R, McQuay H. Opioids in chronic non-cancer pain: systemic review of efficacy and safety. Pain 2004;112:372–80.

[48] Kasch H, Qerama E, Bach FW, Jensen TS. Reduced cold pressor pain tolerance in non-recovered whiplash patients: a 1-year prospective study. Eur J Pain 2005;9:561–9.

[49] Koelbaek-Johansen M, Graven-Nielsen T, Olesen AS, Arendt-Nielsen L. Generalised muscular hyperalgesia in chronic whiplash syndrome. Pain 1999;83:229–34.

[50] Koob G, LeMoal M. Opioids. In: Neurobiology of addiction. Amsterdam: Elsevier; 2006. p. 121–71.

[51] Kosek E, Ekholm J, Hansson P. Sensory dysfunction in fibromyalgia patients with implications for pathogenic mechanisms. Pain 1996;68:375–83.

[52] Kosek E, Hansson P. Modulatory influence on somatosensory perception from vibration and heterotopic noxious conditioning stimulation (HNCS) in fibromyalgia patients and healthy subjects. Pain 1997;70:41–51.

[53] Kosek E, Ordeberg G. Abnormalities of somatosensory perception in patients with painful osteoarthritis normalize following successful treatment. Eur J Pain 2000;4:229–38.

[54] Kosek E, Ordeberg G. Lack of pressure pain modulation by heterotopic noxious conditioning stimulation in patients with painful osteoarthritis before, but not following, surgical pain relief. Pain 2000;88:69–78.

[55] Kosek E, Hansson P. The influence of experimental pain intensity in the local and referred pain area on somatosensory perception in the area of referred pain. Eur J Pain 2002;6:413–25.

[56] Kosek E, Hansson P. Perceptual integration of intramuscular electrical stimulation in the focal and the referred pain area in healthy humans. Pain 2003;105:125–31.

[57] Kosek E, Januszewska A. Mechanisms of pain referral in patients with whiplash associated disorder. Eur J Pain 2008;12:650–60.

[58] Kulkarni B, Bentley DE, Elliott R, Julyan PJ, Boger E, Watson A, Boyle Y, El-Deredy W, Jones AKP. Arthritic pain is processed in brain areas concerned with emotions and fear. Arthritis Rheum 2007;56:1345–54.

[59] Lautenbacher S, Rollman GB. Possible deficiencies of pain modulation in fibromyalgia. Clin J Pain 1997;13:189–96.

[60] Leffler A-S, Kosek E, Hansson P. The influence of pain intensity on somatosensory perception in patients suffering from subacute/chronic lateral epicondylalgia. Eur J Pain 2000;4:57–71.

[61] Leffler A-S, Hansson P, Kosek E. Somatosensory perception in patients suffering from long-term trapezius myalgia at the site overlying the most painful part of the muscle and an area of pain referral. Eur J Pain 2003;7:267–76.

[62] Macefield V, Gandevia S, Henderson L. Discrete changes in cortical activation during experimentally induced referred muscle pain: a single-trial fMRI study. Cereb Cortex 2007;17:2050–9.

[63] Maixner W, Fillingim R, Booker D, Sigurdsson A. Sensitivity of patients with painful temporomandibular disorders to experimentally evoked pain. Pain 1995;63:341–51.

[64] Mao J. Opioid-induced abnormal pain sensitivity. Curr Pain Headache Rep 2006;10:67–70.

[65] Max MB, Lynch SA, Muir J, Shoaf SE, Smoller B, Dubner R. Effects of desipramine, amitriptyline, and fluoxetine on pain in diabetic neuropathy. N Engl J Med 1992;326:1250–6.

[66] McCracken LM. A contextual analysis of attention to chronic pain: what the patient does with their pain might be more important than their awareness of vigilance alone. J Pain 2007;8:230–6.

[67] McCracken LM, Samuel VM. The role of avoidance, pacing and other activity patterns in chronic pain. Pain 2007;130:119–25.

[68] McCracken LM, Vowles KE, Gauntlett-Gilbert J. A prospective investigation of acceptance and control-oriented coping with chronic pain. J Behav Med 2007;30:339–49.

[69] Mease PJ, Russell IJ, Arnold LM, Florian H, Young JP, Martin SA, Sharma U. A randomized, double-blind, placebo-controlled, phase III trial of pregabalin in the treatment of patients with fibromyalgia. J Rheumatol 2008;35:502–14.

[70] Melzack R, Casey K. Sensory, motivational and central control determinants of pain: a new conceptual model. In: Kenshalo D, editor. The skin senses. Springfield: CC Thomas; 1968. p. 423–43.

[71] Merskey H, Bogduk N. Classification of chronic pain. Seattle: IASP Press; 1994.

[72] Meyers S, Flusser D, Brandth K, Heck D. Prevalence of cartilage shards in synovium and their association with synovitis in patients with early and end stage osteoarthritis. J Rheumatol 1992;19:1247–51.

[73] O'Malley PG, Balden E, Tomkins G, Santoro J, Kroenke K, Jackson JL. Treatment of fibromyalgia with antidepressants. A meta-analysis. J Gen Intern Med 2000;15:659–66.

[74] Nicholson B. Benefits of extended-release opioid analgesic formulations in the treatment of chronic pain. Pain Practice 2009;9:71–81.

[75] Pud D, Cohen D, Lawental E, Eisenberg E. Opioids and abnormal pain perception: New evidence from a study of chronic opioid addicts and healthy subjects. Drug Alcohol Depend 2006;82:218–23.

[76] Schug SA, Zech D, Grond S, Jung H, Meuser T, Stobbe B. A long-term survey of morphine in cancer pain patients. J Pain Symptom Manage 1992;7:259–66.

[77] Schug S, Zech D, Grond S. Adverse effects of systemic opioid analgesics. Drug Safety 1992;7:200–13.

[78] Schug S, Gandham N. Opioids: clinical use. In: McMahon S, Koltzenburg M, editors. Textbook of pain. Elsevier; 2006. p. 443–57.

[79] Schweinhardt P, Kalk N, Wartolowska K, Chessell I, Wordsworth P, Tracey I. Investigation into the neural correlates of emotional augmentation of clinical pain. Neuroimage 2008;40:759–66.

[80] Scott D, Jull G, Sterling M. Widespread sensory hypersensitivity is a feature of chronic whiplash-associated disorder but not chronic idiopathic neck pain. Clin J Pain 2005;21:175–81.

[81] Sorensen J, Graven-Nielsen T, Henriksson KG, Bengtsson M, Arendt-Nielsen L. Hyperexcitability in fibromyalgia. J. Rheumatol 1998;25:152–5.

[82] Staud R, Cannon R, Mauderli A, Robinson M, Price D, Vierck C. Temporal summation of pain from mechanical stimulation of muscle tissue in normal controls and subjects with fibromyalgia syndrome. Pain 2003;102:87–95.

[83] Staud R, Vierck CJ, Cannon RL, Mauderli AP, Price DD. Abnormal sensitization and temporal summation of second pain (wind-up) in patients with fibromyalgia syndrome. Pain 2001;91:165–75.

[84] Stein C, Hassan AHS, Lehrberger K, Giefing J, Yassouridis A. Local analgesic effect of endogenous opioid peptides. Lancet 1993;342:321–4.

[85] Sterling M, Jull G, Vicenzino B, Kenardy J. Sensory hypersensitivity occurs soon after whiplash injury and is associated with poor recovery. Pain 2003;104:509–17.

[86] Sterling M, Jull G, Kenardy J. Physical and psychological factors maintain long-term predictive capacity post-whiplash injury. Pain 2006;122:102–8.

[87] Sterling M, Kenardy J. The relationship between sensory and sympathetic nervous system changes and posttraumatic stress reaction following whiplash injury: a prospective study. J Psychosom Res 2006;60:387–93.

[88] Sullivan MJ, Thorn B, Haythornthwaite JA, Keefe F, Martin M, Bradley LA, Lefebvre JC. Theoretical perspectives on the relation between catastrophizing and pain. Clin J Pain 2001;17:52–64.

[89] Thompson P, Carr A. Pain in the rheumatic diseases. Ann Rheum Dis 1997;56:395.

[90] Thomsen A, Becker N, Eriksen J. Opioid rotation in chronic non-malignant pain patients. A retrospective study. Acta Anesthesiol Scand 1999;43:918–23.

[91] Travell J, Simons D. Myofascial pain and dysfunction. In: Travell J, Simons D. The trigger point manual. Baltimore: Williams and Wilkins; 1983.

[92] Treede R-D, Jensen TS, Campbell JN, Cruccu G, Dostrovsky JO, Griffin JW, et al. Neuropathic pain. Redefinition and a grading system for clinical and research purposes. Neurology 2008;70:1630–5.

[93] Turk D, Okifuji A, Sinclair J, Starz T. Differential responses by psychosocial subgroups of fibromyalgia syndrome patients to an interdisciplinary treatment. Arthritis Care Res 1998;11:397–404.

[94] Vecchiet L, Dragani L, Bigontina PD, Obletter G, Giamberardino MA. Experimental referred pain and hyperalgesia from muscles in humans. In: Vecchiet L, Albe-Fessard D, Lindblom U, Giamberardino MA, editors. New trends in referred pain and hyperalgesia. Amsterdam: Elsevier; 1993. p. 239–49.

[95] Vitton O, Gendreau M, Gendreau J, Kranzler J, Rao S. A double-blind placebo-controlled trial of milnacipran in the treatment of fibromyalgia. Hum Psychopharmacol 2004;19:S27–35.

[96] Vlaeyen JW, Linton SJ. Fear-avoidance and its consequences in chronic musculoskeletal pain: a state of the art. Pain 2000;85:317–32.

[97] Waddell G. A new clinical model for the treatment of low back pain. Spine 1987;12:632–44.

[98] Watson C, Chipman M, Monks R. Antidepressant analgesics: a systematic review and comparative study. In: McMahon S, Koltzenburg M, editors. Textbook of pain. Amsterdam: Elsevier; 2006. p. 481–97.

[99] World Health Organization. Cancer pain relief and palliative care. Geneva: World Health Organization; 1996.

[100] World Health Organization. International statistical classification of diseases and related health problems, 10th revision. Geneva: World Health Organization, 1992.

Correspondence to: Associate Prof. Eva Kosek, MD, Department of Clinical Neuroscience, Karolinska Institute, MR-Center N8:00, Karolinska University Hospital, 171 76 Stockholm, Sweden. Email: eva.kosek@ki.se.

Psychological Approaches in Pain Management

Dennis C. Turk and Hilary D. Wilson

Department of Anesthesiology, University of Washington, Seattle, Washington, USA

Effective treatments for patients with chronic pain have not kept pace with advances in understanding of anatomy and neurophysiology. Despite the development of potent medications, sophisticated neuroaugmentation technologies (e.g., spinal cord stimulators), advanced surgical procedures, and a diverse set of somatic treatments (e.g., transcutaneous electric nerve stimulation, diathermy), most people with chronic pain continue to experience significant levels of pain regardless of the treatments they receive [6,44]. Chronic pain, similar to other chronic diseases, makes significant demands on people's lives, and those affected vary widely in how well they cope with the demands that confront them, adapt to the symptoms, and accommodate to the limitations imposed.

An expansive literature demonstrates the important contributions of psychosocial and behavioral factors to symptom onset, magnification, maintenance, accommodation, and response to treatment [13]. Based on current understanding of the roles of cognitive, affective, and behavioral factors, a set of psychological approaches and treatments have been developed to assist in symptom management and to foster adaptation. Many

Mechanisms and Management of Pain for the Physical Therapist
edited by Kathleen A. Sluka
IASP Press, Seattle, © 2009

of these approaches have long histories (e.g., hypnosis, psychotherapy) in the treatment of people with chronic pain. These treatments have been applied to a number of chronic pain diagnoses (Table I).

Although psychological approaches have been used as alternatives to pharmacological and somatic treatments, in most circumstances they are used in conjunction with traditional medical interventions and as integrative components within comprehensive, multidisciplinary rehabilitation programs. In this chapter we will emphasize an important distinction between psychological perspectives on chronic pain and specific psychological treatments, provide a description of the predominant psychological perspectives and most commonly used methods, and review the evidence for the effectiveness of the various techniques for a diverse set of diagnoses (see Table I). Due to space limitations, we will only be able to highlight central features of the perspectives and treatment methods.

Table I
Psychological treatment studies

Diagnosis	No. Studies	No. Patients
RA	13	837
Low back pain	11	601
TMD pain	11	457
Mixed	8	416
OA	5	313
OA/RA	2	1350
Fibromyalgia	2	171
Upper-limb pain	2	193
Disability-related pain	1	33
Sickle cell disease	1	37
Total	56	4378

Source: Adapted from meta-analyses and systematic reviews [8,23,32].
Note: These data do not include studies in which psychological approaches are integrated within comprehensive rehabilitation programs. The primary outcomes in these studies are pain reduction; some also included outcomes related to physical and emotional functioning. OA = osteoarthritis; RA = rheumatoid arthritis; TMD = temporomandibular disorders.

Distinction between Psychological Approaches and Psychosocial Treatments

Several prominent psychological perspectives have guided much of the thinking about chronic pain and subsequent treatments that have evolved, in particular the (1) psychodynamic, (2) operant conditioning (behavioral), and (3) cognitive-behavioral perspectives. In addition to treatments that are directly related to these perspectives, a set of treatment techniques have been developed that are often combined (e.g., biofeedback plus relaxation; hypnosis plus guided imagery plus relaxation) and that may not be directly associated with any one perspective (e.g., hypnosis or biofeedback). The characteristics of these treatments are briefly highlighted in Table II. We will provide an overview of each of these perspectives and treatment

Table II
Psychological interventions

Psychodynamic Therapy: Focus on uncovering unresolved conflicts that are believed to contribute to pain.

Behavior Therapy: A managed approach to behavior change using the basic concepts and principles of behavioral psychology.

Cognitive-Behavioral Therapy (CBT): Primary focus on changing cognitive activity to achieve changes in behavior, thoughts, and emotions. Two broad classes are: (1) coping skills training and (2) cognitive therapy.

Relaxation: Attempts to teach patients how to reduce general levels of physiological arousal or arousal in a specific body part or location (e.g., autogenic training, progressive muscle relaxation).

Biofeedback: Involves measuring an individual's quantifiable bodily functions (e.g., blood pressure, heart rate, skin temperature, sweat gland activity, muscle tension, and electrical activity in the brain) using noninvasive electrical devices that record and amplify physiological signals and conveying the information to the patient in real time. The intent is to raise the patient's awareness and conscious control of his/her unconscious physiological activities. By giving patients access to physiological information about which they are generally unaware, biofeedback allows patients to gain control of physical processes previously considered an automatic response of the autonomic nervous system that may exacerbate their pain.

Hypnosis/Hypnotherapy: The patient is guided by the hypnotherapist to respond to suggestions for changes in subjective experience, perceptions, sensations, thoughts, or behavior. This approach teaches skills that are designed to alter the experience of pain and suffering outside the therapy session.

Meditation: The "intentional self-regulation of attention," a systematic inner focus on particular aspects of inner and outer experience.

strategies and describe the treatments that have been developed that follow from the conceptual models (Table III). However, it is important to acknowledge that the perspectives themselves are quite broad and may include any number of cognitive, behavioral, or psychotherapeutic techniques.

Perhaps more important than the details of each technique are the specific objectives that each of the techniques is used to accomplish (e.g., to increase perception of control, extinguish maladaptive behaviors, or uncover unconscious motivation). The same technique, however, may be used to accomplish different or overlapping objectives. For example, exposure to avoided activities, a common component of operant conditioning treatments, may be conceptualized as a way to help patients learn that the performance of previously avoided activities may not produce the anticipated negative consequences (e.g., promote pain or exacerbate injury). Thus, exposure treatment can provide corrective feedback. From this perspective, the treatment is designed to alter the reinforcement contingencies—activity is not punished by pain, and thus avoidance of activity will be extinguished. However, exposure might also be viewed from a cognitive-behavioral perspective, whereby it is conceptualized as a way to help patients increase their sense of self-efficacy by providing success in performance of previously avoided tasks and reduce anticipation of pain or injury following performance of the activity. In this conceptualization, the use of a behavioral technique is designed not only to change behavior but to change patients' beliefs about themselves and their capabilities. Of course, these two mechanisms are not mutually exclusive.

Table III
Psychological perspectives and illustrative treatments

Perspective	Techniques
Psychodynamic perspective	Insight-orient psychotherapy
Behavioral perspectives	Reinforcement, pacing, goal-setting, exposure, relaxation
Cognitive-behavioral perspective	Cognitive restructuring, problem solving, coping skills training, acceptance
Other	Motivational interviewing, biofeedback, hypnosis, imagery, meditation, supportive counseling

Note: A number of the techniques listed may be used in more than one perspective, with the intent varying. The techniques listed under "other" can be used independently of any particular theoretical perspective or in combination.

Similarly, biofeedback may be viewed as a means of modifying some maladaptive physiological response, but practicing biofeedback may also change patients' perceptions of control over their bodies, whether or not it actually influences physiological mechanisms believed to be associated with the presence of pain. Throughout the remainder of this chapter, it is important to keep in mind the distinction between the psychological perspectives underlying treatment and the details of the treatment modalities themselves.

The Psychodynamic Perspective

Theoretical Perspective

From the psychodynamic perspective, symptoms serve a purpose, and treatment is designed to help the patient identify the unconscious meaning of symptoms that occur in the absence of or in disproportion to physical pathology. Sigmund Freud proposed that the underlying motivational force is the gratification of biologically based, instinctual drives. In classical psychoanalysis, chronic pain that cannot be accounted for by tissue damage can be viewed as the result of an unconscious drive that the individual is unable to gratify in a socially acceptable manner. When such repressed urges threaten to emerge into consciousness, severe anxiety results, and the resolution, however maladaptive it may appear to be, is a psychic compromise that can include the development of physical and emotional symptoms that protect the patient from the trauma created by the awareness of unacceptable drives. In short, symptoms serve a purpose.

Insight-Oriented Treatment

Insight-oriented approaches are predicated on the belief that chronic physical pain may be a somatic presentation of emotional distress and that nonconscious factors will influence both the onset and maintenance of symptoms. Psychodynamic therapy is most commonly used when psychosocial risk factors appear to play a role in pain symptoms, when emotional changes occur during severe and protracted pain, or when the goals of therapy are not only to relieve symptoms of pain, but also to promote long-term adaptation [4].

The overriding goal of psychoanalytic treatment is for patients first to become aware of and later to renounce unconscious impulses and conflicts and then to obtain partial gratification through sublimation in adult roles and relationships. Attempts are made to help patients gain insights into the reasons that pain developed and persists. Maintenance of symptoms may serve as a means of protecting the patient from unacceptable impulses or to obtain some benefit such as support or avoidance of undesirable interactions.

Although insight-oriented psychotherapy may be useful with selected individuals [4], to our knowledge, no randomized controlled trials have been published demonstrating its efficacy for people with chronic pain problems. Although the model described may be applicable in specific circumstances, the usefulness of insight-oriented psychotherapy for patients with chronic pain seems limited.

Operant Conditioning

Theoretical Perspective

In the operant formulation, pain is a subjective experience that can never be viewed directly. Thus, behavioral manifestations of pain—"pain behaviors"—that are observable are key, rather than pain per se. The model proposes that through external contingencies of reinforcement, acute pain behaviors, such as limping to protect a wounded limb from producing additional nociceptive input, can evolve into chronic pain problems. Pain behaviors may be positively reinforced directly, for example, by attention from a spouse or health care provider. They may also be maintained by negative reinforcement through the escape from noxious stimulation by using drugs, resting, or avoiding other activities the patient may consider undesirable, such as work or exercise (Table IV).

In addition, "well behaviors" (e.g., working, exercising) may not be sufficiently reinforced. This lack of reinforcement allows more rewarding pain behaviors to be maintained. Pain behaviors originally elicited by organic factors may respond to reinforcement from environmental events. Fordyce [12] proposed that for this reason, pain behaviors might persist long after the initial cause of the pain is resolved or greatly reduced. The operant conditioning model does not concern itself with the initial cause

Table IV
Operant schedules of reinforcement

Schedule	Consequences	Probability of Behavior Recurring
Positive reinforcement	Reward the behavior	More likely
Negative reinforcement	Prevent or withdraw aversive results	More likely
Punishment	Punish the behavior	Less likely
Neglect	Prevent or withdraw positive results	Less likely

of pain. Rather, it considers pain an internal subjective experience that may be maintained even after its initial physical basis is resolved.

The emphasis on maintaining factors shares some overlap with the psychodynamic perspective. The difference, however, is that from the psychodynamic perspective, symptoms are associated with intrapsychic conflicts, whereas from the operant perspective, maintenance and generalization result from reinforcement contingencies, as described below.

Operant Treatment

Operant approaches focus on the extinction of pain behaviors. Therapists focus on withdrawal of positive attention for pain behaviors while increasing positive reinforcement of well behaviors (e.g., activity). The operant paradigm does not seek to uncover the etiology of symptoms but focuses on the maintenance of pain behaviors and the deficiency of well behaviors. In treatment, pain behaviors are identified, as are their controlling antecedents and consequent reinforcers or punishments [34], such as overly solicitous behaviors by a spouse [37,41].

The efficacy of operant treatment has been demonstrated in a number of studies of persons with various chronic pain disorders, including low back pain [e.g., 51,53] and fibromyalgia syndrome [40]. Based on a meta-analysis of treatment studies for chronic pain, Morley, Eccleston, and Williams [32] reported that the effect size of behavior therapy varied for different outcomes ranging from 0.33 for pain reduction to 0.62 for affective distress, other than depression, where the effect size was quite small and negative (−0.14) compared to control treatments, often standard care (see Tables V and VI).

Table V
Effectiveness of behavior therapy versus a waiting-list
control condition

Domain	N	Mean ES	95% CI	Z
Pain experience	5	0.32	−0.09–0.55	2.73
Mood/depression	4	−0.03	−0.21–0.15	−0.33
Mood/other	2	0.74	0.41–1.08	4.34
Cognitive coping and negative appraisal	1	1.41	(±0.41)*	(3.79)
Cognitive coping and positive appraisal	1	0.56	(±0.37)*	(1.51)
Behavioral expression	5	0.45	0.31–0.59	6.28
Behavioral activity	2	0.54	0.28–0.79	4.12
Social role functioning and interference	4	0.34	0.17–0.51	3.90

Source: Adapted from Morley et al. [32].
Abbreviations: CI = confidence interval; ES = effect size; N = number of studies.
* Figures in parentheses in the 95% CI column are the standard errors for a single effect size.

Table VI
Effectiveness of behavior therapy versus treatment controls

Domain	N	Mean ES	95% CI	Z
Pain experience	4	0.33	−0.04–0.71	1.70
Mood/depression	4	−0.14	−0.38–0.11	−1.07
Mood/other	2	0.62	−0.55–1.79	1.03
Cognitive coping and negative appraisal	2	0.53	−0.16–1.22	1.53
Cognitive coping and positive appraisal	2	−0.13	−0.55–0.29	−0.61
Behavioral expression	2	0.06	−0.02–0.10	3.11
Behavioral activity	0	–	–	–
Social role functioning and interference	4	0.37	0.17–0.58	3.61

Source: Adapted from Morley et al. [32].
Abbreviations: CI = confidence interval; ES = effect size; N = number of studies.

The Cognitive-Behavioral Perspective

Theoretical Perspective

From the cognitive-behavioral perspective, thoughts and emotions are thought to play a key role in potentiating and maintaining stress and physical symptoms (Table VII). Patients are assumed to have negative perceptions regarding their abilities and to lack adequate coping skills to manage both physical and emotional stressors. These ineffective coping mechanisms have been developed over a lifetime of experience and become automatic, and thus the overarching goal of therapy is to help patients identify these negative perceptions, improve their coping skills, and increase self-efficacy beliefs.

Table VII
Assumptions of the cognitive-behavioral perspective

People are active processors of information and not passive reactors

Thoughts (e.g., appraisals, expectancies, and beliefs) can elicit and influence mood, affect physiological processes, have social consequences, and also serve as an impetus for behavior; conversely, mood, physiology, environmental factors, and behavior can influence the nature and content of thought processes

Behavior is reciprocally determined both by the individual and by environmental factors

People can learn more adaptive ways of thinking, feeling, and behaving

People should be active collaborative agents in changing their thoughts, feelings, behavior, and physiology

Source: Adapted from Turk and Meichenbaum [48].

Cognitive-Behavioral Treatment

One of the problems describing cognitive-behavioral therapy (CBT) is that it has become a generic term that includes a range of different cognitive and behavioral techniques. We describe the general approach to treatment from the general cognitive-behavioral perspective; however, while the perspective remains constant, the specific techniques and modalities that are used may vary substantially.

Four key components of CBT have been described [45]: (1) education, (2) skills acquisition, (3) skills consolidation, and (4) generalization and maintenance. The "education" component focuses on helping patients challenge their negative perceptions regarding their abilities. It helps patients to manage pain through "cognitive restructuring," by making them aware of the role that thoughts and emotions play in potentiating and maintaining stress and physical symptoms. Cognitive restructuring includes identification of maladaptive thoughts during problematic situations (e.g., during pain exacerbations or stressful events), introduction and practice of coping thoughts and behaviors, shifting from self-defeating to coping thoughts, practicing positive thoughts, and home practice and follow-up. The therapist encourages patients to test the adaptiveness of their thoughts, beliefs, expectations, and predictions. The crucial element is bringing about a shift in the patient's repertoire from well-established, habitual, and automatic but ineffective responses toward systematic problem-solving and planning, control of affect, behavioral persistence, and disengagement from self-defeating situations when appropriate.

The goal of "skills acquisition" and "consolidation" is to help people learn and, importantly, practice, new pain management behaviors and cognitions, including relaxation, problem solving, distraction methods, activity pacing, and communication. Therapists use education, didactic instruction, Socratic questioning, and role-playing techniques, among other strategies. The techniques, however, are less important than the general message of self-management that is derived from experience using various techniques (some of which are described below). Patients may learn best from observing the outcomes of their own efforts rather than by instruction alone. Often CBT is carried out in a group context, where the therapist can use the support of other patients and also have patients interact with each other to assist in providing alternative ways of thinking and behaving.

Finally, "generalization and maintenance" are geared toward solidifying skills and preventing relapse. Homework is an essential ingredient of CBT. Once patients have been taught and have practiced self-management skills within the therapeutic context, it is essential that they practice them in their home environment where the therapist is not present to guide and support them. The difficulties that will inevitably arise when these attempts are made at home become important topics for discussion and further problem solving during therapeutic encounters. In this phase, therapists assist patients to anticipate future problems and high-risk situations so that they can think about and practice the behavioral responses that may be necessary for adaptive coping. The goal during this phase, then, is to enable patients to develop a problem-solving perspective where they believe that they have the skills and competencies to respond in appropriate ways to problems as they arise. In this manner, attempts are made to help patients learn to anticipate future difficulties, develop plans for adaptive responding, and adjust their behavior accordingly.

A wealth of evidence shows that CBT can help to restore function as well as reduce pain and disability-related behaviors [29,32]. Overall effective sizes compared to treatment controls have ranged from 0.26 for pain reduction to 0.55 for improved coping. Few studies have directly compared the efficacy of CBT with and without standard care, which often consists of medication and physical therapy.

With this overview of the CBT approach, we will discuss specific techniques that can be incorporated with CBT and operant behavior therapy. To reiterate, the primary objective of these techniques is enhancement of patients' sense of self-efficacy by increasing a sense of control to combat the feelings of helplessness and demoralization often felt by people with chronic pain.

Additional Psychological Approaches

Relaxation

Many relaxation techniques exist, and there is a long history of their use in health care. The literature is inconsistent as to which techniques are the most effective, and there is no evidence that any one method is more effective than any other. Moreover, the different components may be synergistic. The key message to the patient is that a broad spectrum of approaches are available, and no particular method is more efficacious. Common approaches involve the use of breathing techniques and guided imagery to help patients obtain a state of relaxation. It is most important to help patients learn which approach will be most helpful by trying a variety of techniques. Clinicians may also note that no one technique is effective for all people all of the time; hence, knowledge of a range of methods may be the best approach. It is important to acknowledge that these methods are skills that require practice to become more proficient. Other than in treatment of chronic headache, relaxation is most commonly used as one modality within a comprehensive treatment plan.

Guided Imagery

Although guided imagery is a common component of relaxation exercises, it is also used to help patients achieve a sense of control and, importantly, distract themselves from pain and accompanying symptoms. This modality involves the generation of different mental images, evoked either by oneself or with the help of the practitioner. When patients with chronic pain are experiencing pain exacerbation, they can use imagery with the goals of redirecting their attention away from their pain and achieving a psychophysiological state of relaxation. The most successful images involve all of the senses (vision, sound, touch, smell, and taste). Some people, however, may have difficulty generating images and may find it helpful to listen to a taped description or purchase a poster on which to focus their attention as a way of assisting their imagination.

Although guided imagery has been advocated as a stand-alone intervention to reduce presurgical anxiety and postsurgical pain, and to accelerate healing [18], it is most often used in conjunction with other treatment interventions such as relaxation and as a coping strategy taught within the context of CBT.

Biofeedback

Biofeedback is a self-regulatory technique. The assumption with regard to biofeedback treatment is that the level of pain is maintained or exacerbated by autonomic nervous system dysregulation, which is believed to be associated with the production of nociceptive stimulation. The primary objective of biofeedback is to teach people to exert control over their physiological processes to assist in re-regulating the autonomic nervous system. When people are treated with biofeedback, they receive information about their physiological processes via biofeedback equipment, and they are taught through this feedback to regulate these processes. These monitored physiological processes may include skin conductance, respiration, heart rate, heart rate variability, skin temperature, brain wave activity, and muscle tension. In addition to the physiological changes that can result from biofeedback, patients gain a sense of control over their bodies. Given the high level of helplessness observed in people with chronic pain problems, the perception of control may be as important as the actual physiological changes observed [e.g., 22].

Biofeedback has been used successfully to treat a number of chronic pain states such as migraine and tension-type headaches, back pain, chronic myofascial pain, temporomandibular disorders, irritable bowel syndrome, and fibromyalgia, either as primary treatment or within the broader context of CBT integrated within rehabilitation programs [3,14,30,33]. In one recent meta-analysis of biofeedback for migraine, Nestoriuc and Martin [33] included 55 studies that they judged to be of relatively high quality and found an effect size of 0.58 for prevention of migraine episodes compared to control conditions. What is particularly impressive is that these results were maintained for up to 17 months following treatment. Several studies have compared biofeedback to prophylactic migraine medication (propranolol) and found that biofeedback was as effective as the medication, with the two treatments having a synergistic effect [20]. The effect sizes for biofeedback for diagnoses other than chronic headache are also impressive, although the number of studies is much smaller. Morley et al. [32] determined that for pain, the effect sizes for biofeedback compared to a control condition were moderate at 0.52 (based on only one study).

Meditation

Meditation is defined as the "intentional self-regulation of attention," a systematic inner focus on particular aspects of inner and outer experience [15]. There are many forms of meditation, although most research has focused on transcendental meditation (TM) and Zen or mindfulness meditation [1].

TM requires concentration; it involves focusing any one of the senses, like a zoom lens, on a specific object. For example, the individual repeats a silent word or phrase ("mantra") with the goal of transcending the ordinary stream of thought [2,3]. Mindfulness meditation is the opposite of TM in that its goal is attempting awareness of the whole perceptual field, like a wide-angle lens. Thus, it incorporates focused attention and whole-field awareness in the present moment. For example, the individual observes without judgment his or her thoughts, emotions, sensations, and perceptions as they arise moment by moment [24,25]. Bonadonna [5] proposed that individuals with chronic illness have an altered ability to concentrate; therefore, TM may be less useful than mindfulness meditation when one is sick. Mindfulness meditation reframes the experience of discomfort in that physical pain or suffering becomes the object of meditation. Attention and awareness of discomfort or suffering is another part of human experience; as such, rather than be avoided it is to be experienced and explored [5].

Meditation has captured the attention of medicine, psychology, and neurocognitive sciences. This interest has arisen in part because experienced meditators demonstrate reduced arousal to daily stress, better performance of tasks that require focused attention, and other health benefits [26,27]. Studies have found that when combined with other therapies, mindfulness-based interventions have decreased pain symptoms, increased healing speed, improved mood, reduced stress, contained health care costs, and decreased visits to primary care [3,16]. However, it is premature to draw any conclusions from the few small outcomes studies that have been reported.

Hypnosis

Hypnosis has been defined as a natural state of aroused, attentive focal concentration coupled with a relative suspension of peripheral awareness. There are three central components in hypnosis: (1) absorption, or the intense involvement in the central object of concentration; (2) dissociation, where experiences that would commonly be experienced consciously occur outside of conscious awareness; and (3) suggestibility, in which persons are more likely to accept outside input without cognitive censoring or criticism [39].

Hypnosis has been used as a treatment intervention for pain control at least since the 1850s. It has been shown to be beneficial in relieving pain for people with headache, burn injury, arthritis, cancer, and chronic back pain [9,23,31,35]. As with relaxation techniques, imagery, and biofeedback, hypnosis is rarely used alone in chronic pain, although it has been used independently with some success with cancer patients [36]; practitioners often use it concurrently with other treatment interventions.

Elkins, Jensen, and Patterson [9] identified 13 controlled studies evaluating the efficacy of hypnosis. In general, hypnosis was significantly more effective than no-treatment comparison groups in reducing pain. However, these reviewers found few studies that compared hypnosis with credible comparison treatments, and so it is impossible to rule out the effects of attention and participation in a study (expectation and regression to the mean). In addition, discrepancies with regard to the methods used to induce hypnosis make it difficult to accurately evaluate efficacy [36].

General Comments about the Efficacy of Psychological Approaches

Early studies evaluating the efficacy of psychological approaches focused on whether treatments were comparable to other therapeutic options, and as suggested above, the clinical outcomes always tended to support the usefulness of psychological approaches and treatment modalities [10,11]. Although only modest improvements in pain-related outcomes were observed, analgesic medication use, physical incapacity, health care utilization, and disability rates showed marked reductions [21,28,38].

More recently, the increased availability of randomized controlled trials, as well as refined analytic techniques, has led to a large number of meta-analyses and systematic reviews (e.g., 7–9,11,17,19,32]. The results of these meta-analyses with adult patients came to somewhat similar conclusions—as a group, psychological treatments have modest benefits in improving pain and physical and emotional functioning.

Although in general the results of the meta-analyses support only modest benefit, it is important to acknowledge once again that any improvement in outcomes from psychological treatments probably occurs in addition to benefits already being realized from standard care. With few exceptions [e.g., 20], investigators providing combination treatments that incorporate both medical and psychological treatments have not attempted to differentiate the synergistic effects.

Effect sizes will also vary depending on what outcome measures are used. There is some debate as to the most appropriate outcomes in clinical trials of chronic pain. At first glance, it might seem obvious that it should be reduction in pain intensity. However, there is growing acknowledgment of the importance of other outcomes such as physical functioning, emotional functioning, health-related quality of life, and patient satisfaction [47]. "Cherry-picking" selected outcomes that support the efficacy of the treatment is not appropriate. Multiple outcomes are important, and investigators evaluating treatment outcomes must consider all that are relevant and balance the results obtained to form their conclusions about treatment success.

Although psychological treatments have been found to be helpful for a number of individuals, there are some for whom they are not beneficial. Investigators are just beginning to explore different aspects of CBT to answer the question "what works for whom?" [43,46,54]. Several studies have begun to explore the characteristics of patients who respond to psychological treatments in general and to specific psychological treatments [42,49].

Recently, Turner, Holtzman, and Mancl [52] found that the mediators of improvement in pain and activity 1 year after completing CBT were cognitive variables including patients' perceptions of control, disability, self-efficacy, harm, and catastrophizing and rumination. Individual patients may learn coping skills and improve feelings of control and self-efficacy through different types of treatments. Identifying factors that allow treatment matching may allow better effect sizes to be realized.

Summary and Conclusions

Pain that persists over time should not be viewed as either solely physical or solely psychological. Rather, the experience of pain is a complex amalgam maintained by an interdependent set of biomedical, psychosocial, and behavioral factors, whose relationships are not static but evolve and change over time. The various interacting factors that affect a person with chronic pain suggest that the phenomenon is quite complex and requires a perspective that takes into consideration cognitive factors (beliefs, attitudes, expectancies, and perceptions of self-efficacy), emotional aspects, and behavioral (social environment) factors and prior learning history, as well as genetic and physical contributors to the pain experience—a biopsychosocial perspective.

From the biopsychosocial perspective, the interaction among the factors enumerated above combines to produce the subjective experience of pain. There is a synergistic relationship whereby psychological and socioenvironmental factors can modulate nociceptive stimulation and the response to treatment. In turn, nociceptive stimulation can influence patients' appraisals of their situation and their treatment, their mood states, and the ways they interact with significant others, including medical practitioners. An integrative, biopsychosocial model of chronic pain needs to incorporate the mutual interrelationships among physical, psychological, and social factors and the changes that occur among these relationships over time [11,50]. A model and treatment approach that focuses on only one of these sets of factors will inevitably be incomplete and inadequate.

Acknowledgments

Preparation of this chapter was supported in part by NIH (NIAMS) grant 2 R01 AR0444724.

References

[1] Alexander CN, Robinson P, Orme-Johnson DW. The effects of transcendental meditation compared to other methods of relaxation and meditation in reducing risk factors, morbidity, and mortality. In: CIANS-ISBM Satellite Conference Symposium: Lifestyle changes in the prevention and treatment of disease. Hannover, 1992. p. 243–63.

[2] Astin JA. Stress reduction through mindfulness meditation. Effects on psychological symptomatology, sense of control, and spiritual experiences. Psychother Psychosom 1997;66:97–106.

[3] Astin JA, Shapiro SL, Eisenberg DM, Forys KL. Mind-body medicine: state of the science, implications for practice. J Am Board Fam Pract 2003;16:131–47.

[4] Basler SC, Grzesiak RC, Dworkin RH. Integrating relational psychodynamic and action-oriented psychotherapies: treating pain and suffering. In: Turk DC, Gatchel R, editors. Psychological approaches to pain management: a practitioner's handbook, 2nd ed. New York: Guilford; 2002. p. 94–127.

[5] Bonadonna R. Meditation's impact on chronic illness. Holistic Nurs Pract 2003;17:309–19.

[6] Breivik H, Collett B, Ventafridda V, Cohen R, Gallacher D. Survey of pain in Europe: prevalence, impact on daily life, and treatment. Eur J Pain 2006;10:287–333.

[7] Campbell JK, Penzien DB, Wall EM; US Headache Consortium. Evidence-based guidelines for migraine headache: behavioral and physical treatments. 2002. Available at: http://www.aan.com/professionals/practice/pdfs/gl0089.pdf.

[8] Dixon KE, Keefe FJ, Scipio CD, Perri LM, Abernethy AP. Psychological interventions for arthritis pain management in adults: a meta-analysis. Health Psychol 2007;26:241–50.

[9] Elkins G, Jensen MP, Patterson DR. Hypnotherapy for the management of chronic pain. Int J Clin Exp Hypn 2007;55:275–87.

[10] Fishbain DA, Cutler RB, Rosomoff HL, Steele-Rosomoff R. Pain facilities: a review of their effectiveness and selection criteria. Curr Rev Pain 1997;1:107–15.

[11] Flor H, Fydrich T, Turk DC. Efficacy of multidisciplinary pain treatment centers: a meta-analytic review. Pain 1992;49:221–30.

[12] Fordyce WE. Behavioral methods for chronic pain and illness. St. Louis: Mosby, 1976.

[13] Gatchel RJ, Peng YB, Peters ML, Fuchs PN, Turk DC. The biopsychosocial approach to chronic pain: scientific advances and future directions. Psychol Bull 2007;133:581–624.

[14] Gevirtz RN, Hubbard DR, Harpin RE. Psychophysiologic treatment of chronic lower back pain. Prof Psychol Res Pr 1996;27:561–6.

[15] Goleman DJ, Schwartz GE. Meditation as an intervention in stress reactivity. J Consult Clin Psychol 1976;44:456–66.

[16] Grossman P, Niemann L, Schmidt S, Walach H. Mindfulness-based stress reduction and health benefits. A meta-analysis. J Psychosom Res 2004;57:35–43.

[17] Guzman J, Esmail R, Karjalainen K, Malmivaara A, Irvin E, Bombardier C. Multidisciplinary rehabilitation for chronic low back pain: systematic review. BMJ 2001;322:1511–6.

[18] Halpin LS, Speir AM, CapoBianco P, Barnett SD. Guided imagery in cardiac surgery. Outcomes Manage 2002;6:132–7.

[19] Hoffman BM, Papas RK, Chatkoff DK, Kerns RD. Meta-analysis of psychological interventions for chronic low back pain. Health Psychol 2007;26:1–9.

[20] Holroyd KA, France JL, Cordingley GE, Holroyd KA, France JL, Cordingley GE. Enhancing the effectiveness of relaxation/thermal biofeedback training with propranolol HCl. J Consult Clin Psychol 1995;63:327–30.

[21] Holroyd KA, Penzien DB. Client variables and the behavioral treatment of recurrent tension headache: a meta-analytic review. J Behav Med 1986;9:515–36.

[22] Holroyd KA, Penzien DB, Hursey KG, Tobin DL, Rogers L, Holm JE. Change mechanisms in EMG biofeedback training: cognitive changes underlying improvements in tension headache. J Consult Clin Psychol 1984;52:1039–53.

[23] Jensen MP, Patterson DR. Hypnotic treatment of chronic pain. J Behav Med 2006;29:95–124.

[24] Kabat-Zinn J. An outpatient program in behavioral medicine for chronic pain patients based on the practice of mindfulness meditation: theoretical considerations and preliminary results. Gen Hosp Psychiatry 1982;4:33–47.

[25] Kabat-Zinn J. Full catastrophe living. New York: Delacorte Press; 1990.

[26] Lazar SW, Kerr CE, Wasserman RH, Gray JR, Greve DN, Treadway MT, McGarvey M, Quinn BT, Dusek JA, Benson H, et al. Meditation experience is associated with increased cortical thickness. Neuroreport 2005;16:1893–7.

[27] Lutz A, Greischar LL, Rawlings NB, Matthieu R, Davidson RJ. Long-term meditators self-induced high-amplitude gamma synchrony during mental practice. Proc Natl Acad Sci USA 2004;101:16369–73.

[28] Malone MD, Strube MJ. Meta-analysis of non-medical treatments for chronic pain. Pain 1988;34:231–44.

[29] McCracken LM, Turk DC. Behavioral and cognitive-behavioral treatment for chronic pain: outcome, predictors of outcome, and treatment process. Spine 2002;27:2564–73.

[30] Medlicott MS, Harris SR. A systematic review of the effectiveness of exercise, manual therapy, electrotherapy, relaxation training, and biofeedback in the management of temporomandibular disorder. Phys Ther 2006;86:955–73.

[31] Montgomery GH, DuHamel KN, Redd WH. A meta-analysis of hypnotically induced analgesia: how effective is hypnosis? Int J Clin Exp Hypnosis 2000;48:138–53.

[32] Morley S, Eccleston C, Williams A. Systematic review and meta-analysis of randomized controlled trials of cognitive behaviour therapy and behaviour therapy for chronic pain in adults, excluding headache. Pain 1999;80:1–13.

[33] Nestoriuc Y, Martin A. Efficacy of biofeedback for migraine: a meta-analysis. Pain 2007;128:111–27.

[34] Novy DM. Psychological approaches for managing chronic pain. J Psychopathol Behav Assess 2004;26:279–88.

[35] Patterson DR, Jensen MP. Hypnosis and clinical pain. Psychol Bull 2003;129:495–521.

[36] Pinnell CM, Covino NA. Empirical findings on the use of hypnosis in medicine: a critical review. Int J Clin Exp Hypnosis 2000;48:170–94.

[37] Romano JM, Turner JA, Jensen MP, Friedman LS, Bulcroft RA, Hops H, Wright SF. Chronic pain patient-spouse behavioral interactions predict patient disability. Pain 1995;63:353–60.

[38] Scheer SJ, Watanabe TK, Radack KL. Randomized controlled trials in industrial low back pain. Part 3. Subacute/chronic pain interventions. Arch Phys Med Rehabil 1997;78:414–23.

[39] Spiegel D, Moore R. Imagery and hypnosis in the treatment of cancer patients. Oncology (Williston Park) 1997;11:1179–89.
[40] Thieme K, Gromnica-Ihle E, Flor H. Operant behavioral treatment of fibromyalgia: a controlled study. Arthritis Rheum 2003;49:314–20.
[41] Thieme K, Spies C, Sinha P, Turk DC, Flor H. Predictors of pain behaviors in fibromyalgia syndrome patients. Arthritis Care Res 2005;53:343–50.
[42] Thieme K, Turk DC, Flor H. Responder criteria for operant and cognitive-behavioral treatment of fibromyalgia syndrome. Arthritis Care Res 2007;57:830–6.
[43] Turk DC. Customizing treatment for chronic pain patients. Who, what and why. Clin J Pain 1990;6:255–70.
[44] Turk DC. Clinical effectiveness and cost effectiveness of treatments for chronic pain patients. Clin J Pain 2002;18:355–65.
[45] Turk DC. Cognitive-behavioral approach to the treatment of chronic pain patients. Reg Anesth Pain Med 2003;28:573–9.
[46] Turk DC. The potential of treatment matching for subgroups of patients with chronic pain: lumping versus splitting. Clin J Pain 2005;21:44–55.
[47] Turk DC, Dworkin RH, Allen RR, Bellamy N, Brandenburg N, et al. Core outcomes domains for chronic pain clinical trials: IMMPACT recommendations. Pain 2003;106:337–45.
[48] Turk DC, Meichenbaum D. A cognitive-behavioral approach to pain management. In: Wall PD, Melzack R. editors. Textbook of pain. London: Churchill Livingstone; 1984. p. 787–94.
[49] Turk DC, Okifuji A, Sinclair JD, Starz TW. Differential responses by psychosocial subgroups of fibromyalgia syndrome patients to an interdisciplinary treatment. Arthritis Care Res 1998;11:397–404.
[50] Turk DC, Rudy TE. Persistent pain and the injured worker: integrating biomedical, psychosocial and behavioral factors. J Occup Rehabil 1991;1:159–79.
[51] Turner JA, Clancy S, McQuade KJ, Cardenas DD. Effectiveness o behavioral therapy for chronic low-back pain: a component analysis. J Consult Clin Psychol 1990;58:573–9.
[52] Turner J, Holtzman S, Mancl L. Mediators, moderators, and predictors of therapeutic change in cognitive-behavioral therapy for chronic pain. Pain 2007;127:276–86.
[53] Vlaeyen JWS, Haazen IWCJ, Schuerman JA, Kole-Snijders AMJ, Van Eek H. Behavioral rehabilitation of chronic low back pain: comparison of an operant, and operant cognitive treatment and an operant respondent treatment. Br J Clin Psychol 1995;34:95–118.
[54] Vlaeyen JWS, Morley S. Cognitive-behavioral treatments for chronic pain: what works for whom? Clin J Pain 2005;21:1–8.

Correspondence to: Dennis C. Turk, PhD, Department of Anesthesiology, Box 356540, University of Washington, Seattle, WA 98195, USA. Tel: 1-206-616-2626; fax: 1-206-543-2958; email: turkdc@u.washington.edu.

Section IV

Pain Syndromes

Myofascial Pain and Fibromyalgia Syndrome

Kathleen A. Sluka

Graduate Program in Physical Therapy and Rehabilitation Science,
The University of Iowa, Iowa City, Iowa, USA

Musculoskeletal pain conditions are common, with regional pain affecting up to 50% and widespread pain affecting up to 10% of the population [9,20]. One of the most common regional pain complaints is myofascial pain syndrome, which has been estimated to be the source of pain in 30% of patients consulting primary care [45] and in up to 85% of patients attending a pain center [13]. Fibromyalgia is a form of chronic widespread musculoskeletal pain that affects 4–10% of the population [9,20]. Myofascial pain syndrome is equally distributed between male and females, whereas fibromyalgia has a greater distribution in females (Table I) [20,44,46]. This chapter will review the diagnostic criteria and treatment strategies for myofascial pain syndrome and fibromyalgia.

Myofascial Pain Syndrome

Epidemiology and Diagnosis

Myofascial pain historically has been considered a localized pain syndrome associated with trigger points in the muscle belly (Table I). However, in some cases, myofascial pain has also been considered a regional

Table I
Characteristics of myofascial pain and fibromyalgia

Myofascial Pain (Trigger Points)	Fibromyalgia
1:1 female to male ratio	4–9:1 female to male ratio
Local or regional pain	Widespread, general pain
Local tenderness	Widespread tenderness
Trigger points	Tender points
Treatment with local therapy: trigger point injections, local stretching and strengthening, ultrasound, TENS*	Treatment with systemic therapy: pharmacological therapy, cognitive-behavioral therapy, aerobic and strengthening exercise, TENS*

* Transcutaneous electrical nerve stimulation.

pain syndrome of muscle origin, as in the case of myofascial pain from the temporomandibular joint. For the purposes of this chapter, myofascial pain will be considered as pain arising from trigger points in the muscle belly, as described by Simons and colleagues [44]. As mentioned above, myofascial pain syndrome is a condition that equally affects males and females. It can be acute or chronic and has been recorded to affect approximately 20–30% of the population [46].

Distinct patterns of pain referral from trigger points have been identified in muscles across the entire body [44]. Trigger points are particularly common in the upper cervical spine and shoulder region and can refer pain to areas of the head and face. However, there are trigger points in most muscles of the body, including the limbs and lower back. Fig. 1 shows examples of trigger points found in the trapezius, extensor digitorum of the forearm, multifidus of the lower back, and piriformis. There are distinct patterns with each trigger point, and adequately understanding and evaluating these patterns is critical to effective treatment.

There is limited consensus on diagnostic criteria for myofascial pain syndrome [55]. The four most common criteria used are: a tender spot in a taut band, recognition of pain by the patient, a predicted pain referral pattern, and a local twitch response. This chapter has adopted the criteria described by Travell and colleagues [44], which generally agree with criteria used in the randomized controlled trials (RCTs) assessed by Tough and colleagues [55]. As stated by Travell and colleagues, the lack of consensus results in a serious impediment to well-controlled research to evaluate the efficacy of treatments [44]. For clinicians who diagnose and treat myofascial pain, the two-volume manual, *Travell & Simons' Myofascial Pain and Dysfunction*, is essential reading [44].

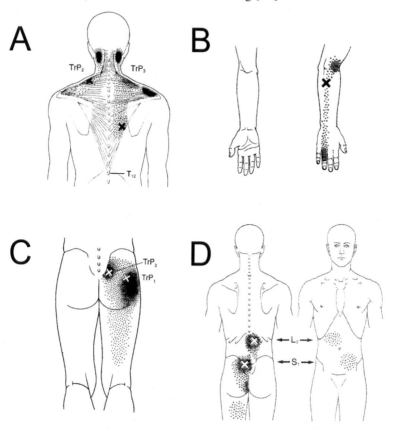

Fig. 1. Examples of trigger points found in the (A) trapezius, (B) extensor digitorum of the forearm, (C) multifidus of the lower back, and (D) piriformis. Reprinted from Simons et al. [44], with permission from Lippincott, Williams, and Wilkins.

Diagnostic criteria as proposed by Travel and Simons [44] are outlined in Table II. In general, myofascial pain is a local or regional pain syndrome occurring in one or two body regions. Four essential criteria must be met to reach a diagnosis of myofascial pain. (1) There should be a palpable taut band in the muscle, with (2) an exquisite spot tenderness of a nodule in the taut band. (3) The patient should recognize the current pain complaint by pressure on the tender nodule. This pressure should reproduce the clinical pain complaint and should not be associated with a new complaint. It should be recognized that it is the *active* trigger points in a

Table II
Diagnostic criteria for myofascial pain and fibromyalgia

Myofascial Pain (Trigger Points)
Major Criteria:
Palpable taut band
Spot tenderness of nodule in taut band
Patient recognition of current pain complaint by pressure on nodule
Limited range of motion with pain
Confirmatory Criteria:
Local twitch response on palpation
Pain in the distribution of the expected trigger point in that muscle on compression of tender nodule
Pain alleviated by stretching muscle or injecting trigger point
Fibromyalgia
Widespread, generalized pain: above and below midline, both sides of body; must include axial distribution
Pain on digital palpation of 11 of 18 tender points
Pain of greater than 3 months' duration

muscle that reproduce the patient's pain complaint. Latent trigger points also exist that have a taut band, spot tenderness, and referral of pain, but do not reproduce a clinical pain complaint. (4) The fourth essential criterion is restricted range of motion as a result of pain. Confirmatory observations include a local twitch response, either visual or on palpation, of the taut band. Although the twitch response is highly specific to myofascial pain syndromes, it is difficult to elicit reliably and has thus been considered a confirmatory observation. Relief of pain by stretching the muscle or trigger point injections also confirms myofascial pain syndrome.

Pathobiology

Increased muscle activity, recorded as endplate noise on electromyography, has been observed in active myofascial trigger points [28]. Spontaneous activity or endplate spikes are observed upon needle insertion into the active trigger points [37]. Furthermore, muscles with active trigger points show changes in biochemical markers—increases in substance P, calcitonin gene-related peptide, bradykinin, interleukin-6, interleukin 1β, tumor necrosis factor-α, serotonin, and norepinephrine, and decreases in pH [42,43]. Interestingly, these changes are located in muscles with active trigger points, but not in those with no trigger points or with latent trigger points. Thus, there are clear changes in muscle activity, and importantly, changes in neurotransmitters, cytokines, and pH that are known to activate and sensitize nociceptors. These changes may explain the underlying pain of myofascial pain syndrome and suggest that peripheral mechanisms are important in the generation of pain.

Assessment Considerations

Evaluation of patients with myofascial pain syndrome should use techniques to evaluate resting pain, pain during palpation of trigger points (e.g., pressure algometry), range of motion, and pain with active range of motion. In addition, the impact of the pain on the patient's overall functional capacity can be assessed with self-efficacy questionnaires or general quality-of-life surveys, as outlined in Chapter 5. The therapist should employ a biopsychosocial approach to the assessment of myofascial pain that accounts for the multidimensional nature of pain and its impact on function and social roles, particularly for patients with chronic myofascial pain.

Medical Management

Treatment of myofascial pain syndrome from a medical perspective involves injection of trigger points. Injections are done with botulism toxin, lidocaine, saline, or dry needling [10,12,14,23]. Trigger point injections typically decrease pain, increase pressure pain threshold, and increase range of motion in people with myofascial pain syndrome [12,14]. The bulk of the evidence suggests that dry needling or saline injections are equivalent to injections of pharmacological agents such as botulism toxin or lidocaine [10,14,23]. There are no RCTs for treatment of myofascial pain with common pharmaceutical agents such as muscle relaxants, nonsteroidal anti-inflammatory drugs (NSAIDs), or antidepressants. Treatment with trigger point injections followed by active physical therapy is generally accepted as the most effective treatment for myofascial pain syndrome [46].

Psychological Management

The use of psychological strategies for the treatment of myofascial pain syndrome has not been assessed in clinical RCTs. It is likely, as with all chronic pain conditions, that cognitive-behavioral therapy aimed at self-management and coping skills would be of great benefit to those with chronic myofascial pain. It is also highly likely that relaxation therapy and biofeedback could reduce any increased muscle activity in the trigger points as a result of myofascial pain.

Physical Therapy

Physical therapy intervention for myofascial pain generally involves multiple techniques including manual therapy, exercise, ultrasound and transcutaneous electrical nerve stimulation (TENS). Passive stretching of the muscle that contains the trigger point is considered a primary treatment for myofascial pain syndrome. In an uncontrolled study, passive stretching along with fluoromethane vapocoolant spray (i.e., spray and stretch) decreased pain and increased pressure pain threshold in people with myofascial pain [26]. Dry needling combined with active stretching exercises (as suggested by Travell and colleagues [44]) produced greater reduction in pain compared to active stretching alone or a no-treatment control condition [11].

Manual therapy generally uses trigger point massage or ischemic pressure application to the trigger point. Hou and colleagues showed that ischemic pressure, applied to the trigger point with a manual massager (Thera Cane), when combined with an active range of motion exercise program, reduces pain, increases pressure pain thresholds, and decreases the amount of time in pain over a 24-hour period to a greater extent than active range of motion exercises alone. In fact, active range of motion exercises alone have no effect on pain measures. Ischemic pressure of the myofascial trigger point has an immediate effect on reducing pain, increasing pressure pain threshold and tolerance, and improving range of motion [24].

The use of conventional ultrasound (continuous, 1.5 W/cm^2) continuously moved over the trigger point provided greater pain relief than placebo ultrasound; however, there was no increased reduction in pain when ultrasound was combined with massage and exercise [15]. In this study, massage and exercise (without ultrasound) reduced the number and pain intensity of myofascial trigger points. In contrast, Sberly and Dickey [47] showed increases in pressure pain thresholds in subjects with myofascial pain treated with conventional ultrasound (continuous, 1.0 W/cm^2, 5 minutes) but not in those treated with lower-intensity ultrasound (continuous, 0.1 W/cm^2, 5 minutes). Majlesi and Unalan [31] suggest better effectiveness with high-power, static ultrasound at the pain threshold, in which the intensity is increased to the level of maximum pain the subject can bear for 4 to 5 seconds and then reduced to 50% of this intensity for another 15 seconds, repeated three times. All subjects in this study had acute myofascial pain, and both groups performed active range of motion exercises. Use of this unconventional mode of ultrasound over the trigger point resulted in a significant reduction in pain and increases in range of motion after the first treatment session that were substantially better than results with conventional ultrasound (continuous, 1.5 W/cm^2, 5 minutes). The number of visits required was significantly lower with high-power ultrasound (2.8 visits) when compared to the group that received conventional ultrasound (11.8 visits). Both groups achieved the same endpoint of normal range of motion and pain at discharge on average between 1 and 2 points on the VAS. Unfortunately, there was no placebo control, and no untreated control, to indicate whether the conventional ultrasound group faired better than those receiving no treatment (normal history) or those using active exercises alone.

Effects of TENS on myofascial pain have been evaluated in several RCTs. Hsueh and colleagues [25] examined the effects of conventional TENS (60 Hz, sensory intensity, 20 minutes) and neuromuscular electrical stimulation (NMES; 10 Hz, motor contraction intensity, 20 minutes) when compared to a placebo on pain, pressure pain thresholds, and range of motion in people with myofascial pain syndrome. Both TENS and NMES reduced pain and increased pressure pain thresholds, with TENS having a greater effect on pain measures. NMES, however, also significantly increased range of motion, on which TENS had no effect. Similarly, high-frequency TENS (100 Hz; pulse width 50 or 250 µs, 10 minutes, sensory intensity) reduced pain, but had no effect on pressure pain thresholds [19]. However, a single treatment with low-frequency TENS (2 Hz, pulse width 250 µs, 10 minutes, strongest tolerable intensity with motor contractions) had no effect on pain or pressure pain thresholds [19]. Interestingly, intramuscular stimulation of the trigger point through a needle electrode (2 Hz, motor contraction, 3 minutes) reduced pain and increased pressure pain thresholds in approximately 50% of subjects [33]. In summary, high-frequency TENS, at adequate intensity and duration, is clearly effective for myofascial pain, and NMES has the greatest effects on range of motion; the effectiveness of electrical stimulation with low frequency is unclear.

Physical therapy usually combines multiple treatments to reduce myofascial pain. One study assessed the addition of combining multiple physical therapy treatments on myofascial trigger points by measuring pain threshold, pain tolerance, and subjective pain scores on a visual analogue scale (VAS). They compared six different treatment paradigms: (1) a hot pack with active range of motion exercises; (2) hot packs, active range of motion exercises, and ischemic pressure; (3) hot packs, active range of motion exercises, ischemic pressure, and TENS; (4) hot packs, active range of motion exercises, ischemic pressure, and spray and stretch; (5) hot packs, active range of motion exercises, ischemic pressure, TENS, and spray and stretch; and (6) hot packs, active range of motion exercises, interferential current, and myofascial release. The group that received hot packs with active range of motion exercises showed significant increases in pain threshold and tolerance and a small decrease in pain (0.77 points on a 10-point scale) [24]. Adding ischemic pressure or spray and stretch to the hot packs and active range of motion treatment showed similar increases in pain thresholds and tolerance but a greater decrease in pain (1.49 points on a 10 point scale). The addition of TENS or interferential therapy to the hot packs and active range of motion similarly increased pain threshold and tolerance and resulted in a further decrease in pain (2.23–3.64 points on a 10-point VAS scale). Addition of spray and stretch had no additional effect when compared to the group that received hot packs, active range of motion, and ischemic pressure without spray and stretch. Thus, it appears that ischemic pressure of the trigger point, applied by the therapist or the patient, reduces symptoms associated with myofascial pain, and the addition of electrical nerve stimulation further decreases pain.

At present there are few data to support the use of active range of motion exercises alone for people with myofascial pain. Active exercises are given with the rationale of maintaining range of motion after treatments aimed at increasing range of motion. There are no studies to date that performed treatments without an active exercise program, suggesting that the inclusion of active range of motion exercises is the standard of care. Stretching exercises have not been systematically evaluated, but a few studies show that there appears to be some effect of stretching alone or combined with trigger point therapy in reducing pain associated with myofascial pain syndrome. Additionally, electrotherapeutic modalities appear to add a greater benefit to the standard treatment protocols, and high-power, high-intensity ultrasound may be a viable therapy for quicker relief of acute myofascial pain than conventional ultrasound alone. Efficacy for the various treatment options for myofascial pain is summarized in Table III.

Table III
Summary of efficacy for myofascial pain treatments

Treatment	Pain	Pressure Pain Threshold	Range of Motion
Trigger point injection	+ (RCT)	+ (RCT)	+ (RCT)
Active ROM exercise*	?	?	?
Ischemic pressure	+ (RCT)	+ (RCT)	+ (RCT)
TENS/interferential therapy	+ (RCT)	+ (RCT)	– (RCT)
NMES	+ (RCT)	+ (RCT)	+ (RCT)
Conventional ultrasound	– (RCT)	– (RCT)	– (RCT)
High-power, high-intensity ultrasound	+ (RCT)	+ (RCT)	+ (RCT)
Hot pack	– (RCT)	– (RCT)	– (RCT)
Spray and stretch	? (uncontr., RCT)	? (uncontr., RCT)	? (uncontr., RCT)

Abbreviations: NMES = neuromuscular electrical stimulation; RCT = randomized controlled trial; ROM = range of motion; TENS = transcutaneous electrical nerve stimulation; uncontr. = uncontrolled trial; +, positive effect; –, no effect; ? unclear if effective, but is a commonly used treatment.
* Usually used in combination with another therapy or as control group; generally not effective in isolation.

Fibromyalgia Syndrome

Epidemiology and Diagnosis

Fibromyalgia syndrome is a generalized widespread pain condition that has a prevalence of 4–10% in the general population. It occurs primarily in women (7:1 female to male ratio), with a peak between 60 and 80 years of age. People with fibromyalgia commonly present with sleep disorders (90%), fatigue (80%), depression (20–40%), and irritable bowel syndrome (12%), and they often have headache, cognitive deficits, chest wall pain, and morning stiffness [40]. It thus is distinctly different from myofascial pain, which is a localized pain condition without associated comorbidities.

Fibromyalgia syndrome classification was formalized in 1990 by the American College of Rheumatology [62]. The criteria are based on symptoms reported by the patient and found on physical examination. Specifically, there must be widespread pain for at least 3 months' duration. The widespread pain is defined as occurring on both sides of the body and above and below the waistline and must include axial pain. On physical examination there should be 11 of 18 tender points to 4 kg of pressure applied by the clinician. These tender points are all bilateral and include the occiput at the suboccipital muscle insertion site; the low cervical at the anterior aspect of the intertransverse spaces of C5–C7; the trapezius at the midpoint of the upper border; the supraspinatus at the origins of the medial border of the scapular spine; the second rib at the upper surfaces just lateral to the costochondral junctions; the lateral epicondyle 2 cm distal to the epicondyles; the gluteal in the upper outer quadrant of buttock in the anterior fold of the muscle; the greater trochanter posterior to the trochanteric prominences; and the knee at the medial fat pad proximal to the joint line (Fig. 2).

Pathobiology

Little is known about the etiology of fibromyalgia syndrome, but it is commonly accepted that central sensitization underlies much of the pain. Increases in substance P and nerve growth factor and decreases in serotonin are found in the cerebrospinal fluid [16,39,41,56]. In addition, there is a generalized decrease in pressure thresholds in people with fibromyalgia outside the site of the tender points, as well as enhanced temporal summation [35,49,50,53,54]. There is also a loss of central inhibition mechanisms, as measured by an ineffective diffuse noxious inhibitory control test [27,29,30,51,54]. Together, these data suggest enhanced excitability in the central nervous system accompanied by decreased inhibition. The contributions of the peripheral nervous system to the central changes are unclear at this point, but some researchers propose

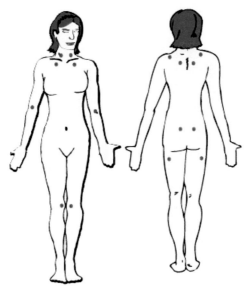

Fig. 2. Diagram illustrating the tender point sites for diagnosis of fibromyalgia syndrome.

abnormal peripheral processing of nociceptive input and autonomic disturbances [48,52,57].

There appears to be a genetic link in some patients with fibromyalgia, with female relatives of patients being more likely to develop the syndrome. Studies show that up to two-thirds of mothers, daughters, and sisters of patients also have fibromyalgia. Genetic analysis of patients with fibromyalgia demonstrate a role for polymorphisms of genes in the serotoninergic, dopaminergic, and catecholaminergic systems in the pathogenesis of the syndrome [3,7,21,34].

Assessment Considerations

Evaluation of patients with fibromyalgia must use a multidisciplinary approach to assess not only the pain, but also its impact on function and quality of life. Patients with fibromyalgia should be referred to both physicians and psychologists to receive effective multidisciplinary treatment. The physical therapist can learn valuable information about pain severity and other dimensions of pain by using standard subjective pain scales and the McGill Pain Questionnaire. Quality of life surveys, self-efficacy questionnaires, and fear-avoidance surveys can give valuable information to the therapist on the impact of the pain on function, and the barriers to treatment with an active exercise program. The Fibromyalgia Impact Questionnaire (FIQ) is a disease-specific tool (Fig. 3) that takes the patient 5 minutes to complete. This simple 20-question survey estimates the impact of fibromyalgia on activities of daily living and work and monitors associated symptoms such as fatigue, stiffness, depression, and anxiety [5]. It is useful not only for research but also in evaluating progress in patients with fibromyalgia.

Medical Management

Treatment of fibromyalgia syndrome requires a multidisciplinary approach involving pharmacological management, psychological treatments, and physical therapy (see Table IV for a summary of the efficacy of various treatments). There is good evidence from RCTs that multidisciplinary treatment combining education, cognitive-behavioral therapy, and exercise is efficacious in improving patient self-efficacy, in lessening the overall impact of the disease on quality of life as measured by the FIQ, and in decreasing pain and improving function, when compared to self-management strategies [18]. Treatment gains are maintained for up to 2 years [18].

    Pharmacological management based on RCTs, and on clinical guidelines published by the American Pain Society, shows efficacy for treatment with tricyclic antidepressants such as amitriptyline for reducing pain,

Table IV
Summary of efficacy of treatments for fibromyalgia syndrome

Strong Evidence	Moderate Evidence	Weak Evidence	No Evidence
Amitriptyline	Tramadol	Growth hormone	Opioids
Cyclobenzaprine	Serotonin reuptake inhibitors	Serotonin	Corticosteroids
Cardiovascular exercise	Dual reuptake inhibitors	Tropisetron	NSAIDs
Cognitive-behavioral therapy	Pregabalin	Manual/massage therapy	Benzodiazepine
Patient education	Strength training	Electrotherapy	Melatonin
Multidisciplinary therapy	Acupuncture	Ultrasound	Calcitonin
	Hypnotherapy		Tender (trigger) point injections
	Biofeedback		Flexibility exercises

Source: Adapted from Goldenberg et al. [18].

improving sleep, decreasing fatigue, and increasing overall well-being and is supported by meta-analysis of existing literature [2,18,32,36]. Similarly, serotonin reuptake inhibitors and dual reuptake inhibitors, aimed at increasing serotonin and norepinephrine, are also effective in reducing pain and improving sleep, fatigue, mood, function, and global well-being in people with fibromyalgia [17]. Recent evidence also suggests that the anti-seizure medications gabapentin and pregabalin are effective in reducing pain and fatigue and improving function and quality of life in people with fibromyalgia [17,32]. Furthermore, there is evidence that the muscle relaxant cyclobenzaprine is effective in treating fibromyalgia [18]. However, NSAIDs have not been shown to be efficacious in treating fibromyalgia [36]. An evidence-based review of the literature published in the *Journal of the American Medical Association,* and supported by the American Pain Society, concluded that there is strong to moderate evidence for the tricyclic antidepressants and cyclobenzaprine; moderate evidence for serotonin reuptake inhibitors, dual reuptake inhibitors, and gabapentin or pregabalin; and no evidence for opioids, NSAIDs or benzodiazepine in the treatment of fibromyalgia syndrome [18].

Psychological Management

Psychological management of fibromyalgia usually involves cognitive-behavioral therapy, relaxation exercises, and instruction in coping skills. Strong evidence to support the effectiveness of cognitive-behavioral therapies for reducing pain and improving quality of life in individuals with fibromyalgia has been confirmed in systematic reviews [18,38,60]. Stress management and relaxation therapy also reduce pain in people with fibromyalgia [59]. In fact, adding cognitive-behavioral therapy to a standard medical care program of exercise and pharmacotherapy provides sustained improvement in physical functioning [61].

Physical Therapy

Physical therapy should emphasize an active protocol aimed primarily at exercise, particularly aerobic conditioning programs. There is strong support for the use of aerobic cardiovascular exercise in the treatment of fibromyalgia syndrome [6,18]. The Cochrane review by Busch and colleagues

FIBROMYALGIA IMPACT QUESTIONNAIRE (FIQ)

Last name: First name: Age :   Todays date :

Duration of FM symptoms (years) :   Years since diagnosis of FM :

Directions: For questions 1 through 11, please check the number that best describes how you did overall for the *past week*. If you don't normally do something that is asked, place an 'X' in the 'Not Applicable' box.

Were you able to:	Always	Most	Occasionally	Never	Not Applicable
1. Do shopping?	□0	□1	□2	□3	□4
2. Do laundry with a washer and dryer?	□0	□1	□2	□3	□4
3. Prepare meals?	□0	□1	□2	□3	□4
4. Wash dishes / cooking utensils by hand?	□0	□1	□2	□3	□4
5. Vacuum a rug?	□0	□1	□2	□3	□4
6. Make beds?	□0	□1	□2	□3	□4
7. Walk several blocks?	□0	□1	□2	□3	□4
8. Visit friends or relatives?	□0	□1	□2	□3	□4
9. Do yard work?	□0	□1	□2	□3	□4
10. Drive a car?	□0	□1	□2	□3	□4
11. Climb stairs?	□0	□1	□2	□3	□4
Sub-total scores *(for internal use only)*	□	□	□	□	□
Total score *(for internal use only)*	□				

12. Of the 7 days in the past week, how many days did you feel good?   Score

□0   □1   □2   □3   □4   □5   □6   □7   □

13. How many days last week did you miss work, including housework, because of fibromyalgia?   Score

□0   □1   □2   □3   □4   □5   □6   □7   □

(Continued)

Fig. 3. Fibromyalgia Impact Questionnaire (FIQ). Possible scores range from 0 (no impact) to 100 (severe impact). To score the FIQ, for Questions 1–11, add the numbers for each checked item and divide by the number of scored items (the number of scored items will be 11 unless some are rated N/A [not applicable]). For Question 12, score the items

(Continuation)

Directions: For the remaining items, mark the point on the line that best indicates how you felt overall for the past week.

14. When you worked how much did pain or other symptoms of your fibromyalgia interfere with your ability to do your work, including housework?

No problem |——————————————————————| Great difficulty
with work   with work

(for internal use only)

[ ] Score

15. How bad has your pain been?

No pain |——————————————————————| Very severe pain

[ ] Score

16. How tired have you been?

No tiredness |——————————————————————| Very tired

[ ] Score

17. How have you felt when you get up in the morning?

Awoke well |——————————————————————| Awoke very
rested   tired

[ ] Score

18. How bad has your stiffness been?

No stiffness |——————————————————————| Very stiff

[ ] Score

19. How nervous or anxious have you felt?

Not anxious |——————————————————————| Very anxious

[ ] Score

20. How depressed or blue have you felt?

Not depressed |——————————————————————| Very
depressed

[ ] Score

[ ] Sub-total

[ ] FIQ TOTAL

in reverse order: 7 = 0, 6 = 1, 5 = 2, etc. Questions 14–20: score the mark on each line on a scale of 0–10; add all scores together. Add the numbers obtained from scoring all the above questions for the total FIQ score. Scores greater than 70 represent severe impact. Reprinted from [5], with permission.

[6] included a total of 2,276 subjects across 34 studies; 1,264 subjects were assigned to exercise interventions. Evidence of moderate quality indicates that aerobic-only exercise training at intensity levels recommended by the American College of Sports Medicine has positive effects on pain, global well-being, and physical function. Strengthening exercises (for 21 weeks), as recommended by the American College of Sports Medicine, also show an increase in global well-being and a reduction in pain, tender points, and possibly depression. In several studies, improvement in pain, FIQ score, function, and depression were maintained for 6 months to 2 years after an aerobic exercise program. There is also evidence for pool therapy, which generally involves active range of motion, stretching, relaxation, and out-of-pool exercises or aerobic exercise and stretching [1,18,22]. These studies generally report a decrease in pain and an increase in quality of life, and one study also noted a decrease in fatigue and improvement in depression [1,22].

Other physical therapy interventions, including manipulation, massage, electrotherapy, and ultrasound, may offer some benefits, as supported by the APS clinical guidelines for fibromyalgia [18]. However, these other therapies are based on limited evidence in RCTs. One RCT showed that connective tissue massage (given in 15 treatments over 10 weeks) reduced pain and analgesic consumption, and improved quality of life as measured by the FIQ when compared to a reference group that was not treated [4]. This effect was not maintained long-term at a 6-month follow-up [4]. In one double-blind RCT, laser therapy applied over acupuncture sites had no effect on pain or function [58]. Thus, physical modalities such as TENS, manual therapy, and ultrasound should be used in combination with aerobic and strength training exercises for people with fibromyalgia. They may be useful to reduce pain in order for patients to better perform their exercise program. Future studies should assess the usefulness of these modalities as an adjunct therapy for people with fibromyalgia.

References

[1]   Altan L, Bingol U, Aykac M, Koc Z, Yurtkuran M. Investigation of the effects of pool-based exercise on fibromyalgia syndrome. Rheumatol Int 2004;24:272–7.
[3]   Arnold LM, Goldenberg DL, Stanford SB, Lalonde JK, Sandhu HS, Keck PE Jr, Welge JA, Bishop F, Stanford KE, Hess EV, et al. Gabapentin in the treatment of fibromyalgia: a randomized, double-blind, placebo-controlled, multicenter trial. Arthritis Rheum 2007;56:1336–44.

[3] Bondy B, Spaeth M, Offenbaecher M, Glatzeder K, Stratz T, Schwarz M, de JS, Kruger M, Engel RR, Farber L, et al. The T102C polymorphism of the 5-HT2A-receptor gene in fibromyalgia. Neurobiol Dis 1999;6:433–9.

[4] Brattberg G. Connective tissue massage in the treatment of fibromyalgia. Eur J Pain 1999;3:235–44.

[5] Burckhardt CS, Clark SR, Bennett RM. The Fibromyalgia Impact Questionnaire: development and validation. J Rheumatol 1991;18:728–33.

[6] Busch AJ, Barber KA, Overend TJ, Peloso PM, Schachter CL. Exercise for treating fibromyalgia syndrome. Cochrane Database Syst Rev 2007;CD003786.

[7] Buskila D, Cohen H, Neumann L, Ebstein RP. An association between fibromyalgia and the dopamine D4 receptor exon III repeat polymorphism and relationship to novelty seeking personality traits. Mol Psychiatry 2004;9:730–1.

[8] Buskila D, Sarzi-Puttini P, Ablin JN. The genetics of fibromyalgia syndrome. Pharmacogenomics 2007;8:67–74.

[9] Clauw DJ, Crofford LJ. Chronic widespread pain and fibromyalgia: what we know, and what we need to know. Best Pract Res Clin Rheumatol 2003;17:685–701.

[10] Cummings TM, White AR. Needling therapies in the management of myofascial trigger point pain: a systematic review. Arch Phys Med Rehabil 2001;82:986–92.

[11] Edwards J, Knowles N. Superficial dry needling and active stretching in the treatment of myofascial pain: a randomised controlled trial. Acupunct Med 2003;21:80–6.

[12] Ferrante FM, Bearn L, Rothrock R, King L. Evidence against trigger point injection technique for the treatment of cervicothoracic myofascial pain with botulinum toxin type A. Anesthesiology 2005;103:377–83.

[13] Fishbain DA, Rosomoff HL, Steele-Rosomoff R, Cutler RB. Pain treatment facilities referral selection criteria. Clin J Pain 1995;11:156–7.

[14] Ga H, Choi JH, Park CH, Yoon HJ. Acupuncture needling versus lidocaine injection of trigger points in myofascial pain syndrome in elderly patients: a randomised trial. Acupunct Med 2007;25:130–6.

[15] Gam AN, Warming S, Larsen LH, Jensen B, Hoydalsmo O, Allon I, Andersen B, Gotzsche NE, Petersen M, Mathiesen B. Treatment of myofascial trigger-points with ultrasound combined with massage and exercise: a randomised controlled trial. Pain 1998;77:73–9.

[16] Giovengo SL, Russell IJ, Larson AA. Increased concentrations of nerve growth factor in cerebrospinal fluid of patients with fibromyalgia. J Rheumatol 1999;26:1564–9.

[17] Goldenberg DL. Pharmacological treatment of fibromyalgia and other chronic musculoskeletal pain. Best Pract Res Clin Rheumatol 2007;21:499–511.

[18] Goldenberg DL, Burckhardt C, Crofford L. Management of fibromyalgia syndrome. JAMA 2004;292:2388–95.

[19] Graff-Radford SB, Reeves JL, Baker RL, Chiu D. Effects of transcutaneous electrical nerve stimulation on myofascial pain and trigger point sensitivity. Pain 1989;37:1–5.

[20] Gran JT. The epidemiology of chronic generalized musculoskeletal pain. Best Pract Res Clin Rheumatol 2003;17:547–61.

[21] Gursoy S, Erdal E, Herken H, Madenci E, Alasehirli B, Erdal N. Significance of catechol-O-methyltransferase gene polymorphism in fibromyalgia syndrome. Rheumatol Int 2003;23:104–7.

[22] Gusi N, Tomas-Carus P, Hakkinen A, Hakkinen K, Ortega-Alonso A. Exercise in waist-high warm water decreases pain and improves health-related quality of life and strength in the lower extremities in women with fibromyalgia. Arthritis Rheum 2006;55:66–73.

[23] Ho KY, Tan KH. Botulinum toxin A for myofascial trigger point injection: a qualitative systematic review. Eur J Pain 2007;11:519–27.

[24] Hou CR, Tsai LC, Cheng KF, Chung KC, Hong CZ. Immediate effects of various physical therapeutic modalities on cervical myofascial pain and trigger-point sensitivity. Arch Phys Med Rehabil 2002;83:1406–14.

[25] Hsueh TC, Cheng PT, Kuan TS, Hong CZ. The immediate effectiveness of electrical nerve stimulation and electrical muscle stimulation on myofascial trigger points. Am J Phys Med Rehabil 1997;76:471–6.

[26] Jaeger B, Reeves JL. Quantification of changes in myofascial trigger point sensitivity with the pressure algometer following passive stretch. Pain 1986;27:203–10.

[27] Kosek E, Ordeberg G. Lack of pressure pain modulation by heterotopic noxious conditioning stimulation in patients with painful osteoarthritis before, but not following, surgical pain relief. Pain 2000;88:69–78.

[28] Kuan TS, Hsieh YL, Chen SM, Chen JT, Yen WC, Hong CZ. The myofascial trigger point region: correlation between the degree of irritability and the prevalence of endplate noise. Am J Phys Med Rehabil 2007;86:183–9.

[29] Lautenbacher S, Rollman GB. Possible deficiencies of pain modulation in fibromyalgia. Clin J Pain 1997;13:189–96.

[30] Leffler AS, Hansson P, Kosek E. Somatosensory perception in a remote pain-free area and function of diffuse noxious inhibitory controls (DNIC) in patients suffering from long-term trapezius myalgia. Eur J Pain 2002;6:149–59.

[31] Majlesi J, Unalan H. High-power pain threshold ultrasound technique in the treatment of active myofascial trigger points: a randomized, double-blind, case-control study. Arch Phys Med Rehabil 2004;85:833–6.

[32] Mease PJ, Russell IJ, Arnold LM, Florian H, Young JP, Jr., Martin SA, Sharma U. A randomized, double-blind, placebo-controlled, phase III trial of pregabalin in the treatment of patients with fibromyalgia. J Rheumatol 2008;35:502–14.

[33] Niddam DM, Chan RC, Lee SH, Yeh TC, Hsieh JC. Central modulation of pain evoked from myofascial trigger point. Clin J Pain 2007;23:440–8.

[34] Offenbaecher M, Bondy B, de JS, Glatzeder K, Kruger M, Schoeps P, Ackenheil M. Possible association of fibromyalgia with a polymorphism in the serotonin transporter gene regulatory region. Arthritis Rheum 1999;42:2482–8.

[35] Price DD, Staud R, Robinson ME, Mauderli AP, Cannon R, Vierck CJ. Enhanced temporal summation of second pain and its central modulation in fibromyalgia patients. Pain 2002;99:49–59.

[36] Rao SG, Bennett RM. Pharmacological therapies in fibromyalgia. Best Pract Res Clin Rheumatol 2003;17:611–27.

[37] Rivner MH. The neurophysiology of myofascial pain syndrome. Curr Pain Headache Rep 2001;5:432–40.

[38] Rossy LA, Buckelew SP, Dorr N, Hagglund KJ, Thayer JF, McIntosh MJ, Hewett JE, Johnson JC. A meta-analysis of fibromyalgia treatment interventions. Ann Behav Med 1999;21:180–91.

[39] Russell IJ. Neurochemical pathogenesis of fibromyalgia. Z Rheumatol 1998;2:63–6.

[40] Russell IJ, Bieber CS. Myofascial pain and fibromyalgia syndrome. In: McMahon SB, Koltzenburg M, editors. Wall and Melzack's textbook of pain. London: Elsevier; 2000. p. 669–81.

[41] Russell IJ, Vaeroy H, Javors M, Nyberg F. Cerebrospinal fluid biogenic amine metabolites in fibromyalgia/fibrositis syndrome and rheumatoid arthritis. Arthritis Rheum 1992;35:550–6.

[42] Shah JP, Danoff JV, Desai MJ, Parikh S, Nakamura LY, Phillips TM, Gerber LH. Biochemicals associated with pain and inflammation are elevated in sites near to and remote from active myofascial trigger points. Arch Phys Med Rehabil 2008;89:16–23.

[43] Shah JP, Phillips TM, Danoff JV, Gerber LH. An in vivo microanalytical technique for measuring the local biochemical milieu of human skeletal muscle. J Appl Physiol 2005;99:1977–84.

[44] Simons DG, Travell JG, Simons LS. Travell & Simons' myofascial pain and dysfunction: the trigger point manual, Vol. 1. Lippincott, Williams and Wilkins; 1999.

[45] Skootsky SA, Jaeger B, Oye RK. Prevalence of myofascial pain in general internal medicine practice. West J Med 1989;151:157–60.

[46] Sola AE, Bonica JJ. Myofascial pain syndromes. In: Loeser JD, Turk DC, Chapman CR, Butler SH, editors. Bonica's management of pain. Philadelphia: Lippincott, Williams and Wilkins; 2000. p. 107–21.

[47] Srbely JZ, Dickey JP. Randomized controlled study of the antinociceptive effect of ultrasound on trigger point sensitivity: novel applications in myofascial therapy? Clin Rehabil 2007;21:411–17.

[48] Staud R. Treatment of fibromyalgia and its symptoms. Expert Opin Pharmacother 2007;8:1629–42.

[49] Staud R, Cannon RC, Mauderli AP, Robinson ME, Price DD, Vierck CJ. Temporal summation of pain from mechanical stimulation of muscle tissue in normal controls and subjects with fibromyalgia syndrome. Pain 2003;102:87–95.

[50] Staud R, Carl KE, Vierck CJ, Price DD, Robinson ME, Cannon RL, Mauderli AP. Repetitive muscle stimuli result in enhanced wind-up of fibromyalgia patients. Arthritis Rheum 2001;44:S395.

[51] Staud R, Robinson ME, Vierck CJ, Price DD. Diffuse noxious inhibitory controls (DNIC) attenuate temporal summation of second pain in normal males but not in normal females or fibromyalgia patients. Pain 2003;101:167–74.

[52] Staud R, Rodriguez ME. Mechanisms of disease: pain in fibromyalgia syndrome. Nat Clin Pract Rheumatol 2006;2:90–8.

[53] Staud R, Vierck CJ, Cannon RL, Mauderli AP, Price DD. Abnormal sensitization and temporal summation of second pain (wind-up) in patients with fibromyalgia syndrome. Pain 2001;91:165–75.

[54] Staud R, Vierck CJ, Mauderli A, Cannon R. Abnormal temporal summation of second pain (wind-up) in patients with the fibromyalgia syndrome. Arthritis Rheum 1998;41:S353.

[55] Tough EA, White AR, Richards S, Campbell J. Variability of criteria used to diagnose myofascial trigger point pain syndrome: evidence from a review of the literature. Clin J Pain 2007;23:278–86.

[56] Vaeroy H, Helle R, Forre O, Kass E, Terenius L. Elevated CSF levels of substance P and high incidence of Raynaud phenomena in patients with fibromyalgia: new features for diagnosis. Pain 1988;31:21–6.

[57] Vierck CJ Jr. Mechanisms underlying development of spatially distributed chronic pain (fibromyalgia). Pain 2006;124:242–63.

[58] Waylonis GW, Wilke S, O'Toole D, Waylonis DA, Waylonis DB. Chronic myofascial pain: management by low-output helium-neon laser therapy. Arch Phys Med Rehabil 1988;69:1017–20.

[59] Wigers SH, Stiles TC, Vogel PA. Effects of aerobic exercise versus stress management treatment in fibromyalgia. A 4.5 year prospective study. Scand J Rheumatol 1996;25:77–86.

[60] Williams DA. Psychological and behavioural therapies in fibromyalgia and related syndromes. Best Pract Res Clin Rheumatol 2003;17:649–65.

[61] Williams DA, Cary MA, Groner KH, Chaplin W, Glazer LJ, Rodriguez AM, Clauw DJ. Improving physical functional status in patients with fibromyalgia: a brief cognitive behavioral intervention. J Rheumatol 2002;29:1280–6.

[62] Wolfe F, Smythe HA, Yunus MB, Bennett RM, Bombardier C, Goldenberg DL, Tugwell P, Campbell SM, Abeles M, Clark P, et al. The American College of Rheumatology 1990 criteria for the classification of fibromyalgia. Report of the multicenter criteria committee. Arthritis Rheum 1990;33:160–72.

Correspondence to: Prof. Kathleen A. Sluka, PT, PhD, Graduate Program in Physical Therapy and Rehabilitation Science, The University of Iowa, 1-252 Medical Education Building, Iowa City, IA 52242-1190, USA. Tel: 1-319-335-9791; fax: 1-319-335-9707; email: kathleen-sluka@uiowa.edu.

Temporomandibular Disorders and Headache

Kathleen A. Sluka

Graduate Program in Physical Therapy and Rehabilitation Science,
The University of Iowa, Iowa City, Iowa, USA

Disorders of the head and face include temporomandibular joint disorder (TMD) and headache (Fig. 1). Headache is the most common pain problem, with a prevalence of 30–78% for tension-type headache and 10–12% for migraine [24,49,53]. There are three classifications of headache: migraine, tension-type headache, and cluster headache [2]. These can be considered primary or secondary, depending on whether they are the result of an organic lesion or a systemic disease. While these types of headaches are defined and described separately, it should be kept in mind that many people have a mixture of migraine and tension-type headache. Most headaches are caused by muscular contraction, vascular dysfunction, or a combination of both.

Temporomandibular disorders involve pain around the temporomandibular joint (TMJ) and the muscles that control jaw movement. TMD conditions fall into three main categories: myofascial conditions, internal derangement of the joint, and arthritis. Many people with TMD also have tension-type headaches, and there is often a mixture of two or three of the TMD conditions in one patient.

TMJ Disorder	Tension HA	Migraine HA

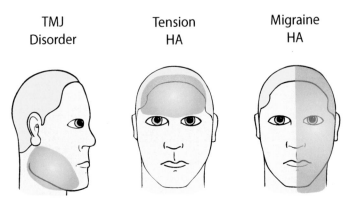

Fig. 1. Schematic diagram showing areas of pain for temporomandibular joint (TMJ) disorders, tension-type headache (HA), and migraine.

Migraine

Epidemiology and Diagnosis

Migraine headaches are associated with recurrent attacks lasting from 4 to 72 hours, which are typically unilateral in adults and are usually located in the frontotemporal region of the head [2,24]. After the attack, the patient is commonly fatigued. Classically, migraine is associated with an aura consisting of visual, sensory, or auditory disturbances that usually precede the headache. However, migraine without aura is more common than migraine with aura by a ratio of 2:1. As is the case for many pain conditions, more females than males (2–3:1) are afflicted with migraine [49]. Interestingly, migraine can start very early in life, affecting approximately 7% of children, and the prevalence increases with age [34]. In a recent survey of the German population, the mean age of onset was 7 years, with some patients reporting age of onset in the range of 1–3 years [34]. The majority of people with migraine have infrequent attacks (one per month), but about 20% of people with migraine have more than one attack per month [49]. Diagnostic criteria for migraine with and without aura are outlined in Table I [28].

Pathobiology

Migraine is considered a neurovascular disorder. The blood vessels supplying the brain and dura mater are innervated largely by unmyelinated C fibers that contain the neuropeptides substance P and calcitonin gene-related peptide [24,44]. Release of these neuropeptides from their peripheral terminals causes vasodilation, with subsequent sensitization of nociceptors and central neurons in the trigeminal system [24]. The clinically effective migraine drugs, the triptans, are serotonin agonists that act peripherally to block neuropeptide release, an effect that has been confirmed both in animal studies and in human subjects with migraine [9,25,44].

Table I
Diagnostic criteria for migraine with and without aura

A. 5 attacks (WITHOUT AURA) or 2 attacks (WITH AURA)

B. Headache lasting 4–72 hours (WITHOUT AURA)

C. Headache with two of the following: unilateral, pulsatory, moderate to severe pain, aggravated by routine physical activity (i.e., walking)

D. During headache one of the following: (1) nausea or vomiting; (2) photophobia or phonophobia

E. Not related to other diseases

F. Fully reversible visual, sensory or speech symptoms (no motor weakness) (WITH AURA)

G. At least two of the following: (1) visual symptoms (i.e. flickering lights, spots or loss of vision), sensory symptoms (i.e., pins and needles, numbness), dysphagic speech disturbance; (2) one symptom gradually develops over 5 minutes, or (3) symptoms last between 5 and 60 minutes

Source: Headache Classification Subcommittee of the International Headache Society [28].

Alterations in the serotonin system also appear to play a role in migraine. Specifically, researchers suspect a depletion in serotonin centrally that contributes to sensitization, as well as an increase in the 5-HT transporter, in patients with migraine [26,54]. Genetic polymorphisms in the 5-HT transporter gene are also observed in migraine and have been linked to susceptibility or predisposition to migraine and to the frequency of attacks [26].

Assessment Considerations

Assessment of pain in people with migraine should include not only the severity of the pain, but also the frequency of the headache. In addition, the impact of the migraine on quality of life and any disability resulting from the migraine should be assessed. The Migraine Disability Assessment Scale (MIDAS) is a simple scale that is validated and easy to use (see Table II) [57]. Based on the total number of days in questions 1–5, the following graded definition can be given to the patient for disability: I, minimal or infrequent disability, score = 0–5; II, mild or infrequent disability, score = 6–10; III, moderate disability, score = 11–20; IV, severe disability, score = 21+.

Table II
Migraine Disability Assessment Scale (MIDAS)

Instructions: Please answer the following questions about ALL your headaches you have had over the last 3 months. Write your answer in the box next to each question. Write zero if you did not do the activity in the last 3 months.

1. On how many days in the last 3 months did you miss work or school because of your headaches? ____ days.

2. How many days in the last 3 months was your productivity at work or school reduced by half or more because of your headaches (not including days in 1)? ___days.

3. On how many days in the last 3 months did you not do household work because of your headache? ____ days.

4. How many days in the last 3 months was your productivity in household work reduced by half or more because of your headaches (do no include days in 3)? ____ days.

5. On how many days in the last 3 months did you miss family, social, or leisure activities because of your headaches? ____ days.

A. On how many days in the last 3 months did you have a headache (if a headache lasted more than one day count each day? ____ days.

B. On a scale of 0–10, on average how painful were these headaches? (0 = no pain; 10 = worst pain imaginable)

Source: Reprinted from [48] with permission from Lippincott, Williams & Wilkins.

Medical Management

Treatment of migraine is primarily managed with pharmacological agents designed either to treat an acute attack or to prevent the frequency of attacks. Patients are also frequently taught nonpharmacological techniques to assist in management of migraines. These treatments include education on how to avoid triggers, relaxation therapy, and biofeedback. Pharmacological and nonpharmacological treatments aimed at managing migraines will generally reduce the frequency of attacks, but not the intensity of the pain during an attack. On the other hand, pharmacological agents aimed at treating acute attacks will reduce the intensity of the pain. The most effective treatment for acute attacks is the use of triptans, the most common of which is sumatriptan, which has been confirmed in systematic reviews to be effective [39]. The triptans are 5-HT$_{1B/1D}$ agonists that act as vasoconstrictors and are aimed at treating the underlying pathology of migraine. Prophylactic treatments include long-term use of beta-blockers, serotonin antagonists, calcium channel blockers, and tricyclic antidepressants. Systematic reviews show that beta-blockers (propranolol) and anticonvulsant drugs reduce the frequency of migraine attacks [8,36,63]. There is good evidence that the intensity and duration of the headache of an acute attack are effectively treated with sumatriptan, and that prophylactic treatments with beta-blockers and anticonvulsant drugs reduce the frequency of attacks. However, data on the use of tricyclic antidepressants for treatment of migraine are inconclusive [43].

Psychological Management

Nonpharmacological approaches include relaxation, biofeedback, and other psychological approaches such as cognitive-behavioral therapies. Systematic reviews show limited evidence of headache improvement with relaxation therapy when compared to wait-list controls, and no evidence for effectiveness of biofeedback when administered in isolation [10]. Combining nonpharmacological approaches results in improvements in headache symptoms when compared to wait-list controls. There is moderate evidence for relaxation combined with biofeedback and limited evidence for relaxation combined with cognitive-behavioral therapy compared with placebo [10,38].

Physical Therapy

Physical therapy aimed at improvement in posture, cervical range of motion (ROM), and strength is essentially ineffective in the treatment of migraine. However, physical therapy is more likely to help subjects who are unresponsive to relaxation and biofeedback techniques [38]. Furthermore, according to systematic reviews, spinal manipulation or mobilization of the cervical spine, delivered by a chiropractor or a physiotherapist, reduces the frequency and severity of attacks and lessens migraine-related disability [3]. However, these conclusions are based on weak evidence, and the treatment is not recommended in practice guidelines [3]. Thus, physical therapy on its own is not effective for treatment of migraine, but it may be effective as an adjunct therapy if combined with relaxation and biofeedback treatments.

Cluster Headache

Cluster headaches occur in the orbital, supraorbital, or temporal areas and are associated with excruciating pain [24]. The headaches are very frequent, occurring between 0.5 and 8 times per day, and are short-lived, lasting between 30 and 180 minutes. The headaches are accompanied by at least one of the following symptoms: lacrimation, nasal congestion or rhinorrhea, eyelid edema, forehead and facial swelling, meiosis and/or ptosis, and a sense of restlessness or agitation. The incidence of cluster headache is very rare, occurring in 0.1–0.4% of the population, with men more likely to be affected than women. The pain associated with cluster headache is typically described as sharp, boring, drilling, stabbing, or piercing, but not throbbing like migraine. The pain is excruciating and typically leaves the person exhausted for some time after the attack. Medical management is essential, and physical therapy is generally not thought to be effective.

Tension-Type Headache

Epidemiology and Diagnosis

Episodic tension-type headaches can be difficult to distinguish from migraine without aura. The lifetime prevalence of tension-type headache is 30–78%, and females are more likely to develop tension-type headaches than males [49]. Tension-type headaches commonly have a muscular component (associated with pericranial tenderness), with tenderness to palpation of the cranium typically found at the base of the skull and around the temporal region.

Diagnostic criteria for tension-type headache were proposed by the International Headache Society in 1988 and are widely used for diagnosis and in research [28]. Tension-type headaches can be classified as episodic, occurring with a frequency of fewer than 15 headaches per

month, or chronic, occurring with a frequency of more than 15 per month
[2]. Episodic tension-type headache has been subdivided into infrequent
(less than 1 day per month) and frequent (1–14 days per month). These
headaches can be further subclassified as those associated with pericranial
tenderness and those without. Diagnostic criteria for tension-type headache are outlined in Table III [28].

Table III
Diagnostic criteria for tension-type headache

A. Episodic: fewer than 15 headaches per month; chronic: more than
15 headaches per month

B. Headache lasting from 30 minutes to 7 days

C. At least 2 of the following: (1) pressing or tightening quality;
(2) mild or moderate intensity; (3) bilateral; (4) not aggravated by
routing physical activity

D. Both of the following: (1) no nausea or vomiting; (2) photophobia
and phonophobia are absent, but may have one of the two

E. Not attributed to another disorder

F. Subtypes: associated with pericranial tenderness or not associated
with pericranial tenderness

Source: Headache Classification Subcommittee of the International
Headache Society [28].

Pathobiology

There is little information on the underlying pathology associated with
tension-type headaches. However, electromyographic (EMG) activity in
the pericranial muscles is higher in people with tension-type headaches
and bears a positive correlation with the intensity of the headache [35].
Further, there is increased cervical muscle co-contraction during cervical
flexion and extension [21], which suggests changes in motor control strategies in people with chronic tension-type headache. There are decreases
in pressure pain thresholds in the pericranial area, as well as in sites distinct from this area, such as the hands or lower legs [53]. Further, people
with chronic tension-type headaches have a greater number of active trigger points and greater pain intensity on palpation of the trigger points [9].
Together, these data suggest that there may be local changes that result in
peripheral sensitization, which in turn leads to alterations in central neuron processing of nociceptive stimuli and central sensitization.

Assessment Considerations

Assessment of tension-type headache should include standard pain measures, the visual analogue scale and McGill Pain Questionnaire. In addition, assessments of self-efficacy and quality of life should be considered because there can be a significant impact on daily function in this group of patients. Understanding the frequency of headaches, the duration of each headache, and the intensity of headaches is important in examining and assessing the outcome of treatment. Palpation for tenderness over muscle groups will help guide manual therapy treatments.

Medical Management

The first choice of pharmacological treatment for tension-type headaches are the nonsteroidal anti-inflammatory drugs (NSAIDs); this class of drugs reduces the intensity of the headache [48,53]. If NSAIDs are ineffective, or if patients have chronic headaches, tricyclic antidepressants are a common pharmacological therapy [53]. Systematic reviews do not, however, support the use of selective serotonin reuptake inhibitors (SSRIs) for prophylactic treatment of tension-type headache [43].

Psychological Management

Nonpharmacological treatments include relaxation therapy, biofeedback, cognitive-behavioral therapy, and physical therapy. There is good evidence that psychological therapies (relaxation therapy or cognitive-behavioral therapy) are effective, with long-term improvements, for treatment of children and adolescents with chronic headache, as confirmed in systematic reviews and a meta-analysis [19,20,60]. In adults, treatment with stress management therapy reduces headache frequency, analgesic use, and disability but produces a greater effect when combined with tricyclic antidepressants [30]. The efficacy of cognitive-behavioral therapy (stress management), relaxation therapy, and biofeedback has been confirmed in a meta-analysis [4,5].

Physical Therapy Management

Physical therapy is typically not effective for people with cluster or migraine headaches. However, tension-type headaches, which are typically of muscular origin, are effectively treated with physical therapy. Physical therapy for tension-type headache typically involves education regarding posture and biomechanics, as well as an exercise program aimed at improving posture of the cervical spine [27,59]. Manual therapy is also commonly used to reduce muscle contraction in the upper cervical spine and the temporalis muscles and to reduce pain [27,59]. According to the systematic review by Bronfort and colleagues, there is weak evidence to support the use of spinal manipulation and mobilization as a prophylactic treatment, producing short-term effects [6]. The use of other physical pain-relieving modalities, such as transcutaneous electrical nerve stimulation (TENS) or thermal treatments, is unclear and has not been studied in randomized controlled trials (RCTs). However, because they are easy to use, inexpensive, and have negligible side effects, their use should be tried to reduce pain and muscle tension.

There is limited research to support the use of physical therapy in tension-type headache (see Table IV). However, evidence from RCTs is generally favorable. Torelli et al. [59] examined the effect of 8 weeks of physical therapy on subjects with episodic or chronic tension-type headache. The physical therapy group received treatment consisting of massage, relaxation, stretching, and a home exercise program twice a week for 4 weeks. The last 4 weeks consisted of an exercise program only. A second group received an 8-week observation period by a neurologist, followed by physical therapy. The main measurement outcome was headache frequency, and the goal of treatment was to instruct the subjects how to manage the condition on their own. In both episodic and chronic tension-type headache, the frequency of headache and consumption of analgesics were reduced with physical therapy treatment after 8 weeks and maintained at a 12-week follow-up period, with the effect being greater in patients with chronic tension-type headache. The intensity and duration of headaches were unaffected by physical therapy treatment. Similarly, Hammill and colleagues [27] showed a reduction in the frequency of headache and an improvement in the Sickness Impact Profile, a quality-of-life measure, with a physical therapy treatment consisting of education for posture at home and in the workplace, isotonic home exercises, massage, and stretching of the cervical spine muscles. A long-term follow-up at 12 months showed that this effect continued through the follow-up period.

Table IV
Evidence for physical therapy treatments for headache and TMD

Disease	Treatment	Refs.	Type of Study	Results
Migraine	Postural, cervical range of motion, strengthening exercises	[38]	RCT	Effective only when used if unresponsive to relaxation and biofeedback
Migraine	Manipulation of cervical spine	[3]	Cochrane review	Reduces frequency, severity and disability; weak evidence
Tension-type headache	Massage, relaxation, stretching, and home exercise	[27,59]	RCT and CT	Reduces frequency of attacks, reduces analgesic consumption, and improves quality of life
TMD	Postural exercises	[40,41]	Systematic review	Reduces pain and improves ROM
TMD	Home exercise and manual therapy	[23,31, 42,64]	RCT	Reduces pain and improves jaw function
TMD	High-frequency TENS	[32]	RCT	Reduces pain and EMG activity
TMD	Low-level laser therapy	[24,47]	RCT	Reduces pain

Abbreviations: CT = controlled trial; EMG = electromyography; RCT = randomized controlled trial; ROM = range of motion; TMD = temporomandibular joint dysfunction.

Therefore, a multimodal approach incorporating education, exercise, and manual therapy is probably the most effective physical therapy approach for people with tension-type headaches.

Temporomandibular Disorders

Epidemiology and Diagnosis

Temporomandibular disorders (TMD) involve pain around the temporomandibular joint (TMJ) and the muscles that control jaw movement [46,61]. TMD is more common in women than men; incidence rates vary between 10% and 20% of the population [61]. TMD conditions fall into three main categories: myofascial pain, internal derangement, and arthritis [46,61]. Myofascial pain involves pain in the muscles that control jaw function. Myofascial pain associated with TMD is a general term used to describe pain associated with muscles and does not necessarily include trigger points, as defined for myofascial pain below the head (described in Chapter 14) [46,61].

TMD can be acute, is generally cyclical, and usually goes away with little or no treatment. In some conditions, however, the pain can become chronic and may result in significant disability and loss of function [46,61]. Pain is generally worse with movement, and there is tenderness over the muscles surrounding the jaw and neck [46,61]. The pain is poorly localized, dull, aching, and bilateral. It is often referred to the ear, mandible, and temporal areas but can also be located in the teeth and face [46,61]. There is decreased function of the jaw, measured as a decrease in bite force, limited jaw opening, and asymmetrical mandibular movement [46,61]. Headache is also commonly associated with TMD, and there is a higher incidence of tension-type headache (but not migraine) in people with TMD. EMG analysis of the masticatory muscles shows hyperactivity, as well as an asymmetrical recruitment of the temporal and masseter muscles (which are normally symmetrical) [50].

Internal derangement of the TMJ is thought to be an abnormal relationship between the articular disk and the mandible, fossa, and articular eminence [61]. Symptoms include pain, limited mouth opening, deviation of mouth opening, and clicking, cracking, or snapping when opening the jaw [61]. Diagnosis is typically made by magnetic resonance imaging (MRI), along with assessment of signs and symptoms [61]. The etiology of internal derangement is thought to be a result of trauma, muscle hyperactivity, or hyperextension of the mandible. Arthritis, both osteoarthritis and rheumatoid arthritis, can occur at the TMJ joint and can result in similar conditions to those outlined in Chapter 18.

Pathobiology

Data from animal and human studies suggest that there are alterations in the peripheral and central nervous systems in TMD [15,61]. Myofascial pain of the muscles of mastication, and arthritis of the TMJ, are forms of musculoskeletal pain with similar underlying mechanisms to those associated with the spine or extremities [61]. Inflammation of the masticatory muscles, or of the TMJ, results in peripheral and central sensitization, including changes in brainstem facilitatory and inhibitory pathways [55]. These changes probably underlie the pain and hyperalgesia observed in people with TMD [55].

In a prospective study that followed subjects for at least 3 years, Maixner and colleagues showed that polymorphisms in the catechol-amine-O-methyltransferase (*COMT*) gene and the β_2-adrenergic receptor gene underlie the susceptibility to development of TMD [12,13]. The *COMT* gene codes for the COMT enzyme, which regulates levels of catecholamines and enkephalins, and the β_2-adrenergic receptor is activated by catecholamines. In normal subjects, three major *COMT* haplotypes (LPS, APS, and HPS) determine COMT enzymatic activity [13]. The LPS haplotype is associated with low pain sensitivity, APS with average pain sensitivity, and HPS with the highest pain sensitivity. Individuals who develop TMD show a higher incidence of the HPS haplotype of the *COMT* gene [13]. There is also increased incidence of development of TMD in individuals with a genetic polymorphism in the β_2-adrenergic receptor gene that is associated with high expression of the receptor [12]. Thus, alterations in the catecholamine pathway influence the likelihood that an individual will develop TMD.

Assessment Considerations

As with all pain conditions, particularly those that are chronic, adequate assessment of pain using subjective pain measures and the McGill Pain Questionnaire is essential. In addition, ROM of the jaw (jaw-opening distance) should be measured in all subjects. Assessment of the pain's effect on function through a self-efficacy questionnaire, and of its impact on quality of life, are also valuable to guide the treatment plan and to assess treatment success.

Medical Management

Treatment of patients with TMJ varies depending on the underlying problems. Therapy generally involves pharmacological management, self-care, cognitive-behavioral therapy, physical therapy, and splint therapy. In some cases, particularly for internal derangement of the TMJ, arthroscopic surgery is used. Few studies have assessed the effectiveness of current pharmacological treatment for chronic TMDs and orofacial pain. Pharmacological management using NSAIDs (ibuprofen or piroxicam) has been shown in several controlled trials to be ineffective when compared to placebo [15,37]. However one study using the NSAID naproxen showed a positive reduction in pain compared with placebo [15,58]. Systematic reviews have shown that amitriptyline, clonazepam, and diazepam are effective treatments for TMD [37,56]. More recent evidence from RCTs shows effectiveness of cyclobenzaprine and gabapentin for patients with TMD [29]. Lastly, direct corticosteroid injection into the TMJ in patients with rheumatoid arthritis is more effective than placebo treatment [37]. Thus, treatment with antidepressants, anticonvulsants, muscle relaxants, and possibly NSAIDs appears to reduce pain in patients with TMD and orofacial pain.

For painful limited jaw opening, successful treatment with arthrocentesis (TMJ lavage and placement of medications into the joint) is reported in 70–90% of cases [16]. For internal derangement, surgery is used only after unsuccessful nonsurgical treatment, in patients with significant pain and dysfunction, and if there is imaging evidence of pathology [16]. Surgical interventions include arthroscopy, condylotomy, and disk repositioning or diskectomy [16].

For patients with internal derangement of the TMJ, one common treatment is a splint to correct jaw alignment. However, there is inconclusive evidence on the use of splints or occlusional adjustment (bite modification) for the treatment of TMD to reduce pain, at rest and on palpation, when compared to no treatment or placebo treatment [1,33]. As with all TMDs, conservative physical therapy treatment is recommended, involving exercise to increase the ROM and strength of the jaw muscles and modalities to reduce pain (see below). In advanced cases that are unresponsive to conservative treatment, surgery is often recommended [16].

Psychological Management/Self-Care

Self-care management is a common treatment for people with TMD. Self-care strategies include education, resting during pain, relaxation techniques, massage, hot and/or cold packs, stretching, and exercise. Positive effects for a self-care strategy to reduce pain and activity interference have been observed in several RCTs [17,45,51].

Brief cognitive-behavioral therapy for TMD is also efficacious in reducing pain, improving coping skills, and lessening activity interference. Effectiveness of therapy is increased when combining self-care management with cognitive-behavioral therapy, and some treatment effects are maintained at a 1-year follow-up assessment [18,62].

Physical Therapy Management

Physical therapy treatment for TMD involves education on posture, exercise, stretching, and soft-tissue massage. Use of heat, cold, or TENS can help to reduce pain to allow the patient to exercise and stretch the soft tissue. While these therapies are recommended treatments for people with TMD, there are minimal RCTs, and thus few systematic reviews, to support the effectiveness of these treatments (see Table IV).

Recommendations for stretching exercises and manual therapy are generally aimed at increasing ROM. Clinical trials show that home stretching exercises and manual therapy aimed at stretching soft tissue around the jaw muscles increase jaw opening and in some cases decrease pain [23,31,42]. Postural exercise training by physical therapists also significantly improves pain and increases pain-free ROM of the jaw [64]. Although the most common physical therapy treatments are aimed at increasing flexibility (stretching), strengthening, and endurance, there are currently no studies examining the effects of strengthening or endurance exercises on pain associated with TMD [14]. Systematic reviews confirm the effectiveness of active and passive oral exercises that improve posture in reducing pain and improving ROM [40,41]. As other musculoskeletal pain conditions respond well to a strengthening program, these exercises may be an important component of the exercise program.

For control of pain, hot and cold packs are inexpensive and can be self-administered. However, there is no research to support or refute their effectiveness for TMD. High-frequency, conventional TENS also reduces pain and decreases EMG activity of the masticatory muscles in people with TMD [52], and low-frequency TENS reduces EMG activity [32]. A systematic review confirmed the effectiveness of TENS [41]. Two RCTs show that low-level laser therapy (10 J/cm2 or 15 J/cm2) reduces pain in people with TMJ syndrome when compared to a placebo treatment [22,47]. Addition of ultrasound, massage, and stretching by a physical therapist, or heat, massage, and stretching by the patient in a self-care program, provided no additional effect on pain, pressure pain thresholds, or function; both treatments worked equally well [11,42]. Thus, physical therapy should be aimed at improving function and posture with the use of education, exercises, and manual therapy. Modalities such as laser therapy, TENS, heat, and cold should be used as necessary to reduce pain. Evidence from a limited number of RCTs supports the efficacy of TENS and laser therapy, as well as education, exercise, and manual therapy. Future clinical trials will need to expand these studies by defining optimal treatment parameters and examining the effects of endurance and strengthening exercises.

References

[1]   Al-Ani MZ, Davies SJ, Gray RJ, Sloan P, Glenny AM. Stabilisation splint therapy for temporomandibular pain dysfunction syndrome. Cochrane Database Syst Rev 2004;CD002778.
[2]   Bigal ME, Lipton RB. Headache. In: McMahon SB, Koltzenburg M, editors. Wall and Melzack's textbook of pain. London: Elsevier; 2006. p. 837–50.
[3]   Biondi DM. Physical treatments for headache: a structured review. Headache 2005;45:738–46.
[4]   Blanchard EB, Appelbaum KA, Guarnieri P, Morrill B, Dentinger MP. Five year prospective follow-up on the treatment of chronic headache with biofeedback and/or relaxation. Headache 1987;27:580–3.
[5]   Bogaards MC, ter Kuile MM. Treatment of recurrent tension headache: a meta-analytic review. Clin J Pain 1994;10:174–90.
[6]   Bronfort G, Nilsson N, Haas M, Evans R, Goldsmith CH, Assendelft WJ, Bouter LM. Noninvasive physical treatments for chronic/recurrent headache. Cochrane Database Syst Rev 2004;CD001878.
[7]   Buzzi MG, Carter WB, Shimizu T, Heath H, III, Moskowitz MA. Dihydroergotamine and sumatriptan attenuate levels of CGRP in plasma in rat superior sagittal sinus during electrical stimulation of the trigeminal ganglion. Neuropharmacology 1991;30:1193–200.
[8]   Chronicle E, Mulleners W. Anticonvulsant drugs for migraine prophylaxis. Cochrane Database Syst Rev 2004;CD003226.
[9]   Couppe C, Torelli P, Fuglsang-Frederiksen A, Andersen KV, Jensen R. Myofascial trigger points are very prevalent in patients with chronic tension-type headache: a double-blinded controlled study. Clin J Pain 2007;23:23–7.
[10] Damen L, Bruijn J, Koes BW, Berger MY, Passchier J, Verhagen AP. Prophylactic treatment of migraine in children. Part 1. A systematic review of non-pharmacological trials. Cephalalgia 2006;26:373–83.
[11] De Laat A, Stappaerts K, Papy S. Counseling and physical therapy as treatment for myofascial pain of the masticatory system. J Orofac Pain 2003;17:42–9.
[12] Diatchenko L, Anderson AD, Slade GD, Fillingim RB, Shabalina SA, Higgins TJ, Sama S, Belfer I, Goldman D, Max MB, et al. Three major haplotypes of the beta-2 adrenergic receptor define psychological profile, blood pressure, and the risk for development of a common musculoskeletal pain disorder. Am J Med Genet B Neuropsychiatr Genet 2006;141:449–62.
[13] Diatchenko L, Nackley AG, Slade GD, Bhalang K, Belfer I, Max MB, Goldman D, Maixner W. Catechol-O-methyltransferase gene polymorphisms are associated with multiple pain-evoking stimuli. Pain 2006;125:216–24.

[14] Di Fabio RP. Physical therapy for patients with TMD: a descriptive study of treatment, disability, and health status. J Orofac Pain 1998;12:124–35.

[15] Dionne RA, Kim H, Gordon SM. Acute and chronic dental and orofacial pain. In: McMahon SB, Koltzenburg M, editors. Wall and Melzack's textbook of pain. London: Elsevier; 2006. p. 819–35.

[16] Dolwick MF. Temporomandibular joint surgery for internal derangement. Dent Clin North Am 2007;51:195–08, vii–viii.

[17] Dworkin SF, Turner JA, Mancl L, Wilson L, Massoth D, Huggins KH, LeResche L, Truelove E. A randomized clinical trial of a tailored comprehensive care treatment program for temporomandibular disorders. J Orofac Pain 2002;16:259–76.

[18] Dworkin SF, Turner JA, Wilson L, Massoth D, Whitney C, Huggins KH, Burgess J, Sommers E, Truelove E. Brief group cognitive-behavioral intervention for temporomandibular disorders. Pain 1994;59:175–87.

[19] Eccleston C, Morley S, Williams A, Yorke L, Mastroyannopoulou K. Systematic review of randomised controlled trials of psychological therapy for chronic pain in children and adolescents, with a subset meta-analysis of pain relief. Pain 2002;99:157–65.

[20] Eccleston C, Yorke L, Morley S, Williams AC, Mastroyannopoulou K. Psychological therapies for the management of chronic and recurrent pain in children and adolescents. Cochrane Database Syst Rev 2003;CD003968.

[21] Fernandez-de-las-Penas C, Falla D, Arendt-Nielsen L, Farina D. Cervical muscle co-activation in isometric contractions is enhanced in chronic tension-type headache patients. Cephalalgia 2008;28:744–51.

[22] Fikackova H, Dostalova T, Navratil L, Klaschka J. Effectiveness of low-level laser therapy in temporomandibular joint disorders: a placebo-controlled study. Photomed Laser Surg 2007;25:297–303.

[23] Furto ES, Cleland JA, Whitman JM, Olson KA. Manual physical therapy interventions and exercise for patients with temporomandibular disorders. Cranio 2006;24:283–91.

[24] Goadsby PJ. Primary neurovascular headache. In: McMahon SB, Koltzenburg M, editors. Textbook of pain. Philadelphia: Elsevier; 2006. p. 851–74.

[25] Goadsby PJ, Edvinsson L. The trigeminovascular system and migraine: studies characterizing cerebrovascular and neuropeptide changes seen in humans and cats. Ann Neurol 1993;33:48–56.

[26] Hamel E. Serotonin and migraine: biology and clinical implications. Cephalalgia 2007;27:1293–300.

[27] Hammill JM, Cook TM, Rosecrance JC. Effectiveness of a physical therapy regimen in the treatment of tension-type headache. Headache 1996;36:149–53.

[28] Headache Classification Subcommittee of the International Headache Society. The international classification of headache disorders: 2nd edition. Cephalgia 2004;1:9–160.

[29] Herman CR, Schiffman EL, Look JO, Rindal DB. The effectiveness of adding pharmacologic treatment with clonazepam or cyclobenzaprine to patient education and self-care for the treatment of jaw pain upon awakening: a randomized clinical trial. J Orofac Pain 2002;16:64–70.

[30] Holroyd KA, O'Donnell FJ, Stensland M, Lipchik GL, Cordingley GE, Carlson BW. Management of chronic tension-type headache with tricyclic antidepressant medication, stress management therapy, and their combination: a randomized controlled trial. JAMA 2001;285:2208–15.

[31] Ismail F, Demling A, Hessling K, Fink M, Stiesch-Scholz M. Short-term efficacy of physical therapy compared to splint therapy in treatment of arthrogenous TMD. J Oral Rehabil 2007;34:807–13.

[32] Kamyszek G, Ketcham R, Garcia R, Jr., Radke J. Electromyographic evidence of reduced muscle activity when ULF-TENS is applied to the Vth and VIIth cranial nerves. Cranio 2001;19:162–8.

[33] Koh H, Robinson PG. Occlusal adjustment for treating and preventing temporomandibular joint disorders. Cochrane Database Syst Rev 2003;CD003812.

[34] Kroner-Herwig B, Heinrich M, Morris L. Headache in German children and adolescents: a population-based epidemiological study. Cephalalgia 2007;27:519–27.

[35] Levine RL, Levy LA. Relationship between self-reported intensity of headache and magnitude of surface EMG. Psychol Rep 2006;98:91–4.

[36] Linde K, Rossnagel K. Propranolol for migraine prophylaxis. Cochrane Database Syst Rev 2004;CD003225.

[37] List T, Axelsson S, Leijon G. Pharmacologic interventions in the treatment of temporomandibular disorders, atypical facial pain, and burning mouth syndrome. A qualitative systematic review. J Orofac Pain 2003;17:301–10.

[38] Marcus DA, Scharff L, Mercer S, Turk DC. Nonpharmacological treatment for migraine: incremental utility of physical therapy with relaxation and thermal biofeedback. Cephalalgia 1998;18:266–72.

[39] McCrory DC, Gray RN. Oral sumatriptan for acute migraine. Cochrane Database Syst Rev 2003;CD002915.

[40] McNeely ML, Armijo OS, Magee DJ. A systematic review of the effectiveness of physical therapy interventions for temporomandibular disorders. Phys Ther 2006;86:710–25.

[41] Medlicott MS, Harris SR. A systematic review of the effectiveness of exercise, manual therapy, electrotherapy, relaxation training, and biofeedback in the management of temporomandibular disorder. Phys Ther 2006;86:955–73.

[42] Michelotti A, de WA, Steenks M, Farella M. Home-exercise regimes for the management of nonspecific temporomandibular disorders. J Oral Rehabil 2005;32:779–85.

[43] Moja PL, Cusi C, Sterzi RR, Canepari C. Selective serotonin re-uptake inhibitors (SSRIs) for preventing migraine and tension-type headaches. Cochrane Database Syst Rev 2005;CD002919.

[44] Moskowitz MA. Genes, proteases, cortical spreading depression and migraine: impact on pathophysiology and treatment. Funct Neurol 2007;22:133–6.

[45] Mulet M, Decker KL, Look JO, Lenton PA, Schiffman EL. A randomized clinical trial assessing the efficacy of adding 6 × 6 exercises to self-care for the treatment of masticatory myofascial pain. J Orofac Pain 2007;21:318–28.

[46] National Institute of Dental and Craniofacial Research. TMJ disorders. 2008. Available at: http://www.nidcr.nih.gov/OralHealth/Topics/TMJ/TMJDisorders.htm.

[47] Nunez SC, Garcez AS, Suzuki SS, Ribeiro MS. Management of mouth opening in patients with temporomandibular disorders through low-level laser therapy and transcutaneous electrical neural stimulation. Photomed Laser Surg 2006;24:45–9.

[48] Ramacciotti AS, Soares BG, Atallah AN. Dipyrone for acute primary headaches. Cochrane Database Syst Rev 2007;CD004842.

[49] Rasmussen BK. Epidemiology of headache. Cephalalgia 2001;21:774–7.

[50] Ries LG, Alves MC, Berzin F. Asymmetric activation of temporalis, masseter, and sternocleidomastoid muscles in temporomandibular disorder patients. Cranio 2008;26:59–64.

[51] Riley JL, III, Myers CD, Currie TP, Mayoral O, Harris RG, Fisher JA, Gremillion HA, Robinson ME. Self-care behaviors associated with myofascial temporomandibular disorder pain. J Orofac Pain 2007;21:194–202.

[52] Rodrigues D, Siriani AO, Berzin F. Effect of conventional TENS on pain and electromyographic activity of masticatory muscles in TMD patients. Braz Oral Res 2004;18:290–5.

[53] Schoenen J. Tension-type Headache. In: McMahon SB, Koltzenburg M, editors. Melzack and Wall's textbook of pain. London: Elsevier; 2006. p. 875–86.

[54] Schuh-Hofer S, Richter M, Geworski L, Villringer A, Israel H, Wenzel R, Munz DL, Arnold G. Increased serotonin transporter availability in the brainstem of migraineurs. J Neurol 2007;254:789–96.

[55] Sessle BJ. Peripheral and central mechanisms of orofacial pain and their clinical correlates. Minerva Anestesiol 2005;71:117–36.

[56] Sommer C. Pharmacotherapy of orofacial pain. Schmerz 2002;16:381–8.

[57] Stewart WF, Lipton RB, Kolodner KB, Sawyer J, Lee C, Liberman JN. Validity of the Migraine Disability Assessment (MIDAS) score in comparison to a diary-based measure in a population sample of migraine sufferers. Pain 2000;88:41–52.

[58] Ta LE, Dionne RA. Treatment of painful temporomandibular joints with a cyclooxygenase-2 inhibitor: a randomized placebo-controlled comparison of celecoxib to naproxen. Pain 2004;111:13–21.

[59] Torelli P, Jensen R, Olesen J. Physiotherapy for tension-type headache: a controlled study. Cephalalgia 2004;24:29–36.

[60] Trautmann E, Lackschewitz H, Kroner-Herwig B. Psychological treatment of recurrent headache in children and adolescents: a meta-analysis. Cephalalgia 2006;26:1411–26.

[61] Truelove EJ, Dworkin SF, Burgess JA, Bonica JJ. Facial and head pain caused by myofascial and temporomandibular disorders. In: Loeser JD, Butler SH, Chapman CR, Turk DC, editors. Bonica's management of pain. Philadelphia: Lippincott, Williams and Wilkins; 2001. p. 895–908.

[62] Turner JA, Mancl L, Aaron LA. Short- and long-term efficacy of brief cognitive-behavioral therapy for patients with chronic temporomandibular disorder pain: a randomized, controlled trial. Pain 2006;121:181–94.

[63] Victor S, Ryan SW. Drugs for preventing migraine headaches in children. Cochrane Database Syst Rev 2003;CD002761.
[64] Wright EF, Domenech MA, Fischer JR, Jr. Usefulness of posture training for patients with temporomandibular disorders. J Am Dent Assoc 2000;131:202–10.

Correspondence to: Prof. Kathleen A. Sluka, PT, PhD, Graduate Program in Physical Therapy and Rehabilitation Science, The University of Iowa, 1-252 Medical Education Building, Iowa City, IA 52242-1190, USA. Tel: 1-319-335-9791; fax: 1-319-335-9707; email: kathleen-sluka@uiowa.edu.

Spinal Pain

16

Steven Z. George

Center for Pain Research and Behavioral Health and Brooks Center for Rehabilitation Studies, Department of Physical Therapy, University of Florida, Gainesville, Florida, USA

Spinal pain has an adverse societal impact because it is a common source of persistent pain and disability. This chapter reviews spinal pain syndromes, which will be operationally defined as pain originating from either the cervical or lumbar region. This chapter will review the clinical presentation and epidemiology of spinal pain and discuss common treatments. Current reports from the peer-reviewed literature will be emphasized. The overall goal of this chapter is to provide an appropriate context for effective management of spinal pain.

Low back pain (LBP) has been operationally defined as painful symptoms between T12 and the gluteal fold [19]. When these parameters are met, LBP is often referred to as "local." LBP can also occur together with leg pain, which has been operationally defined as painful symptoms distal to the gluteal fold or the knee. Clinically, the two primary patterns of leg pain are "referred," in which structures other than a lumbar nerve root are implicated as the source of symptoms, and "radicular," in which a specific lumbar nerve root is implicated. A subgroup of LBP that occurs following injury at work is "work-related" or "occupational" LBP.

Neck pain is operationally defined as painful symptoms between C1 and T1 [35]. When these parameters are met, neck pain is referred to as "local." Neck pain can occur with arm pain, which has been operationally defined as painful symptoms distal to the acromion process or the elbow. The two primary patterns of arm pain are "referred" pain, in which structures other than a cervical nerve root are implicated as the source of symptoms, and "radicular" pain, in which a specific cervical nerve root is implicated. Neck pain that occurs at work is "work-related" or "occupational," and neck pain following a motor vehicle accident is known as "whiplash-associated disorder" (WAD).

Definitive and specific anatomical diagnostic criteria for LBP and neck pain are currently unavailable in the peer-reviewed literature. As a result, the term "nonspecific" has been applied to pain in the low back or neck that is not related to underlying pathology (i.e., related to a tumor, infection, or fracture) [19,35]. It has been estimated that up to 90% of LBP and neck pain is nonspecific, and it is these nonspecific syndromes that have a substantial adverse impact on society [19,35]. Therefore, this chapter will focus on issues related to nonspecific spinal pain syndromes, and will not include information related to conditions associated with specific spinal pathology (e.g., spinal stenosis or spondylolisthesis).

General Presentation of Spinal Pain

Causes of Low Back Pain

Definitive causes of LBP are lacking in the literature. The development of LBP is believed to be multifactorial, potentially related to combinations of physical loading, physical characteristics, and genetic, behavioral, psychological, anatomical, and societal factors [88]. It is beyond the scope of this chapter to review this entire literature, so only the example of lumbar anatomy and imaging studies will be used to demonstrate the difficulty in determining definitive causes of LBP.

Traditionally, abnormal lumbar anatomy (a herniated disk, spinal stenosis, or exaggerated lumbar lordosis) was believed to be causative of LBP. However, subsequent imaging studies have indicated that abnormal lumbar anatomy is not always associated with LBP, and that LBP can occur when lumbar anatomy is normal. Specifically, Stadnik et al. [74] report that 81% of asymptomatic patients have evidence of a bulging disk at some spinal level. Furthermore, Savage et al. [71] reported that 32% of asymptomatic subjects have abnormal lumbar anatomy, while only 47% of subjects who are experiencing LBP have abnormal lumbar anatomy, as identified on imaging studies. Abnormal lumbar anatomy is also not strongly linked with severity of symptoms in those experiencing LBP. Herno et al. [41] demonstrated a poor correlation between LBP symptoms and the degree of lumbar stenosis identified on magnetic resonance imaging (MRI). George et al. [32] report no difference in severity of LBP or in functional limitations caused by LBP based on the amount of lumbar lordosis measured on a radiograph.

The lack of a definitive relationship between LBP and lumbar anatomy is only one example of the difficulty in identifying specific causes of LBP. Similar problems exist for other risk factors. For example, there is a promising link between certain genetic factors and lumbar disk degeneration; however, a strong genetic link to the clinical presentation of LBP has not been identified [2]. Therefore, many different risk factors have the potential to cause LBP, without any single primary factor being currently identified in the literature.

Epidemiology and Course of Low Back Pain

The prevalence of LBP is well documented in the literature, although estimates vary widely due to methodological differences. A population-based study from the Netherlands found that LBP was the most common form of musculoskeletal pain reported by adults 25 years of age and older, with a point prevalence of 26.9% (95% CI: 25.5–28.3) [68]. One systematic review pooled higher-quality studies and provided point prevalence estimates ranging from 12% to 33%, 1-year prevalence estimates ranging from 22% to 65%, and lifetime prevalence estimates ranging from 11% to 84% [89]. Women tend to have a higher prevalence of LBP than men. In the Netherlands study, the point prevalence of LBP was 28.1% for women (95% CI = 26.1–30.1) and 25.6% for men (95% CI = 23.5–27.7) [68]. Older age is also associated with higher prevalence of LBP [54,78], but the prevalence of LBP eventually levels off and declines in later decades [68].

The course of LBP is often viewed as one with discrete acute and chronic stages, with complete symptom resolution as a common occurrence.

However, prospective studies indicate that recurrence is often experienced [87]. For example, 65% of patients with acute LBP who are followed for 1 year reported one or more additional episodes [5]. Von Korff has suggested operational definitions to help clinicians and researchers to better describe the course of LBP (Table I) [86]. Although these definitions have not been universally adopted, they are a better reflection of the course of LBP, rather than simply indicating acute and chronic phases of the disease.

Table I
Operational definitions for describing the course of low back pain

Descriptor	Operational Definition of an Episode of Low Back Pain
Transient back pain	Present for no more than 90 consecutive days and does not recur over a 12-month period
Recurrent back pain	Present for less than half the days in a 12-month period and occurs in multiple episodes over the year
Chronic back pain	Present for at least half the days in a 12-month period in single or multiple episodes
Acute back pain	Onset is recent and sudden and does not meet the previously defined criteria for recurrent or chronic pain
First onset	First occurrence in the patient's lifetime
Flare-up	Distinct phase (with definable beginning and end points) of pain superimposed on a chronic or recurrent course; refers to a period when the pain is markedly more severe than is usual for the patient

Source: Von Korff [86].

Prognostic factors for persistent LBP have also been investigated in the literature, and several factors are consistently associated with poor outcome. The co-occurrence of leg pain with LBP is an indicator of poor outcome, as are high initial pain and disability scores [11,73,80]. Psychological distress is also predictive of poor outcome [57,69]. Last, while obesity has not been linked to causing LBP, it is associated with poor outcomes following onset of LBP [55]. Specific to studies of work-related LBP, severe leg pain, high disability, poor general health, and unavailability of light duties are all associated with still receiving compensation 3 months after an injury [23,60]. A systematic review of factors found that longer sick leave is associated with higher disability levels, older age, female gender, more social dysfunction or isolation, heavier work, and receiving higher compensation [76].

Causes of Neck Pain

As with LBP, definitive causes of neck pain are not reported in the literature, and the development of neck pain is believed to be multifactorial [35]. The identification of abnormal cervical anatomy is not conclusive to the cause of neck pain. For example, there is no evidence that degenerative changes in the cervical spine are a risk factor for neck pain [43]. A recent best-evidence review that investigated risk factors for neck pain indicated several potential unmodifiable risk factors including middle age, being female, and specific genetic factors [43]. The review also highlighted several modifiable risk factors for neck pain, including smoking, exposure to environmental tobacco smoke, and psychological health [43]. Few definitive risk factors have been identified for WAD [44]. For neck pain in the workplace, high quantitative job demands, low social support at work, a sedentary work position, and repetitive or precision work are all risk factors [14]. However, none of these factors alone are predictive of neck pain, lending support to the overall conclusion that neck pain has many potential causes [14,43,44].

Epidemiology and Course of Neck Pain

The prevalence of neck pain has not been reported as much as LBP, but the available reports suggest that neck pain is also commonly experienced. The previously mentioned population-based study from the Netherlands indicated that the point prevalence of neck pain is 20.6% (95% CI = 19.3–21.9) [68]. Population-based studies estimate the annual cumulative incidence of an episode of neck pain at 17.9% (95% CI: 16.0–19.7%) in the United Kingdom [15] and 14.6% (95% CI: 11.3–17.9%) in Canada [13]. Higher rates are reported in working populations; for example, about 40% of workers complained of neck pain in a French cohort study [56]. In general, women reported higher rates of neck pain, with an incidence rate ratio of 1.7, a relative risk ratio of 1.3, and an odds ratio of 1.6 in comparison to men [13,15,56].

Available population studies suggest that, as in LBP, patterns of chronic and recurrent neck pain exist. The Canadian cohort study followed 587 subjects with neck pain at the time of the baseline survey and found that only 37% reported symptom resolution 12 months later [13]. In the French cohort study, 11% of subjects had neck pain symptoms lasting more than 30 days [56]. A recent best-evidence summary suggests a similar pattern, with estimates that 50–85% of those experiencing neck pain will experience it again 1–5 years later, regardless of the original cause [7–9].

Prognostic factors for persistent neck pain have been investigated, and individual studies suggest that women are at greater risk for poor outcomes [13,56]. A recent best-evidence summary also indicates that older age, poor overall health, and prior neck pain episodes are all predictive of poor outcome [8]. Furthermore, poor outcome is also associated with several psychological factors such as general psychological distress, worrying, anger, or frustration [8]. In the work setting, physical job demands were not strongly linked to outcome, but having little influence on one's work situation, being a white collar worker, and participating in general exercise or sport were associated with a better outcome [7]. Specific to WAD, poor recovery is associated with high initial pain and disability, psychological distress, passive coping styles, and availability of compensation [9].

Societal Impact of Low Back and Neck Pain

In Australia, 53% of adults reported some disability from LBP during a 6-month period [90]. Persistent LBP significantly influences the capacity to work and is associated with the inability to obtain or maintain employment [75] and with reduced productivity at work [77]. Neck pain with disability is reported as high as 11.5% in the general population [43], and up to 14% of workers report being limited at work due to neck pain [14]. It is not surprising then that LBP and neck pain are common reasons to seek health care from physical therapists [18], accounting for approximately 25% and 12% of all patients discharged from outpatient clinics, respectively [47]. Effective management of LBP and neck pain is a high priority for physical therapists so that the societal burden of these pain syndromes is lessened.

Physical Therapy Treatment of Spinal Pain

Physical Therapy Examination of Patients with Spinal Pain

Examination of spinal pain should start with red flag screening. The goal of this part of the process is to determine if physical therapy treatment of spinal pain is appropriate. Red flags are signs and symptoms that spinal pain may be related to serious medical pathology such as a tumor,

fracture, or infection. Positive red flags are an indication that additional information is warranted before treatment can begin, and patients
should be referred to the appropriate professional for additional diagnostic testing. Red flag screening typically starts with a medical questionnaire followed by a medical history to confirm positive answers [3].
Common red flags for spinal pain include constant pain, unexplained
weight loss, concurrent fever, a history of cancer, and changes in bowel
and bladder function.

Examination of spinal pain should then proceed to screening for
yellow flags. The goal of this part of the process is to determine if the patient has factors indicative of a poor prognosis. The identification of psychological factors has been advocated most consistently for yellow flag
screening in spinal pain [40,58]. The specific psychological factors used in
yellow flag screening vary, but depression, fear-avoidance beliefs, and pain
catastrophizing are currently recommended [30,37,79]. Chapter 5 outlines
the Fear Avoidance Questionnaire as a measure for psychological factors.
Patients with elevated scores during the acute pain phase may be considered at risk for developing chronic spinal pain [29,30], and those with high
scores during the chronic pain phase may have a poor prognosis [91,92].
Thus, individuals with elevated scores should be targeted with an interdisciplinary approach that includes psychological management to enhance
treatment outcomes.

Evidence Supporting Common Physical Therapy
Treatments for Spinal Pain

After red and yellow flag screening is completed, specific treatment options are then considered. Treatment of spinal pain will differ for patients
having acute pain versus those with chronic pain. Treatment goals for
those with acute spinal pain are pain relief through appropriately matched
interventions and early return to normal activities. Treatment goals for
those with chronic spinal pain are reduced physical impairment, improved
conditioning through exercise, and improved tolerance of functional or
occupational activities.

Numerous systematic reviews [1,21,24,31,36,39,42,52,64,66,67]
have investigated the efficacy of treatments for LBP. Furthermore, a clinical practice guideline from the American College of Physicians and the

American Pain Society was recently published; these recommendations (Table II) will serve as the primary reference on treatment efficacy for this chapter [10]. For patients with acute LBP, the strongest evidence for commonly used physical therapy treatments (Grade B evidence) is for advice to remain active, evidence-based patient education, superficial heat, and spinal manipulation. For patients with acute LBP, there is insufficient evidence (lower than Grade B) supporting the use of ultrasound, superficial cold, TENS, traction, exercise therapy, massage, acupuncture, yoga, or back school [10,24,42,66]. For patients with chronic LBP, the strongest evidence for commonly used physical therapy treatments (Grade B) is for advice to remain active, evidence-based patient education, spinal manipulation, exercise therapy, massage, acupuncture, and yoga [10]. For patients with chronic LBP, there is moderate evidence supporting back schools for many outcomes, but the methodological quality of existing studies is a concern [42]. For patients with chronic LBP, there is insufficient evidence (lower than Grade B) supporting the use of ultrasound, superficial cold, TENS, or traction [10,24,42,66].

Several systematic reviews [33,34,38,48,49,53,67,82] have also investigated the efficacy of treatments for neck pain. A best-evidence summary from the Task Force on Neck Pain and its Associated Disorders was recently published, and these recommendations will serve as the primary reference on treatment efficacy for this chapter [6,45]. This summary did not distinguish between acute and chronic neck pain, but it did make recommendations for noninvasive interventions used by physical therapists. For WAD, there is some evidence that educational videos, joint mobilization, and exercises are more effective than usual medical care (medication, advice, and rest) or physical modalities (superficial heat or cold and ultrasound) [45]. Treatment focused on regaining function and returning to work is more effective than treatments without such a focus for patients with WAD. For nonspecific neck pain, exercise interventions, low-level laser therapy, and acupuncture were more effective than no, sham, or comparison treatments [45]. There is insufficient evidence to support the use of ultrasound, superficial heat or cold, TENS, magnets, iontophoresis, traction, or massage [38,45,53,67]. Poor methodology is a common comment in the review articles that considered the efficacy of treatments for neck pain [34,38,45,49,53].

Table II
Current treatment recommendations
for acute and chronic low back pain

Acute Low Back Pain	Chronic Low Back Pain
Self-Care Methods	
Advice to remain active	Advice to remain active
Books, handouts	Books, handouts
Superficial heat	
Pharmacological Therapies	
Acetaminophen	Acetaminophen
NSAIDs	NSAIDs
Skeletal muscle relaxants	Antidepressants
Benzodiazepines	Benzodiazepines
Tramadol, opioids	Tramadol, opioids
Nonpharmacological Therapies	
Spinal manipulation	Spinal manipulation
	Exercise therapy
	Massage
	Yoga
	Cognitive-behavioral therapy
	Progressive relaxation
	Intensive interdisciplinary
	rehabilitation

Source: Adapted from Chou et al. [10].
Abbreviations: NSAIDs = nonsteroidal anti-inflammatory
drugs.

Treatment-Based Classification for Acute Spinal Pain

Physical therapy treatment of acute spinal pain has recently emphasized identifying patient subgroups based on clinical characteristics that are linked to positive clinical outcome, as opposed to identification of spinal pathology. Traditionally, physical therapy treatment of acute spinal pain was guided by the identification of specific pathology, whether through palpation based on biomechanical theory (structural or movement faults) or through imaging findings (evidence of a herniated disk). There is compelling evidence that knowledge of specific pathology does not improve patient outcomes, and in some cases worsens them [50,51]. For example, the presence of static or dynamic pelvic asymmetry did not improve the outcome from a specific manipulative technique [22], and knowledge of lumbar imaging did not improve patient outcomes from LBP [61].

Treatment-based classification (TBC) approaches are one way in which spinal pain subgroups have been described in the literature [70]. TBC systems for spinal pain attempt to (1) identify patients for whom conservative treatment is inappropriate, (2) define discrete clinical syndromes based on key historical and physical examination findings, and (3) provide matched treatment that is most likely to be associated with an optimal clinical outcome. TBC approaches consider the role of pathology in determining appropriateness of treatment, but do not emphasize the identification of specific pathology as a prerequisite to treatment. Instead, TBC emphasizes the identification of patient characteristics that indicate a favorable response to a specific treatment (Fig. 1).

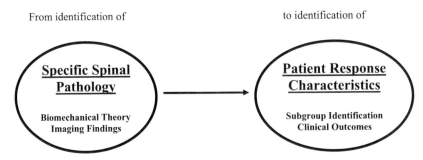

Fig. 1. Paradigm shift in physical therapy treatment philosophy.

There are several TBC systems for LBP and neck pain, and it is beyond the scope of this chapter to review them all [70,84]. Instead, this chapter provides a focused review of a TBC system for LBP described by Delitto et al. [16] and of a TBC for neck pain recently described by Fritz and Brennan [25]. These systems were selected based on their availability in the peer-reviewed literature. Readers interested in more details on these, or other, TBC systems are encouraged to consult the original sources. TBC systems for chronic spinal pain have not yet been described in the literature, and therefore are not included in this chapter.

Treatment-Based Classification for Acute Low Back Pain

Delitto et al. [16] described a TBC system for LBP in 1995. This system was modified in 2000 by Fritz and George [28] by collapsing the seven original treatment categories to four categories due to treatment similarities.

The resulting treatment classification subgroups were specific exercise, manipulation, stabilization, and traction. The decision-making process for classifying patients into the three most common groups (specific exercise, manipulation, and stabilization) is summarized in Fig. 2 [26].

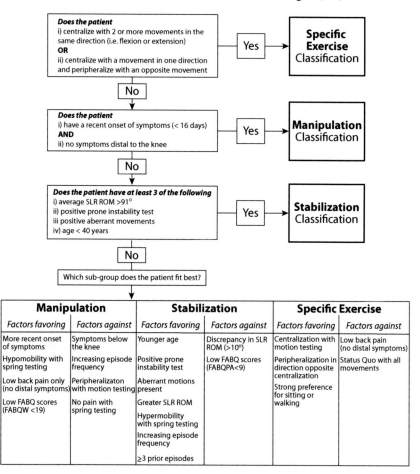

Fig. 2. Algorithm for clinical decision making using a treatment-based classification for low back pain [26]. FABQ = Fear Avoidance Beliefs Questionnaire; FABQPA = FABQ physical activity subscale; FABQW = FABQ work subscale; LBP = low back pain; ROM = range of motion; SLR = straight leg raise; sx = symptoms. Reprinted from Fritz et al. [26] with permission from Wolters Kluwer Health.

Although preliminary, the evidence to support the use of this TBC system for LBP is compelling. Separate studies have reported acceptable levels of reliability ranging from κ = 0.4 to 0.6, which does not vary based on clinical experience [26,28]. There are two randomized controlled trials demonstrating prescriptive validity for this TBC system. The first trial, by Fritz et al. [27], shows that patients assigned to TBC physical therapy report improvements in disability, physical function, and return-to-work rates at 4 weeks in comparison to guideline-based physical therapy. The second trial, by Brennan et al. [4], shows that treatment matched to the classification system is more effective at reducing self-report of disability at 4 weeks and 6 months, in comparison to unmatched treatment.

Treatment-Based Classification for Acute Neck Pain

Fritz and Brennan [25] reported a TBC system for neck pain in 2007. The treatment classification subgroups were mobility, centralization (symptoms that move toward the spine or abate in intensity with cervical spine motion), exercise and conditioning, pain control, and headache. The decision-making process for classifying patients into these subgroups is summarized in Fig. 3 [25].

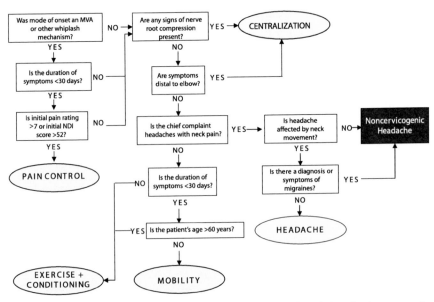

Fig. 3. Algorithm for clinical decision making using a treatment-based classification system for neck pain [25]. MVA = motor vehicle accident; NDI = Neck Disability Index. Reprinted from Fritz and Brennan [25], with permission from the American Physical Therapy Association.

The one available report on this TBC system for neck pain suggests that the reliability of this system is high, with $\kappa = 0.95$ [25]. This report also provides descriptive data on the different neck pain classification categories as follows: centralization (34.7%), exercise and conditioning (32.8%), mobility (17.5%), headache (9.1%), and pain control (5.8%) [25]. In an analysis of clinical outcome, patients receiving treatment matched by the TBC system fare better in disability and pain ratings compared to those receiving unmatched treatment [25]. While this information is promising, it is important to note that no randomized trials of this system have been completed. Therefore, additional studies are needed before the TBC for neck pain is validated.

Medical Management

Medical Management of Spinal Pain

Spinal pain is a common reason for people to seek health care, not only from physical therapists, but also from physicians and alternative and complimentary practitioners [12,17,20,59,72,81,85,93]. Only 25–50% of individuals who experience spinal pain seek treatment [12,46], and these patients have greater disability and pain intensity in comparison to those who do not seek health care [12,46,62]. Because of the common use of other medical services, physical therapists must be aware of general trends in medical management of spinal pain.

Medical management parallels the trend in physical therapy management of spinal pain. Commonalities include a de-emphasis of the recognition of specific pathology, unless serious medical causes are suspected, and the consideration of psychological factors in determining prognosis. The importance of recognizing subgroups of spinal pain, self-care options, and the consideration of a wide range of potential treatments for those who do not improve as expected have recently been stressed in the medical management of spinal pain.

Guidelines for Diagnosis and Treatment of Low Back Pain

As previously mentioned, the American College of Physicians/American Pain Society clinical guidelines serve as the primary source of recommendations for this chapter [10]. The guideline recommendations for diagnosis of LBP include the performance of a focused examination with the primary purpose of placing patients into one of three subgroups [10]. The subgroups are nonspecific LBP, LBP potentially associated with stenosis or radiculopathy, and LBP potentially associated with another specific spinal cause. Assessment of psychological risk factors is recommended for all subgroups, to serve the purpose of identifying those at risk for developing persistent LBP. Routine imaging or other diagnostic testing is not recommended for patients with nonspecific LBP. Diagnostic imaging is recommended for patients who have severe or progressive neurological deficits or when serious underlying conditions (red flags) are suspected from the history. MRI is the recommended diagnostic imaging technique for patients with lumbar spinal stenosis or suspected radiculopathy. Computed tomography (CT) is recommended for diagnostic imaging for candidates for surgery or epidural steroid injection.

The guideline recommendations for treatment of LBP include educational options of providing facts about the course of LBP, encouraging patients to return to normal activities, and providing information about self-care options [10]. Medication should start with acetaminophen (paracetamol) or nonsteroidal anti-inflammatory drugs (NSAIDs) for those with acute LBP, although the use of skeletal muscle relaxants, benzodiazepines, and opioids is also acceptable for acute LBP. Medication for chronic LBP can include acetaminophen, NSAIDs, antidepressants, benzodiazepines, and opioids. Medical practice guidelines typically suggest nonpharmacological treatment options only for those patients whose symptoms do not improve. The nonpharmacological options have been reviewed above and are reported in Table II.

Clinical Practice Guidelines for Neck Pain

As previously mentioned, the Task Force on Neck Pain and Its Associated Disorders recently published a best-evidence synthesis, and their management recommendations serve as the primary source for the recommendations in this chapter [6,45,63]. Emergency room assessment of neck pain is of special interest because this is where patients with traumatic neck injuries (i.e., WAD) are first evaluated, and identification of fracture is a high management priority [63]. The recommendations of the task force are that fracture assessment for neck pain is primarily indicated for patients with severe trauma or cervical radiculopathy. Available screening protocols have high predictive value in detecting cervical fracture for low-risk trauma patients. CT scans are a better choice for identifying cervical fracture for high-risk or multiple injury trauma patients. Furthermore, a clinical physical examination is acceptable in ruling out neurological compression or structural lesion. However, many commonly used assessment tools such as electrophysiology, imaging, anesthetic facet injections, medial branch block, diskography, functional tests, and blood tests have unproven roles in the assessment of neck pain [63]. A four-grade classification system for assessment of neck pain severity has been suggested (Table III), as such ratings have not been standardized in the past [35].

Table III
Classification system for severity of neck pain

Stage of Neck Pain	Operational Definition
Grade I	No signs or symptoms suggestive of major structural pathology and no or minor interference with activities of daily living; will probably respond to minimal intervention such as reassurance and pain control; does not require intensive investigations or ongoing treatment
Grade II	No signs or symptoms suggestive of major structural pathology, but major interference with activities of daily living; requires pain relief and early activation/intervention aimed at preventing long-term disability
Grade III	No signs or symptoms suggestive of major structural pathology, but presence of neurological signs such as decreased deep tendon reflexes, weakness, and/or sensory deficits; might require investigation and occasionally more invasive treatments
Grade IV	Signs or symptoms of major structural pathology such as fracture, myelopathy, neoplasm, or systemic disease; requires prompt investigation and treatment

Source: Guzman et al. [35].

Minimal data have been published on pharmacological management of neck pain. A Cochrane review shows that for acute whiplash, administering intravenous methylprednisolone within 8 hours of injury reduces pain at 1 week but has no effect on pain at 6 months compared to placebo [65]. Furthermore, the review shows limited evidence and unclear benefits in patients with subacute and chronic neck disorders for muscle relaxants, analgesics, and NSAIDs [65]. Short-term relief is associated with epidural or corticosteroid nerve root injection, but injection does not seem to decrease the chances of having surgery [6]. The best-evidence summary does not support the use of intra-articular steroid injections, radiofrequency neurotomy, or cervical disk arthroplasty for patients with local neck pain [6]. In comparison to conservative treatment, surgical treatment for cervical radiculopathy is associated with better short-term outcomes, but long-term outcomes are similar [6]. Cervical disk arthroplasty has similar long-term outcomes to anterior fusion surgery for patients with cervical radiculopathy [6].

Interdisciplinary Management of Chronic Spinal Pain

Chronic spinal pain has a multifactorial etiology, so optimal management may be best provided by an interdisciplinary team promoting an active approach to pain management. There are many potential members of this team, but most teams consist of a core unit including a physician, psychologist, and physical therapist. For more details on interdisciplinary pain management, see Chapter 11. In this setting, the physician is responsible for overall medical management, including pharmacological therapies. Psychological management includes treatments that use cognitive strategies, either alone or in combination with behavioral approaches, that are supported by evidence for treatment of chronic LBP [10]. Physical therapy management includes improvement in physical impairments and tolerance of functional activities. Interdisciplinary pain rehabilitation programs are an intensive approach, sometimes keeping patients in treatment for up to 8 hours a day. There is compelling information that such approaches provide cost-effective alternatives for the treatment of chronic pain [10,83], although this evidence is not absolute [48,64].

References

[1]   Assendelft WJ, Morton SC, Yu EI, Suttorp MJ, Shekelle PG. Spinal manipulative therapy for low back pain. Cochrane Database Syst Rev 2004;CD000447.
[2]   Battie MC, Videman T, Parent E. Lumbar disc degeneration: epidemiology and genetic influences. Spine 2004;29:2679–90.
[3]   Boissonnault WG, Badke MB. Collecting health history information: the accuracy of a patient self-administered questionnaire in an orthopedic outpatient setting. Phys Ther 2005;85:531–43.
[4]   Brennan GP, Fritz JM, Hunter SJ, Thackerary A, Delitto A, Erhard RE. Identifying sub-groups of patients with "non-specific" low back pain: results of a randomized clinical trial. Spine 2006;31:623–31.
[5]   Carey TS, Garrett JM, Jackman A, Hadler N. Recurrence and care seeking after acute back pain: results of a long-term follow-up study. North Carolina Back Pain Project. Med Care 1999;37:157–64.

[6]   Carragee EJ, Hurwitz EL, Cheng I, Carroll LJ, Nordin M, Guzman J, Peloso P, Holm LW, Côté P,
      Hogg-Johnson S, et al. Treatment of neck pain: injections and surgical interventions: results of
      the Bone and Joint Decade 2000–2010 Task Force on Neck Pain and Its Associated Disorders.
      Spine 2008;33:S153–69.

[7]   Carroll LJ, Hogg-Johnson S, Côté P, van der Velde G, Holm LW, Carragee EJ, Hurwitz EL, Peloso
      PM, Cassidy JD, Guzman J, et al. Course and prognostic factors for neck pain in workers: results
      of the Bone and Joint Decade 2000-2010 Task Force on Neck Pain and Its Associated Disorders.
      Spine 2008;33:S93–100.

[8]   Carroll LJ, Hogg-Johnson S, Côté P, van der Velde G, Holm LW, Carragee EJ, Hurwitz EL, Peloso
      PM, Cassidy JD, Guzman J, et al. Course and prognostic factors for neck pain in the general
      population: results of the Bone and Joint Decade 2000–2010 Task Force on Neck Pain and Its
      Associated Disorders. Spine 2008;33:S75–82.

[9]   Carroll LJ, Holm LW, Hogg-Johnson S, Côté P, Cassidy JD, Haldeman S, Nordin M, Hurwitz EL,
      Carragee EJ, van der Velde G, et al. Course and prognostic factors for neck pain in whiplash-
      associated disorders (WAD): results of the Bone and Joint Decade 2000–2010 Task Force on
      Neck Pain and Its Associated Disorders. Spine 2008;33:S83–92.

[10] Chou R, Qaseem A, Snow V, Casey D, Cross JT Jr, Shekelle P, Owens DK; Clinical Efficacy As-
      sessment Subcommittee of the American College of Physicians; American College of Physicians;
      American Pain Society Low Back Pain Guidelines Panel. Diagnosis and treatment of low back
      pain: a joint clinical practice guideline from the American College of Physicians and the Ameri-
      can Pain Society. Ann Intern Med 2007;147:478–91.

[11] Coste J, Delecoeuillerie G, Cohen DL, Le Parc JM, Paolaggi JB. Clinical course and prognos-
      tic factors in acute low back pain: an inception cohort study in primary care practice. BMJ
      1994;308:577–80.

[12] Côté P, Cassidy JD, Carroll L. The treatment of neck and low back pain: who seeks care? who goes
      where? Med Care 2001;39:956–67.

[13] Côté P, Cassidy JD, Carroll LJ, Kristman V. The annual incidence and course of neck pain in the
      general population: a population-based cohort study. Pain 2004;112:267–73.

[14] Côté P, van der Velde G, Cassidy JD, Carroll LJ, Hogg-Johnson S, Holm LW, Carragee EJ, Hal-
      deman S, Nordin M, Hurwitz EL, et al. The burden and determinants of neck pain in workers:
      results of the Bone and Joint Decade 2000–2010 Task Force on Neck Pain and Its Associated
      Disorders. Spine 2008;33:S60–74.

[15] Croft PR, Lewis M, Papageorgiou AC, Thomas E, Jayson MI, Macfarlane GJ, Silman AJ. Risk fac-
      tors for neck pain: a longitudinal study in the general population. Pain 2001;93:317–25.

[16] Delitto A, Erhard RE, Bowling RW. A treatment-based classification approach to low
      back syndrome: identifying and staging patients for conservative treatment. Phys Ther
      1995;75:470–85.

[17] Deyo RA, Phillips WR. Low back pain. A primary care challenge. Spine 1996;21:2826–32.

[18] Di Fabio RP, Boissonnault W. Physical therapy and health-related outcomes for patients with
      common orthopaedic diagnoses. J Orthop Sports Phys Ther 1998;27:219–30.

[19] Dionne CE, Dunn KM, Croft PR, Nachemson AL, Buchbinder R, Walker BF, Wyatt M, Cassidy
      JD, Rossignol M, Leboeuf-Yde C, et al. A consensus approach toward the standardization of back
      pain definitions for use in prevalence studies. Spine 2008;33:95–03.

[20] Eisenberg DM, Davis RB, Ettner SL, Appel S, Wilkey S, Van Rompay M, Kessler RC. Trends in
      alternative medicine use in the United States, 1990–1997: results of a follow-up national survey.
      JAMA 1998;280:1569–95.

[21] Engers A, Jellema P, Wensing M, van der Windt DA, Grol R, van Tulder MW. Individual patient
      education for low back pain. Cochrane Database Syst Rev 2008;CD004057.

[22] Flynn T, Fritz J, Whitman J. A clinical prediction rule for classifying patients with low
      back pain who demonstrate short-term improvement with spinal manipulation. Spine
      2002;27:2835–43.

[23] Fransen M, Woodward M, Norton R, Coggan C, Dawe M, Sheridan N. Risk factors associated
      with the transition from acute to chronic occupational back pain. Spine 2002;27:92–8.

[24] French SD, Cameron M, Walker BF, Reggars JW, Esterman AJ. Superficial heat or cold for low
      back pain. Cochrane Database Syst Rev 2006;CD004750.

[25] Fritz JM, Brennan GP. Preliminary examinszation of a proposed treatment-based classifica-
      tion system for patients receiving physical therapy interventions for neck pain. Phys Ther
      2007;87:513–24.

[26] Fritz JM, Brennan GP, Clifford SN, Hunter SJ, Thackeray A. An examination of the reliability of a classification algorithm for subgrouping patients with low back pain. Spine 2006;31:77–82.

[27] Fritz JM, Delitto A, Erhard RE. Comparison of classification-based physical therapy with therapy based on clinical practice guidelines for patients with acute low back pain: a randomized clinical trial. Spine 2003;28:1363–71.

[28] Fritz JM, George S. The use of a classification approach to identify subgroups of patients with acute low back pain. Interrater reliability and short-term treatment outcomes. Spine 2000;25:106–14.

[29] Fritz JM, George S, Delitto A. The role of fear avoidance beliefs in acute low back pain: relationships with current and future disability and work status. Pain 2001;94:7–15.

[30] Fritz JM, George SZ. Identifying psychosocial variables in patients with acute work-related low back pain: the importance of fear-avoidance beliefs. Phys Ther 2002;82:973–83.

[31] Furlan AD, Brosseau L, Imamura M, Irvin E. Massage for low back pain. Cochrane Database Syst Rev 2002;CD001929.

[32] George SZ, Hicks GE, Nevitt MA, Cauley JA, Vogt MT. The relationship between lumbar lordosis and radiologic variables and lumbar lordosis and clinical variables in elderly, African-American women. J Spinal Disord Tech 2003;16:200–6.

[33] Gross AR, Aker PD, Goldsmith CH, Peloso P. Patient education for mechanical neck disorders. Cochrane Database Syst Rev 2000;CD000962.

[34] Gross AR, Hoving JL, Haines TA, Goldsmith CH, Kay T, Aker P, Bronfort G; Cervical Overview Group. Manipulation and mobilisation for mechanical neck disorders. Cochrane Database Syst Rev 2004;CD004249.

[35] Guzman J, Hurwitz EL, Carroll LJ, Haldeman S, Côté P, Carragee EJ, Peloso PM, van der Velde G, Holm LW, Hogg-Johnson S, Nordin M, Cassidy JD. A new conceptual model of neck pain: linking onset, course, and care: the Bone and Joint Decade 2000–2010 Task Force on Neck Pain and Its Associated Disorders. Spine 2008;33:S14–23.

[36] Hagen KB, Hilde G, Jamtvedt G, Winnem M. Bed rest for acute low-back pain and sciatica. Cochrane Database Syst Rev 2004;CD001254.

[37] Haggman S, Maher CG, Refshauge KM. Screening for symptoms of depression by physical therapists managing low back pain. Phys Ther 2004;84:1157–66.

[38] Haraldsson BG, Gross AR, Myers CD, Ezzo JM, Morien A, Goldsmith C, Peloso PM, Bronfort G; Cervical Overview Group. Massage for mechanical neck disorders. Cochrane Database Syst Rev 2006;3:CD004871.

[39] Hayden JA, van Tulder MW, Malmivaara A, Koes BW. Exercise therapy for treatment of nonspecific low back pain. Cochrane Database Syst Rev 2005;CD000335.

[40] Hazard RG, Haugh LD, Reid S, Preble JB, MacDonald L. Early prediction of chronic disability after occupational low back injury. Spine 1996;21:945-951.

[41] Herno A, Airaksinen O, Saari T, Pitkanen M, Manninen H, Suomalainen O. Computed tomography findings 4 years after surgical management of lumbar spinal stenosis. No correlation with clinical outcome. Spine 1999;24:2234–9.

[42] Heymans MW, van Tulder MW, Esmail R, Bombardier C, Koes BW. Back schools for non-specific low-back pain. Cochrane Database Syst Rev 2004;CD000261.

[43] Hogg-Johnson S, van der Velde G, Carroll LJ, Holm LW, Cassidy JD, Guzman J, Côté P, Haldeman S, Ammendolia C, Carragee E, et al. The burden and determinants of neck pain in the general population: results of the Bone and Joint Decade 2000–2010 Task Force on Neck Pain and Its Associated Disorders. Spine 2008;33:S39–51.

[44] Holm LW, Carroll LJ, Cassidy JD, Hogg-Johnson S, Côté P, Guzman J, Peloso P, Nordin M, Hurwitz E, van der Velde G, et al. The burden and determinants of neck pain in whiplash-associated disorders after traffic collisions: results of the Bone and Joint Decade 2000–2010 Task Force on Neck Pain and Its Associated Disorders. Spine 2008;33:S52–9.

[45] Holm LW, Carroll LJ, Cassidy JD, Hogg-Johnson S, Côté P, Guzman J, Peloso P, Nordin M, Hurwitz E, van der Velde G, et al. Treatment of neck pain: noninvasive interventions: results of the Bone and Joint Decade 2000–2010 Task Force on Neck Pain and Its Associated Disorders. Spine 2008;33:S123–52.

[46] IJzelenberg W, Burdorf A. Patterns of care for low back pain in a working population. Spine 2004;29:1362–8.

[47] Jette AM, Smith K, Haley SM, Davis KD. Physical therapy episodes of care for patients with low back pain. Phys Ther 1994;74:101–10.

[48] Karjalainen K, Malmivaara A, van Tulder M, Roine R, Jauhiainen M, Hurri H, Koes B. Multidis-ciplinary biopsychosocial rehabilitation for neck and shoulder pain among working age adults. Cochrane Database Syst Rev 2003;CD002194.

[49] Kay TM, Gross A, Goldsmith C, Santaguida PL, Hoving J, Bronfort G. Exercises for mechanical neck disorders. Cochrane Database Syst Rev 2005;CD004250.

[50] Kendrick D, Fielding K, Bentley E, Kerslake R, Miller P, Pringle M. Radiography of the lumbar spine in primary care patients with low back pain: randomised controlled trial. BMJ 2001;322:400–5.

[51] Kendrick D, Fielding K, Bentley E, Miller P, Kerslake R, Pringle M. The role of radiography in primary care patients with low back pain of at least 6 weeks duration: a randomised (unblinded) controlled trial. Health Technol Assess 2001;5:1–69.

[52] Khadilkar A, Milne S, Brosseau L, Robinson V, Saginur M, Shea B, Tugwell P, Wells G. Transcu-taneous electrical nerve stimulation (TENS) for chronic low-back pain. Cochrane Database Syst Rev 2005;CD003008.

[53] Kroeling P, Gross A, Houghton PE. Electrotherapy for neck disorders. Cochrane Database Syst Rev 2005;CD004251.

[54] Leboeuf-Yde C, Kyvik KO. At what age does low back pain become a common problem? A study of 29,424 individuals aged 12–41 years. Spine 1998;23:228–34.

[55] Leboeuf-Yde C, Kyvik KO, Bruun NH. Low back pain and lifestyle. Part II: Obesity. Information from a population-based sample of 29,424 twin subjects. Spine 1999;24:779–83.

[56] Leclerc A, Niedhammer I, Landre MF, Ozguler A, Etore P, Pietri-Taleb F. One-year predictive factors for various aspects of neck disorders. Spine 1999;24:1455–62.

[57] Linton SJ. A review of psychological risk factors in back and neck pain. Spine 2000;25:1148–56.

[58] Linton SJ, Hallden K. Can we screen for problematic back pain? A screening questionnaire for predicting outcome in acute and subacute back pain. Clin J Pain 1998;14:209–15.

[59] Mäntyselkä P, Kumpusalo E, Ahonen R, Kumpusalo A, Kauhanen J, Viinamäki H, Halonen P, Takala J. Pain as a reason to visit the doctor: a study in Finnish primary health care. Pain 2001;89:175–80.

[60] McIntosh G, Frank J, Hogg-Johnson S, Bombardier C, Hall H. Prognostic factors for time receiving workers' compensation benefits in a cohort of patients with low back pain. Spine 2000;25:147–57.

[61] Modic MT, Obuchowski NA, Ross JS, Brant-Zawadzki MN, Grooff PN, Mazanec DJ, Benzel EC. Acute low back pain and radiculopathy: MR imaging findings and their prognostic role and effect on outcome. Radiology 2005;237:597–604.

[62] Mortimer M, Ahlberg G. To seek or not to seek? Care-seeking behaviour among people with low-back pain. Scand J Public Health 2003;31:194–203.

[63] Nordin M, Carragee EJ, Hogg-Johnson S, Weiner SS, Hurwitz EL, Peloso PM, Guzman J, van der Velde G, Carroll LJ, Holm LW, et al. Assessment of neck pain and its associated disorders: results of the Bone and Joint Decade 2000–2010 Task Force on Neck Pain and Its Associated Disorders. Spine 2008;33:S101–22.

[64] Ostelo RW, van Tulder MW, Vlaeyen JW, Linton SJ, Morley SJ, Assendelft WJ. Behavioural treat-ment for chronic low-back pain. Cochrane Database Syst Rev 2005;CD002014.

[65] Peloso P, Gross A, Haines T, Trinh K, Goldsmith CH, Burnie S. Medicinal and injection therapies for mechanical neck disorders. Cochrane Database Syst Rev 2007;CD000319.

[66] Philadelphia Panel. Philadelphia Panel evidence-based clinical practice guidelines on selected rehabilitation interventions for low back pain. Phys Ther 2001;81:1641–74.

[67] Philadelphia Panel. Philadelphia Panel evidence-based clinical practice guidelines on selected rehabilitation interventions for neck pain. Phys Ther 2001;81:1701–17.

[68] Picavet HS, Schouten JS. Musculoskeletal pain in the Netherlands: prevalences, consequences and risk groups, the DMC(3)-study. Pain 2003;102:167–78.

[69] Pincus T, Burton AK, Vogel S, Field AP. A systematic review of psychological factors as predic-tors of chronicity/disability in prospective cohorts of low back pain. Spine 2002;27:E109–20.

[70] Riddle DL. Classification and low back pain: a review of the literature and critical analysis of selected systems. Phys Ther 1998;78:708–37.

[71] Savage RA, Whitehouse GH, Roberts N. The relationship between the magnetic resonance im-aging appearance of the lumbar spine and low back pain, age and occupation in males. Eur Spine J 1997;6:106–14.

[72] Sherman KJ, Cherkin DC, Connelly MT, Erro J, Savetsky JB, Davis RB, Eisenberg DM. Comple-mentary and alternative medical therapies for chronic low back pain: what treatments are pa-tients willing to try? BMC Complement Altern Med 2004;4:9.

[73] Smedley J, Inskip H, Cooper C, Coggon D. Natural history of low back pain. A longitudinal study in nurses. Spine 1998;23:2422–6.

[74] Stadnik TW, Lee RR, Coen HL, Neirynck EC, Buisseret TS, Osteaux MJ. Annular tears and disk herniation: prevalence and contrast enhancement on MR images in the absence of low back pain or sciatica. Radiology 1998;206:49–55.

[75] Stang P, Von Korff M, Galer BS. Reduced labor force participation among primary care patients with headache. J Gen Intern Med 1998;13:296–302.

[76] Steenstra IA, Verbeek JH, Heymans MW, Bongers PM. Prognostic factors for duration of sick leave in patients sick listed with acute low back pain: a systematic review of the literature. Occup Environ Med 2005;62:851–60.

[77] Stewart WF, Ricci JA, Chee E, Morganstein D, Lipton R. Lost productive time and cost due to common pain conditions in the US workforce. JAMA 2003;290:2443–54.

[78] Stranjalis G, Tsamandouraki K, Sakas DE, Alamanos Y. Low back pain in a representative sample of Greek population: analysis according to personal and socioeconomic characteristics. Spine 2004;29:1355–60.

[79] Sullivan MJ, Stanish WD. Psychologically based occupational rehabilitation: the Pain-Disability Prevention Program. Clin J Pain 2003;19:97–104.

[80] Thomas E, Silman AJ, Croft PR, Papageorgiou AC, Jayson MI, MacFarlane GJ. Predicting who develops chronic low back pain in primary care: a prospective study. BMJ 1999;318:1662–7.

[81] Tindle HA, Davis RB, Phillips RS, Eisenberg DM. Trends in use of complementary and alternative medicine by US adults: 1997–2002. Altern Ther Health Med 2005;11:42–9.

[82] Trinh KV, Graham N, Gross AR, Goldsmith CH, Wang E, Cameron ID, Kay T; Cervical Overview Group. Acupuncture for neck disorders. Cochrane Database Syst Rev 2006;3:CD004870.

[83] Turk DC. Clinical effectiveness and cost-effectiveness of treatments for patients with chronic pain. Clin J Pain 2002;18: 355–65.

[84] Van Dillen LR, Sahrmann SA, Norton BJ, Caldwell CA, McDonnell MK, Bloom NJ. Movement system impairment-based categories for low back pain: stage 1 validation. J Orthop Sports Phys Ther 2003;33:126–42.

[85] Vingård E, Mortimer M, Wiktorin C, Pernold RPTG, Fredriksson K, Németh G, Alfredsson L; Musculoskeletal Intervention Center-Norrtälje Study Group. Seeking care for low back pain in the general population: a two-year follow-up study: results from the MUSIC-Norrtalje Study. Spine 2002;27:2159–65.

[86] Von Korff M. Studying the natural history of back pain. Spine 1994;19:2041S–6S.

[87] Von Korff M, Deyo RA, Cherkin D, Barlow W. Back pain in primary care. Outcomes at 1 year. Spine 1993;18:855–62.

[88] Waddell G. 1987 Volvo award in clinical sciences. A new clinical model for the treatment of low-back pain. Spine 1987;12:632–44.

[89] Walker BF. The prevalence of low back pain: a systematic review of the literature from 1966 to 1998. J Spinal Disord 2000;13:205–17.

[90] Walker BF, Muller R, Grant WD. Low back pain in Australian adults: prevalence and associated disability. J Manipulative Physiol Ther 2004;27:238–44.

[91] Woby SR, Watson PJ, Roach NK, Urmston M. Adjustment to chronic low back pain: the relative influence of fear-avoidance beliefs, catastrophizing, and appraisals of control. Behav Res Ther 2004;42:761–74.

[92] Woby SR, Watson PJ, Roach NK, Urmston M. Are changes in fear-avoidance beliefs, catastrophizing, and appraisals of control, predictive of changes in chronic low back pain and disability? Eur J Pain 2004;8:201–10.

[93] Wolsko PM, Eisenberg DM, Davis RB, Kessler R, Phillips RS. Patterns and perceptions of care for treatment of back and neck pain: results of a national survey. Spine 2003;28:292–7.

Correspondence to: Steven Z. George, PT, PhD, Center for Pain Research and Behavioral Health and Brooks Center for Rehabilitation Studies, Department of Physical Therapy, University of Florida, Gainesville, Florida, USA. Email: szgeorge@phhp.ufl.edu.

Neuropathic Pain and Complex Regional Pain Syndrome

Kathleen A. Sluka

Graduate Program in Physical Therapy and Rehabilitation Science,
The University of Iowa, Iowa City, Iowa, USA

Epidemiology and Diagnosis

Neuropathic Pain

Neuropathic pain is defined by the International Association for the Study of Pain (IASP) as pain arising as a direct consequence of a lesion or disease affecting the somatosensory system (www.iasp-pain.org). Peripheral neuropathic pain is a direct consequence of a lesion or disease affecting the peripheral somatosensory system, whereas central neuropathic pain is a direct consequence of a lesion or disease affecting the central somatosensory system. Neuropathic pain can occur as a result of numerous conditions, some of which are listed in Table I, and can be considered a mononeuropathy or a polyneuropathy [39]. Neuropathies, with or without pain, affect up to 8% of the population, with estimates as high as 5% for painful neuropathies [39].

Complex Regional Pain Syndrome

Complex regional pain syndrome type I (CRPS-I, also known as reflex sympathetic dystrophy) is a condition that occurs after a trauma to the distal part of the extremity such as a fracture, surgery, or sprain, and CRPS-II (also known as causalgia) occurs after direct injury to a nerve [43]. CRPS

Mechanisms and Management of Pain for the Physical Therapist
edited by Kathleen A. Sluka
IASP Press, Seattle, © 2009

Table I
Origins of neuropathic pain

Mononeuropathy	Polyneuropathy
Trauma from amputation, nerve injury, entrapment, neuroma, thoracotomy	Trauma from spinal cord injury, stroke
	Metabolic causes or malnutrition: alcoholism, diabetes, pellagra
Other causes: diabetes, herpes zoster, herpes simplex, vasculitis, trigeminal neuralgia	Drugs: cisplatin, ethambutol, nitrofurantoin, vincristine
	Toxins: acrylamide, arsenic, ethylene oxide, pentachlorophenol, thallium
	Heredity: amyloid neuropathy, Fabry's disease, Charcot-Marie-Tooth disease
	Malignancy: myeloma, carcinoma
	Infection: Guillain-Barré syndrome, HIV

can therefore be considered as a form of peripheral neuropathic pain. CRPS-I occurs most commonly after a distal fracture; it is more common in women than men (with a 3:1 ratio), and the greatest incidence occurs between 60 and 69 years of age [10]. Incidence rates in the general population are generally low, with estimates of 26.2 per 100,000 person years [10]. CRPS is associated with distal extremity pain and swelling, with the pain being disproportionate to the injury. Allodynia is common in CRPS, with patients describing difficulty wearing socks or gloves. The pain, hyperalgesia, and allodynia are not related to a nerve territory. Other changes include (1) autonomic effects such as increased blood flow and sweating; (2) trophic changes such as abnormal nail growth, decreased hair growth, glossy skin, and osteoporosis; and (3) loss of range of motion, weakness, and functional motor disturbances (such as decreased proprioception, loss of fine motor control, dystonia, or tremor) [2]. The IASP diagnostic criteria [43] are outlined in Table II for types I and II. In general, CRPS-I occurs after an initiating noxious event and CRPS-II occurs after nerve injury, with the other criteria being nearly identical.

Pathology

A number of animal models have been developed to assess the pathological changes that occur after nerve injury [3,11,25]. These models involve injury to a peripheral nerve or to the dorsal root and result in long-lasting

Table II
Diagnostic criteria for complex regional pain syndrome (CRPS)

CRPS-I	CRPS-II
1. Develops after an initiating noxious event.	1. Develops after nerve injury.
2. Spontaneous pain or allodynia/ hyperalgesia occurs but is not limited to the territory of a single nerve, and is disproportionate to the inciting event.	2. Spontaneous pain or allodynia/ hyperalgesia occurs but is not limited to the territory of the injured nerve.
3. There is or has been evidence of edema, skin blood flow abnormality, or abnormal sudomotor activity in the region of the pain since the inciting event.	3. There is or has been evidence of edema, skin blood flow abnormality, or abnormal sudomotor activity in the region of the pain since the nerve injury.
4. The diagnosis is excluded by the existence of conditions that would otherwise account for the degree of pain and dysfunction.	4. The diagnosis is excluded by the existence of conditions that would otherwise account for the degree of pain and dysfunction.

mechanical and heat hyperalgesia. Studies using these models have identified clear alterations in the sympathetic nervous system, changes in peripheral and central glial cells, increased activity in peripheral nociceptors, and central sensitization [33]. Both injured and uninjured nerve fibers located within the same nerve show increased spontaneous firing, presumably as a result of upregulation of specific sodium channels ($Na_V1.3$ and $Na_V1.8$) in both injured and uninjured axons after nerve injury [18,33]. Dorsal horn neurons in the spinal cord show enhanced responsiveness to peripherally applied stimuli, including nonpainful Aβ-fiber stimuli [33,35]. Descending facilitation from the brainstem has been proposed to maintain the changes in the spinal cord and the hyperalgesia associated with nerve injury [4,33,36,45]. Thus, both peripheral and central mechanisms contribute to the pain and allodynia associated with neuropathic pain syndromes.

The role of the sympathetic nervous system can be inferred from the results of sympathectomy (a surgical or chemical procedure that destroys nerves in the sympathetic nervous system). The sympathetic nervous system seems to play an important role in the hyperexcitability and ectopic discharges of axotomized dorsal root ganglion (DRG) neurons, because blockade of sympathetic activity decreases these discharges.

Sprouting of sympathetic fibers and an upregulation of adrenergic receptors also occur in the DRG after axotomy [7–9,24]. Further, animal studies show that sympathectomy reverses hyperalgesia in some models of neuropathic pain [7–9,24]. In some cases of clinical neuropathic pain, sympathectomy—chemical or surgical—reduces the pain and associated symptoms of neuropathic injury. However, systematic reviews show weak or no evidence for the effectiveness of sympathectomy [28].

Management

Medical Management

Medical management of neuropathic pain is aimed at reducing pain and improving function through the use of pharmacological, surgical, and interventional techniques. Pharmacological approaches generally involve the use of opioids, anticonvulsants, or antidepressants to manage neuropathic pain. The use of opioid agonists is common for the management of neuropathic pain, and their efficacy has been confirmed in meta-analysis and systematic reviews. Specifically, opioid agonists lead to a greater reduction in pain when compared to placebo [13,14,21,22]. Further, the pain associated with dynamic mechanical allodynia and cold allodynia are also reduced to a greater extent by opioid agonists when compared to placebo [14,15]. Both gabapentin and carbamazepine are effective in treatment of neuropathic pain; both drugs are similarly effective [13,21,47–49]. Tricyclic antidepressants and selective serotonin reuptake inhibitors are also utilized to treat neuropathic pain, and their efficacy has been confirmed in a systematic reviews of up to 61 randomized controlled trials (RCTs) for diabetic neuropathy and postherpetic neuralgia [13,21,38]. However, for postherpetic neuralgia, systematic reviews show that N-methyl D-aspartate (NMDA) antagonists (ketamine, dextromethorphan, and memantine) are no more effective than placebo [13,21].

Topically administered creams such as capsaicin, lidocaine, and anti-inflammatories can also be used to manage neuropathic pain, particularly in peripheral neuropathies such as postherpetic neuralgia. Capsaicin cream and lidocaine are more effective than placebo for reduction in pain associated with postherpetic neuralgia, as confirmed in a meta-analysis and one systematic review [13,21].

Spinal cord stimulation is a technique in which an electrical stimulator is implanted epidurally over the dorsal column of the spinal cord and electrical current is applied (usually at 60 Hz) directly to the dorsal columns to produce an analgesic effect. A systematic review of the literature found evidence to support the use of spinal cord stimulation in patients with refractory neuropathic back and leg pain from failed back surgery syndrome based on one RCT and 72 case studies (Grade B evidence), as measured by pain reduction of more than 50% [43]. Spinal cord stimulation also decreases pain and analgesic use in people with CRPS-I (Grade A evidence) [44].

The use of sympathectomy for treatment of CRPS is historically based on the concept that the pain is "sympathetically maintained." However, a systematic review of the literature on chemical or surgical sympathectomy concluded that there is weak evidence to support the use of sympathectomy and that the complications of the procedure can be significant [28]. Further, the literature to support the use of sympathetic blockade for people with CRPS is inconclusive, and analgesic effects could not be determined in meta-analysis or systematic reviews [5,17].

In summary, there is good evidence for the use of systemically administered antidepressants, anticonvulsants, and opioids and for the use of topical capsaicin and lidocaine for patients with neuropathic pain. There is also good to moderate evidence for the use of spinal cord stimulation for the treatment of neuropathic pain and CRPS. However there is inconclusive or no evidence for the use of NMDA antagonists or sympathectomy for the management of neuropathic pain and CRPS.

Psychological Management

There is limited evidence for the efficacy of psychological treatment in neuropathic pain, despite its common use in patients with painful neuropathic disorders such as CRPS [20]. One trial investigated the effects of cognitive-behavioral therapy in the treatment of HIV-induced peripheral neuropathy as compared to treatment with supportive psychotherapy; both groups showed improvement in pain and functioning after 6 weeks of therapy, but there were higher dropout rates in the supportive psychotherapy group [16]. However, chronic pain conditions in general respond well to psychological interventions, including cognitive-behavioral therapy, relaxation, and education on coping skills [20] (see Chapter 13).

Physical Therapy Management

Evidence for effectiveness of physical therapy treatments for neuropathic pain conditions, including CRPS, is limited, particularly with respect to high-quality RCTs (Table III). However, treatments usually involve the use of (1) exercise therapy to improve range of motion, strength, and coordination; (2) sensory and motor re-education to reduce pain and improve function; and (3) modalities such as transcutaneous electrical nerve stimulation (TENS) to reduce pain (for review [19,41]).

Table III
Evidence for physical therapy treatments of neuropathic pain, including CRPS

Treatment	Type of Study	Results
Exercise	RCT, CT	Reduces pain at rest and with movement, improves range of motion and function
TENS	RCT	Reduces pain and allodynia
Motor imagery/ mirror therapy	RCT	Reduces pain, analgesic consumption, swelling, and disability
Desensitization therapy	Systematic review based on 1 RCT	Reduces allodynia and improves hand sensibility

Abbreviations: CRPS = complex regional pain syndrome; CT = controlled trial; RCT = randomized controlled trial; TENS = transcutaneous electrical nerve stimulation.

Exercise therapy should be used to improve and restore function in patients with neuropathic pain. Several studies have included exercise as part of the protocol for treatment of neuropathic pain and in particular CRPS. However, there is a general lack of RCTs evaluating the effectiveness of physical therapy for acute or chronic neuropathic pain conditions other than CRPS. The literature evaluating the effects for acute or chronic CRPS includes a few controlled trials, some of which were randomized to other treatments for comparison. For adults with CRPS-I, a controlled trial was performed involving a stress-loading program of scrubbing, carrying, and functional hand-loading activities. The program results in a decrease in pain and trophic changes, along with improvements in grip strength and range of motion [46]. For children with CRPS, an uncontrolled study found that exercise results in a complete resolution of pain and return of function in nearly all patients [40]. However, in both of the above studies, there was no control comparison group, and thus subjects were not randomized. When physical therapy, defined as exercise using graded activity to improve function, strength and mobility, was combined with spinal cord stimulation in patients with chronic CRPS, there was no difference compared to a group that only received spinal cord stimulation [23]. However, all patients had received prior physical therapy, and a large number of patients (approximately 50%) did not complete the study, mostly due to a change in treatment plan by the therapist or because of a worsening condition. These problems make it difficult to draw any conclusions of effectiveness in this study. In another study of acute CRPS of the upper extremity, physical therapy was compared to occupational therapy, and a control condition that included education and social work. The experimenter selected treatments based on the following objectives: physical therapy objectives were to increase pain control, optimize coping skills, and extinguish the source of pain, and occupational therapy objectives were to reduce inflammation, protect and support the hands, normalize sensation, improve hand function, and improve activities of daily living. Physical therapy improved pain, both at rest and with movement, and increased range of motion of the upper extremity to a greater extent than occupational therapy or the control condition [32].

Durmus and colleagues [12] assessed the efficacy of electromagnetic therapy combined with exercise therapy and calcitonin treatment as compared to a combination of placebo, exercise therapy, and calcitonin in patients with CRPS-I. Positive outcomes were reported for both groups, with decreases in pain at rest and with movement, and reductions in swelling; however, the lack of group differences suggests that treatment with exercise and calcitonin is effective and that the addition of electromagnetic therapy provides no benefit [12]. One RCT utilized cognitive-behavioral therapy in combination with physical therapy delivered once or three times per week. Both groups show similar improvements in physical function [27]. It is difficult from this study to assess the efficacy of psychological treatments, or that of physical therapy, as there were no control groups that received individual treatments or no treatment. In summary, there is weak evidence, based on poor-quality trials, to support the use of a general exercise program for people with neuropathic pain, in particular CRPS.

TENS, when used for treatment of neuropathic pain, is typically applied either over the affected nerve, or if the pain is too severe for the patient to tolerate direct stimulation, the electrodes can be placed around the painful area. High-frequency TENS, assessed in RCTs and one case study, reduces pain in people with diabetic neuropathy or mixed peripheral neuropathies (caused by amputation or nerve injury) [1,6,26,42]. Effects of high-frequency TENS in randomized placebo-controlled trials show reductions in both resting pain and allodynia when compared to placebo [1,6,26]. Thus, there is good evidence from RCTs that TENS is effective in patients with neuropathic pain.

Motor imagery and mirror feedback exercises have been assessed in people with neuropathic pain and CRPS. Mirror therapy involves movement of the affected limb inside a mirror-box to provide visual feedback of the affected hand to replace that of the (reflected) unaffected hand. Pain was reduced in people with acute or chronic CRPS-I following treatment with mirror therapy in RCTs when compared to standard treatment [29–31]. There was also an associated decrease in analgesic consumption, reduced swelling, improvement on the neuropathic pain scale, and decreased disability following treatment in acute and intermediate CRPS (with onset within 1 year); the effects of treatment were long-lasting [29–31]. This technique is similarly effective for patients with phantom limb pain [31,37]. Thus, there is good evidence from RCTs that motor imagery using mirror therapy reduces pain and disability in people with CRPS-I and phantom limb pain.

Similarly, graded sensory stimuli are often used to extinguish the allodynia associated with CRPS. Sensory re-education, also referred to as desensitization therapy, relies on controlled stimuli aimed at desensitizing the affected limb. Graded stimuli are applied to the allodynic area of the affected limb starting with soft stimuli, such as a cotton wisp, and increasing to a rough stimulus, such as sandpaper. Kits can be purchased through hand therapy catalogues and include graded textures that are rubbed on the skin, or buckets of graded sensory particles in which the limb can be placed. One high-quality RCT supports the use of sensory re-education for people with neuropathic pain to reduce allodynia and improve cutaneous sensibility [34].

In summary, there is moderate evidence from controlled trials, both randomized and non-randomized, to support the use of exercise for treatment of CRPS. There is good evidence to support the use of TENS and mirror image therapy for neuropathic pain and CRPS and limited evidence to support to support the use of sensory re-education therapy for CRPS.

References

[1] Alvaro M, Kumar D, Julka IS. Transcutaneous electrostimulation: emerging treatment for diabetic neuropathic pain. Diabetes Technol Ther 1999;1:77–80.
[2] Baron R. Complex regional pain syndrome. In: McMahon SB, Koltzenburg M, editors. Melzack and Wall's textbook of pain. London: Elsevier; 2006. p. 1011–27.
[3] Bennett GJ, Xie YK. A peripheral mononeuropathy in rat that produces disorders of pain sensation like those seen in man. Pain 1988;33:87–107.
[4] Burgess SE, Gardell LR, Ossipov MH, Malan TP, Vanderah TW, Lai J, Porreca F. Time-dependent descending facilitation from the rostral ventromedial medulla maintains, but does not initiate, neuropathic pain. J Neurosci 2002;22:5129–36.
[5] Cepeda MS, Carr DB, Lau J. Local anesthetic sympathetic blockade for complex regional pain syndrome. Cochrane Database Syst Rev 2005;CD004598.
[6] Cheing GL, Luk ML. Transcutaneous electrical nerve stimulation for neuropathic pain. J Hand Surg (Br) 2005;30:50–5.
[7] Choi Y, Yoon YW, Na HS, Kim SH, Chung JM. Behavioral signs of ongoing pain and cold allodynia in a rat model of neuropathic pain. Pain 1994;59:369–76.
[8] Chung JM, Chung K. Importance of hyperexcitability of DRG neurons in neuropathic pain. Pain Pract 2002;2:87–97.
[9] Chung K, Lee BH, Yoon YW, Chung JM. Sympathetic sprouting in the dorsal root ganglia of the injured peripheral nerve in a rat neuropathic pain model. J Comp Neurol 1996;376:241–52.
[10] de Mos M, de Bruijn AG, Huygen FJ, Dieleman JP, Stricker BH, Sturkenboom MC. The incidence of complex regional pain syndrome: a population-based study. Pain 2007;129:12–20.
[11] Decosterd I, Woolf CJ. Spared nerve injury: an animal model of persistent peripheral neuropathic pain. Pain 2000;87:149–58.
[12] Durmus A, Cakmak A, Disci R, Muslumanoglu L. The efficiency of electromagnetic field treatment in Complex Regional Pain Syndrome Type I. Disabil Rehabil 2004;26:537–45.
[13] Dworkin RH, O'Connor AB, Backonja M, Farrar JT, Finnerup NB, Jensen TS, Kalso EA, Loeser JD, Miaskowski C, Nurmikko TJ, et al. Pharmacologic management of neuropathic pain: evidence-based recommendations. Pain 2007;132:237–51.
[14] Eisenberg E, McNicol E, Carr DB. Opioids for neuropathic pain. Cochrane Database Syst Rev 2006;3:CD006146.
[15] Eisenberg E, McNicol ED, Carr DB. Efficacy of mu-opioid agonists in the treatment of evoked neuropathic pain: systematic review of randomized controlled trials. Eur J Pain 2006;10:667–76.
[16] Evans S, Fishman B, Spielman L, Haley A. Randomized trial of cognitive behavior therapy versus supportive psychotherapy for HIV-related peripheral neuropathic pain. Psychosomatics 2003;44:44–50.
[17] Finegold AA, Perez FM, Iadarola MJ. In vivo control of NMDA receptor transcript level in motoneurons by viral transduction of a short antisense gene. Brain Res Mol Brain Res 2001;90:17–25.
[18] Gold MS, Weinreich D, Kim CS, Wang R, Treanor J, Porreca F, Lai J. Redistribution of $Na_v1.8$ in uninjured axons enables neuropathic pain. J Neurosci 2003;23:158–66.

[19] Harden RN, Swan M, King A, Costa B, Barthel J. Treatment of complex regional pain syndrome: functional restoration. Clin J Pain 2006;22:420–4.

[20] Haythornthwaite JA, Benrud-Larson LM. Psychological assessment and treatment of patients with neuropathic pain. Curr Pain Headache Rep 2001;5:124–9.

[21] Hempenstall K, Nurmikko TJ, Johnson RW, A'Hern RP, Rice AS. Analgesic therapy in postherpetic neuralgia: a quantitative systematic review. PLoS Med 2005;2:e164.

[22] Hollingshead J, Duhmke RM, Cornblath DR. Tramadol for neuropathic pain. Cochrane Database Syst Rev 2006;3:CD003726.

[23] Kemler MA, Rijks CP, de Vet HC. Which patients with chronic reflex sympathetic dystrophy are most likely to benefit from physical therapy? J Manipulative Physiol Ther 2001;24:272–8.

[24] Kim SH, Chung JM. Sympathectomy alleviates mechanical allodynia in an experimental animal model for neuropathy in the rat. Neurosci Lett 1991;134:131–4.

[25] Kim SH, Chung JM. An experimental-model for peripheral neuropathy produced by segmental spinal nerve ligation in the rat. Pain 1992;50:355–63.

[26] Kumar D, Alvaro MS, Julka IS, Marshall HJ. Diabetic peripheral neuropathy. Effectiveness of electrotherapy and amitriptyline for symptomatic relief. Diabetes Care 1998;21:1322–5.

[27] Lee BH, Scharff L, Sethna NF, McCarthy CF, Scott-Sutherland J, Shea AM, Sullivan P, Meier P, Zurakowski D, Masek BJ, et al. Physical therapy and cognitive-behavioral treatment for complex regional pain syndromes. J Pediatr 2002;141:135–40.

[28] Mailis A, Furlan A. Sympathectomy for neuropathic pain. Cochrane Database Syst Rev 2003;CD002918.

[29] McCabe CS, Haigh RC, Ring EF, Halligan PW, Wall PD, Blake DR. A controlled pilot study of the utility of mirror visual feedback in the treatment of complex regional pain syndrome (type 1). Rheumatology (Oxford) 2003;42:97–01.

[30] Moseley GL. Graded motor imagery is effective for long-standing complex regional pain syndrome: a randomised controlled trial. Pain 2004;108:192–8.

[31] Moseley GL. Graded motor imagery for pathologic pain: a randomized controlled trial. Neurology 2006;67:2129–34.

[32] Oerlemans HM, Oostendorp RA, de Boo T, Goris RJ. Pain and reduced mobility in complex regional pain syndrome I: outcome of a prospective randomised controlled clinical trial of adjuvant physical therapy versus occupational therapy. Pain 1999;83:77–83.

[33] Ossipov MH, Lai J, Porreca F. Mechanisms of experimental neuropathic pain: integration from animal models. In: McMahon SB, Koltzenburg M, editors. Wall and Melzack's textbook of pain. London: Elsevier; 2006. p. 929–46.

[34] Oud T, Beelen A, Eijffinger E, Nollet F. Sensory re-education after nerve injury of the upper limb: a systematic review. Clin Rehabil 2007;21:483–94.

[35] Palecek J, Paleckova V, Dougherty PM, Carlton SM, Willis WD. Responses of spinothalamic tract cells to mechanical and thermal- stimulation of skin in rats with experimental peripheral neuropathy. J Neurophysiol 1992;67:1562–73.

[36] Porreca F, Burgess SE, Gardell LR, Vanderah TW, Malan TP, Ossipov MH, Lappi DA, Lai J. Inhibition of neuropathic pain by selective ablation of brainstem medullary cells expressing the mu-opioid receptor. J Neurosci 2001;21:5281–8.

[37] Ramachandran VS, Rogers-Ramachandran D, Cobb S. Touching the phantom limb. Nature 1995;377:489–90.

[38] Saarto T, Wiffen PJ. Antidepressants for neuropathic pain. Cochrane Database Syst Rev 2007;CD005454.

[39] Scadding JW, Koltzenburg M. Painful peripheral neuropathies. In: McMahon SB, Koltzenburg M, editors. Textbook of pain. London: Elsevier; 2006. p. 973–1010.

[40] Sherry DD, Wallace CA, Kelley C, Kidder M, Sapp L. Short- and long-term outcomes of children with complex regional pain syndrome type I treated with exercise therapy. Clin J Pain 1999;15:218–23.

[41] Smith TO. How effective is physiotherapy in the treatment of complex regional pain syndrome type I? A review of the literature. Musculoskeletal Care 2005;3:181–200.

[42] Somers DL, Somers MF. Treatment of neuropathic pain in a patient with diabetic neuropathy using transcutaneous electrical nerve stimulation applied to the skin of the lumbar region. Phys Ther 1999;79:767–75.

[43] Stanton-Hicks M, Janig W, Hassenbusch S, Haddox JD, Boas R, Wilson P. Reflex sympathetic dystrophy: changing concepts and taxonomy. Pain 1995;63:127–33.

[44] Taylor RS. Spinal cord stimulation in complex regional pain syndrome and refractory neuropathic back and leg pain/failed back surgery syndrome: results of a systematic review and meta-analysis. J Pain Symptom Manage 2006;31:S13–9.

[45] Vera-Portocarrero LP, Zhang ET, Ossipov MH, Xie JY, King T, Lai J, Porreca F. Descending facilitation from the rostral ventromedial medulla maintains nerve injury-induced central sensitization. Neuroscience 2006;140:1311–20.

[46] Watson HK, Carlson L. Treatment of reflex sympathetic dystrophy of the hand with an active "stress loading" program. J Hand Surg (Am) 1987;12:779–85.

[47] Wiffen PJ, McQuay HJ, Edwards JE, Moore RA. Gabapentin for acute and chronic pain. Cochrane Database Syst Rev 2005;CD005452.

[48] Wiffen PJ, McQuay HJ, Moore RA. Carbamazepine for acute and chronic pain. Cochrane Database Syst Rev 2005;CD005451.

[49] Wiffen PJ, Rees J. Lamotrigine for acute and chronic pain. Cochrane Database Syst Rev 2007;CD006044.

Correspondence to: Prof. Kathleen A. Sluka, PT, PhD, Graduate Program in Physical Therapy and Rehabilitation Science, The University of Iowa, 1-252 Medical Education Building, Iowa City, IA 52242-1190, USA. Tel: 1-319-335-9791; fax: 1-319-335-9707; email: Kathleen-sluka@uiowa.edu.

Osteoarthritis and Rheumatoid Arthritis

Kathleen A. Sluka

Graduate Program in Physical Therapy and Rehabilitation Science,
The University of Iowa, Iowa City, Iowa, USA

Epidemiology

Arthritic conditions can generally be classified into inflammatory or non-inflammatory conditions. Inflammatory conditions are the least prevalent, with rheumatoid arthritis affecting approximately 1% of the population [50]. Other inflammatory conditions include systemic lupus erythematosus (with a prevalence of 0.5%), ankylosing spondylitis (1.0%), and gout (1.0%). The prevalence of osteoarthritis, or degenerative joint disease, increases with age, affecting approximately 30% of those over the age of 65 years [50]. This chapter will focus on rheumatoid arthritis and osteoarthritis because they are commonly treated by physical therapists.

Diagnostic Criteria

Osteoarthritis

Osteoarthritis, also termed degenerative joint disease, is a chronic disease that affects the cartilage and subchondral bone. Radiological studies generally confirm a loss of articular cartilage and the formation of new bone and cartilage. The severity of osteoarthritis is scored on the Kellgren-Lawrence scale: 0 = no features of OA; 1 = doubtful OA with minute osteophytes (bone spurs); 2 = minimal OA with definite osteophytes but unimpaired joint space; 3 = moderate OA with osteophytes and moderate loss of joint space; and 4 = severe OA with greatly impaired joint space and sclerosis of subchondral bone [50]. Diagnostic criteria by the American College of Rheumatology combine symptoms along with radiographic evidence of joint destruction [1]. Diagnostic criteria for primary osteoarthritis of the knee are outlined in Table I; similar criteria are available for the hand and hip [2,3]. Although osteoarthritis is traditionally thought to be non-inflammatory, recent evidence suggests mild inflammation of the synovium [4,5]. Osteoarthritis is associated with pain, stiffness, functional limitations, and decreased quality of life [50]. Localized osteoarthritis generally occurs in the knees or hips but can also occur in other joints such as the hand or shoulder. Osteoarthritis can also be generalized, occurring in multiple joints (e.g., knees, hips, and hands). Pain is the major reason an individual seeks medical attention and is the major determinant of functional loss and decreased quality of life in people with osteoarthritis.

Table I
The American College of Rheumatology
diagnostic criteria for primary osteoarthritis

1. Localized
a. Hip
b. Knee
c. Hand
d. Other: shoulder, elbow, wrist, ankle

2. Generalized: multiple joints

3. Pain and 5 of the following criteria
a. age >50 years
b. stiffness <30 minutes
c. crepitus
d. bony tenderness
e. bony enlargement
f. no palpable warmth
g. erythrocyte sedimentation rate <40 mm/h
h. rheumatoid factor <1:40
i. synovial fluid signs of osteoarthritis
j. osteophytes

Source: Altman et al. [1–3].

Rheumatoid Arthritis

Rheumatoid arthritis is an immune-mediated chronic inflammatory condition that affects multiple joints, usually in a symmetrical pattern [50]. The cause is unknown but probably involves both genetic and environmental factors [51]. Inflammatory synovitis, the key pathological feature in rheumatoid arthritis, results in inflammatory cell infiltration and hypertrophy of the synovium. Increased levels of the proinflammatory cytokines tumor necrosis factor-α (TNF-α) and interleukin-1, as well as destructive matrix metalloproteinase enzymes, are produced by the synoviocytes [11,27]. In addition to inflammatory signs in the joints, patients complain of fatigue, and 20–40% of patients have signs of systemic disease outside the joint, including pulmonary, cardiac or vascular, ocular, and neurological symptoms [43,50]. Laboratory findings include an abnormal X-ray showing soft-tissue swelling, loss of joint space, and bony erosions; an abnormal erythrocyte sedimentation rate (ESR); and a positive serum rheumatic factor [50]. General criteria for diagnosis, usually performed by a rheumatologist, are outlined in Table II.

Rheumatoid arthritis has a distinctly different pain pattern than osteoarthritis. In general, inflammatory conditions such as rheumatoid arthritis get worse with rest, result in stiffness in the morning lasting more than 1 hour, get better with low-grade activity, and are associated with swelling. In contrast, people with osteoarthritis generally feel better with rest, have progressively worse symptoms throughout the day with activity, and have minimal signs of inflammation [50].

Table II
The American College of Rheumatology diagnostic
criteria for rheumatoid arthritis

1. Morning stiffness >1 hour
2. Involvement in three or more joints
3. Involvement in hands
4. Symmetrical
5. Rheumatoid nodules
6. Positive serum rheumatoid factor
7. Radiographic evidence of rheumatoid arthritis

Source: Arnett et al. [7].

Pathology

Osteoarthritis

Osteoarthritis is associated with loss of cartilage, remodeling of bone, and intermittent inflammation [50]. Changes in the synovium, bone, and ligaments begin early in the disease process [51]. Release of inflammatory cytokines such as interleukin-1 and TNF from chondrocytes and synoviocytes contributes to the cartilage destruction [6]. These inflammatory substances, when released into osteoarthritic joints, sensitize peripheral nociceptors and lead to central sensitization of dorsal horn neurons [49]. There is also a loss of inhibitory control mechanisms in osteoarthritis [32]. Together, the peripheral and central changes observed in people with osteoarthritis contribute to the pain and loss of function.

Rheumatoid Arthritis

Rheumatoid arthritis is an inflammatory joint disease with synovitis as the key feature [50]. The disease is associated with inflammatory cell infiltration into the joint and joint tissues, which results in hyperplasia of the synovial lining, as well as fibrin deposition. There is release of inflammatory cytokines, particularly TNF-α and interleukin-1, in the synovial fluid [50,51]. As noted below, targeting the effects of TNF-α and interleukin-1 has become the standard of care, giving rise to a class of disease-modifying drugs.

Assessment Considerations

Special considerations for the assessment of pain in people with osteoarthritis and rheumatoid arthritis include analyzing the nature of the pain across the day, assessing pain with functional activities, and gauging the impact of pain on daily function. The Knee Injury and Osteoarthritis Outcome Score (KOOS) was developed as an extension to the Western Ontario and McMaster Osteoarthritis Index (WOMAC). The KOOS and WOMAC are commonly used in patients with osteoarthritis to assess the impact of pain on function and have proven valid and reliable [9,48]. For rheumatoid arthritis, assessments should also include examining for signs of inflammation, swelling, and pain in multiple joints. Overall, assessment of pain should include standard pain scales, self-efficacy questionnaires, quality-of-life questionnaires, and measurement of functional deficits. The same group that developed the KOOS devised a questionnaire aimed at people with rheumatoid and osteoarthritis of the lower extremities, called the Rheumatoid and Arthritis Outcome Score (RAOS) [48]. Both the KOOS and RAOS are freely available (www.koos.nu).

Medical Management

Management of osteoarthritis and rheumatoid arthritis requires a multidisciplinary approach that includes pharmacology, psychology, physical therapy, and surgery. Treatment of patients with osteoarthritis is generally aimed at managing painful symptoms and improving functional capacity. On the other hand, treatment of rheumatoid arthritis uses disease-modifying drugs and anti-inflammatory medications to reduce the disease process and the accompanying symptoms.

Osteoarthritis

The goals for medical management of osteoarthritis are to reduce the pain and other symptoms, either through systemic pharmacological treatments or local intra-articular injections. Systematic reviews show that opioid agonists (tramadol), acetaminophen (paracetamol), NSAIDs, and interleukin-1 inhibitors reduce pain and in some cases improve function in people with osteoarthritis [20,22,24,58,59]. Local treatments generally include intra-articular injection of corticosteroids or hyaluronic acid. Intra-articular corticosteroid injection is more effective than placebo for pain reduction and global self-assessment scores, producing decreases in pain for up to 4 weeks [10]. Further, intra-articular injection of hyaluronic acid is more effective than corticosteroids for changes in pain, WOMAC score, and range of motion [10]. Total joint replacement is considered when pain and functional limitations result in a diminished quality of life, when there is radiographic evidence of joint damage, and when there is moderate to severe pain that is not adequately relieved by an nonsurgical approaches [38]. Total joint replacement, generally of the hip or knee, is the primary surgical approach and clearly reduces pain and improves function and quality of life in people with osteoarthritis, as confirmed by the National Institutes of Health (NIH) consensus statement. According to the consensus statement, there is a rapid and substantial improvement in pain, functional status, and overall health-related quality of life in about 90% of patients; about 85% of patients are satisfied with the results of surgery [38].

Rheumatoid Arthritis

Disease-modifying antirheumatic drugs (DMARDs) are drugs that have a beneficial effect on the course of rheumatoid arthritis by slowing the progression of the disease. They also decrease symptoms such as pain and swelling and improve function and quality of life. There are a number of agents in this category, including those aimed at reducing TNF-α effects (etanercept, adalimumab), inhibiting activated lymphocytes (leflunomide), or inhibiting folic acid synthesis (methotrexate), as well as immunosuppressive agents (cyclophosphamide, azathioprine, cyclosporine) and gold salts. The effectiveness of these DMARDs has been confirmed in numerous systematic reviews and meta-analyses [13,14,37,39,52–57,61], and thus drugs of this category should be prescribed for all patients with moderate to severe rheumatoid arthritis.

Drugs aimed at reducing the inflammatory process serve as analgesics as well as anti-inflammatories. Corticosteroids and NSAIDs can be used to reduce symptoms as an adjunct to DMARDs [25,50,63]. For relief of pain, acetaminophen is also an effective treatment, producing results similar to those of NSAIDs [50,63]. Intra-articular treatment with steroid injections reduces pain and swelling associated with rheumatoid arthritis and improves function [41,60]. Lastly, the effectiveness of local treatments such as topical NSAIDs or capsaicin has been confirmed in randomized controlled trials (RCTs) [21,44]. Local treatments are useful for patients who cannot tolerate systemic therapy or as an adjunct to DMARDs.

Psychological Management

The pain and loss of function in individuals with osteoarthritis and rheumatoid arthritis have a significant impact on quality of life. Therefore, psychological management can be helpful in these chronic pain conditions. Cognitive-behavioral approaches are aimed at teaching coping skills and preventing fear of further injury. These therapies typically incorporate coping strategies, relaxation therapy, education on disease and treatments, and stress management skills. Such therapy reduces pain, lessens joint tenderness and swelling, and improves self-efficacy in people with rheumatoid arthritis (for review see [15,31]). When compared to routine care, cognitive-behavioral therapy for patients with rheumatoid arthritis yields improvements in pain affect, coping, and emotional stability [see 31]. Long-term effects of cognitive behavioral therapy are observed for at least 12–15 months after treatment, as evidenced by decreased use of medical service and reductions in pain [15,31]. Similarly, in people with osteoarthritis, cognitive-behavioral therapy reduces pain, with effects that are maintained through a 6-month follow-up [15,29,30,31].

Physical Therapy Management

The goals of physical therapy management of osteoarthritis and rheumatoid arthritis are to maintain or improve function and decrease pain. Exercise, including both aerobic and strengthening programs, works to improve function and, along with other modalities, helps to decrease pain. Given that rheumatoid arthritis has a strong inflammatory component, treatment with anti-inflammatory modalities, such as ice, is also beneficial. Education is also a key component of treatment of both conditions, focusing on the disease process, the benefits of routine physical exercise, and home management of pain with heat and ice.

Osteoarthritis

The Osteoarthritis Research Society International and the American Pain Society have developed evidence-based guidelines for the management of osteoarthritis with nonpharmacological treatments [64]. Physical therapy interventions include those aimed at reducing pain, i.e., transcutaneous electrical nerve stimulation (TENS) and thermotherapy, and those aimed at improving both function and pain, i.e., exercise programs. There is good evidence that either land-based or aquatic exercise reduces pain and improves physical function for people with osteoarthritis [8,23]. Either low- or high-intensity aerobic exercise will improve pain and function in people with osteoarthritis to a similar extent; home-based exercise programs and group exercise programs are equally effective [17,47]. According to a meta-analysis, both aerobic and strengthening exercises are

effective in reducing pain and decreasing disability in people with osteoarthritis [47]. Recommendations from systematic reviews suggest that effective exercise programs should include advice and education to promote
increased physical activity [47].

In the physical therapy management of pain in people with osteoarthritis, a number of treatments show effectiveness for reducing pain
and improving function (Table III). Both conventional, high-frequency
TENS and acupuncture-like, low-frequency TENS, as well as low-level laser therapy, reduce pain associated with osteoarthritis [12,40]. Cryotherapy improves range of motion, edema, and function, but not pain [18].
However, ultrasound is ineffective in people with osteoarthritis [12]. One
RCT shows that a Grade III accessory joint mobilization of the knee reduces pain and improves function immediately after treatment in people
with knee osteoarthritis when compared to a placebo control group [35].
Thus, TENS, low-level laser therapy, and joint mobilization reduce pain
in people with osteoarthritis, and ice improves functional outcomes with
short-term effects.

Table III
Evidence for physical therapy treatments for osteoarthritis

Treatment	Pain	Function
Aerobic exercise	+ (SR)	+ (SR)
Strengthening exercise	+ (SR)	+ (SR)
TENS	+ (SR)	Not examined
Cryotherapy	– (SR)	+ (SR)
Heat therapy	? (SR) (recommended)	Not examined
Joint mobilization	+ (RCT)	+ (RCT)
Ultrasound	– (SR)	Not examined
Low-level laser therapy	+ (SR)	Not examined

Abbreviations: RCT = randomized controlled trial; SR =
systematic review; TENS = transcutaneous electrical nerve
stimulation; +, evidence of benefit; –, no evidence of benefit.

Rheumatoid Arthritis

Patient education improves disability, joint tenderness and swelling, global
assessment scores, and psychological status in people with rheumatoid

arthritis; the effects of education on pain are inconclusive [45]. Education for patients with rheumatoid arthritis can increase compliance with an exercise program, but the effects are short-term [33].

Exercise is generally recommended to improve function, decrease fatigue, and decrease pain, and its effects have been confirmed in systematic reviews [26,28,34,42,62]. High- or low-intensity strengthening programs as well as aerobic exercises decrease pain and improve function and health status in people with osteoarthritis, as confirmed in systematic reviews (Evidence Ia; Strength B) and recommended in evidence-based guidelines [17,28,34]. However, high-intensity, load-bearing exercise should be applied with caution because during acute inflammatory arthritic conditions it may aggravate the disease process in patients with pre-existing extreme joint damage [36].

Table IV
Evidence for physical therapy treatments
for rheumatoid arthritis

Treatment	Pain	Function
Aerobic exercise	+ (SR)	+ (SR)
Strengthening exercise	+ (SR)	+ (SR)
TENS	+ (SR)	Not examined
Cryotherapy	(SR)	– (SR)
Superficial heat therapy	? (SR)	Not examined
Ultrasound	+ (SR)	+ (SR)
Joint mobilization	Not studied	Not studied

Abbreviations: SR = systematic review; TENS = transcutaneous electrical nerve stimulation. +, evidence of benefit; –, no evidence of benefit.

The use of electrical stimulation (TENS) significantly improves hand function, pain at rest, joint tenderness, and patient assessment of joint pain, but not pain with grip when compared to placebo or no-treatment controls [16]. The use of thermal modalities to treat pain in people with rheumatoid arthritis is supported by minimal data from relatively low-quality RCTs. However, deep heating with ultrasound applied to the hand improves range of motion of the wrist, grip strength, and morning stiffness and decreases the number of swollen and painful joints [19]. Although no significant effects of superficial heat or cold therapy are observed in people with rheumatoid arthritis for pain, range of motion, or function, Robinson and colleagues recommend thermal modalities as a palliative therapy [46]. At present there are no data on manual therapy techniques to support or refute their effectiveness in rheumatoid arthritis. In summary, evidence suggests that relief of pain can be accomplished with a number of nonpharmacological treatments including exercise, TENS, and thermal therapy. Further, function can be improved with strengthening and aerobic exercises, which are recommended treatments (Table IV).

References

[1]   Altman R, Asch E, Bloch D, Bole G, Borenstein D, Brandt K, Christy W, Cooke TD, Greenwald R, Hochberg M. Development of criteria for the classification and reporting of osteoarthritis. Classification of osteoarthritis of the knee. Diagnostic and Therapeutic Criteria Committee of the American Rheumatism Association. Arthritis Rheum 1986;29:1039–49.

[2]   Altman R, Alarcón G, Appelrouth D, Bloch D, Borenstein D, Brandt K, Brown C, Cooke TD, Daniel W, Gray R,, et al. The American College of Rheumatology criteria for the classification and reporting of osteoarthritis of the hand. Arthritis Rheum 1990;33:1601–10.

[3]   Altman R, Alarcón G, Appelrouth D, Bloch D, Borenstein D, Brandt K, Brown C, Cooke TD, Daniel W, Feldman D, et al. The American College of Rheumatology criteria for the classification and reporting of osteoarthritis of the hip. Arthritis Rheum 1991;34:505–14.

[4]   Altman RD. Structure-/disease-modifying agents for osteoarthritis. Semin Arthritis Rheum 2005;34:3–5.

[5]   Altman RD, Gray R. Inflammation in osteoarthritis. Clin Rheum Dis 1985;11:353–65.

[6]   Amin AR. Regulation of tumor necrosis factor-alpha and tumor necrosis factor converting enzyme in human osteoarthritis. Osteoarthritis Cartilage 1999;7:392–4.

[7]   Arnett FC, Edworthy SM, Bloch DA, McShane DJ, Fries JF, Cooper NS, Healey LA, Kaplan SR, Liang MH, Luthra HS, et al. The American Rheumatism Association 1987 revised criteria for the classification of rheumatoid arthritis. Arthritis Rheum 1988;31:315–24.

[8]   Bartels EM, Lund H, Hagen KB, Dagfinrud H, Christensen R, Danneskiold-Samsoe B. Aquatic exercise for the treatment of knee and hip osteoarthritis. Cochrane Database Syst Rev 2007;CD005523.

[9]   Bellamy N, Buchanan WW, Goldsmith CH, Campbell J, Stitt LW. Validation study of WOMAC: a health status instrument for measuring clinically important patient relevant outcomes to antirheumatic drug therapy in patients with osteoarthritis of the hip or knee. J Rheumatol 1988;15:1833–40.

[10] Bellamy N, Campbell J, Robinson V, Gee T, Bourne R, Wells G. Intraarticular corticosteroid for treatment of osteoarthritis of the knee. Cochrane Database Syst Rev 2006;CD005328.

[11] Bingham CO, III. The pathogenesis of rheumatoid arthritis: pivotal cytokines involved in bone degradation and inflammation. J Rheumatol Suppl 2002;65:3–9.

[12] Bjordal JM, Johnson MI, Lopes-Martins RA, Bogen B, Chow R, Ljunggren AE. Short-term efficacy of physical interventions in osteoarthritic knee pain. A systematic review and meta-analysis of randomised placebo-controlled trials. BMC Musculoskelet Disord 2007;8:51.

[13] Blumenauer B, Judd M, Cranney A, Burls A, Coyle D, Hochberg M, Tugwell P, Wells G. Etanercept for the treatment of rheumatoid arthritis. Cochrane Database Syst Rev 2003;CD004525.

[14] Blumenauer B, Judd M, Wells G, Burls A, Cranney A, Hochberg M, Tugwell P. Infliximab for the treatment of rheumatoid arthritis. Cochrane Database Syst Rev 2002;CD003785.

[15] Bradley LA, Alberts KR. Psychological and behavioral approaches to pain management for patients with rheumatic disease. Rheum Dis Clin North Am 1999;25:215–32, viii.

[16] Brosseau L, Judd MG, Marchand S, Robinson VA, Tugwell P, Wells G, Yonge K. Transcutaneous electrical nerve stimulation (TENS) for the treatment of rheumatoid arthritis in the hand. Cochrane Database Syst Rev 2003;CD004377.

[17] Brosseau L, MacLeay L, Robinson V, Wells G, Tugwell P. Intensity of exercise for the treatment of osteoarthritis. Cochrane Database Syst Rev 2003;CD004259.

[18] Brosseau L, Yonge KA, Robinson V, Marchand S, Judd M, Wells G, Tugwell P. Thermotherapy for treatment of osteoarthritis. Cochrane Database Syst Rev 2003;CD004522.

[19] Casimiro L, Brosseau L, Robinson V, Milne S, Judd M, Well G, Tugwell P, Shea B. Therapeutic ultrasound for the treatment of rheumatoid arthritis. Cochrane Database Syst Rev 2002;CD003787.

[20] Cepeda MS, Camargo F, Zea C, Valencia L. Tramadol for osteoarthritis. Cochrane Database Syst Rev 2006;3:CD005522.

[21] Deal CL, Schnitzer TJ, Lipstein E, Seibold JR, Stevens RM, Levy MD, Albert D, Renold F. Treatment of arthritis with topical capsaicin: a double-blind trial. Clin Ther 1991;13:383–95.

[22] Fidelix TS, Soares BG, Trevisani VF. Diacerein for osteoarthritis. Cochrane Database Syst Rev 2006;CD005117.

[23] Fransen M, McConnell S, Bell M. Therapeutic exercise for people with osteoarthritis of the hip or knee. A systematic review. J Rheumatol 2002;29:1737–45.

[24] Garner S, Fidan D, Frankish R, Judd M, Towheed T, Wells G, Tugwell P. Rofecoxib for the treatment of rheumatoid arthritis. Cochrane Database Syst Rev 2002;CD003685.

[25] Garner SE, Fidan DD, Frankish RR, Judd MG, Towheed TE, Wells G, Tugwell P. Rofecoxib for rheumatoid arthritis. Cochrane Database Syst Rev 2005;CD003685.

[26] Gaudin P, Leguen-Guegan S, Allenet B, Baillet A, Grange L, Juvin R. Is dynamic exercise beneficial in patients with rheumatoid arthritis? Joint Bone Spine 2008;75:11–7.

[27] Gearing AJ, Beckett P, Christodoulou M, Churchill M, Clements J, Davidson AH, Drummond AH, Galloway WA, Gilbert R, Gordon JL. Processing of tumour necrosis factor-alpha precursor by metalloproteinases. Nature 1994;370:555–7.

[28] Gossec L, Pavy S, Pham T, Constantin A, Poiraudeau S, Combe B, Flipo RM, Goupille P, Le Loët X, Mariette X, et al. Treatments in early rheumatoid arthritis: clinical practice guidelines based on published evidence and expert opinion. Joint Bone Spine 2006;73:396–402.

[29] Keefe FJ, Caldwell DS, Williams DA, Gil KM, Mitchel D, Robertson C. Pain coping skills training in the management of osteoarthritic knee pain: a comparative study. Behavior Therapy 1990;21:49–62.

[30] Keefe FJ, Caldwell DS, Williams DA, Gil KM, Robertson C. Pain coping skills training in the management of osteoarthritic knee pain: II. Follow-up results. Behavior Therapy 1990;21:435–47.

[31] Keefe FJ, Smith SJ, Buffington AL, Gibson J, Studts JL, Caldwell DS. Recent advances and future directions in the biopsychosocial assessment and treatment of arthritis. J Consult Clin Psychol 2002;70:640–55.

[32] Kosek E, Ordeberg G. Lack of pressure pain modulation by heterotopic noxious conditioning stimulation in patients with painful osteoarthritis before, but not following, surgical pain relief. Pain 2000;88:69–78.

[33] Mayoux-Benhamou A, Giraudet-Le Quintrec JS, Ravaud P, Champion K, Dernis E, Zerkak D, Roy C, Kahan A, Revel M, Dougados M. Influence of patient education on exercise compliance in rheumatoid arthritis: a prospective 12-month randomized controlled trial. J Rheumatol 2008;35:216–23.

[34] Metsios GS, Stavropoulos-Kalinoglou A, Veldhuijzen van Zanten JJ, Treharne GJ, Panoulas VF, Douglas KM, Koutedakis Y, Kitas GD. Rheumatoid arthritis, cardiovascular disease and physical exercise: a systematic review. Rheumatology (Oxford) 2008;47:239–48.

[35] Moss P, Sluka KA, Wright A. The initial effects of knee joint mobilization on osteoarthritic hyperalgesia. Man Ther 2007;12:109–18.

[36] Munneke M, de Jong Z, Zwinderman AH, Ronday HK, van SD, Dijkmans BA, Kroon HM, Vliet Vlieland TP, Hazes JM. Effect of a high-intensity weight-bearing exercise program on radiologic damage progression of the large joints in subgroups of patients with rheumatoid arthritis. Arthritis Rheum 2005;53:410–7.

[37] Navarro-Sarabia F, Ariza-Ariza R, Hernandez-Cruz B, Villanueva I. Adalimumab for treating rheumatoid arthritis. Cochrane Database Syst Rev 2005;CD005113.

[38] NIH Consensus Statement on total knee replacement. NIH Consens State Sci Statements 2003;20:1–34.

[39] Osiri M, Shea B, Robinson V, Suarez-Almazor M, Strand V, Tugwell P, Wells G. Leflunomide for treating rheumatoid arthritis. Cochrane Database Syst Rev 2003;CD002047.

[40] Osiri M, Welch V, Brosseau L, Shea B, McGowan J, Tugwell P, Wells G. Transcutaneous electrical nerve stimulation for knee osteoarthritis. Cochrane Database Syst Rev 2000;CD002823.

[41] Ostergaard M, Halberg P. Intra-articular corticosteroids in arthritic disease: a guide to treatment. BioDrugs 1998;9:95–103.

[42] Ottawa Panel. Ottawa Panel evidence-based clinical practice guidelines for therapeutic exercises in the management of rheumatoid arthritis in adults. Phys Ther 2004;84:934–72.

[43] Pouchot J, Kherani RB, Brant R, Lacaille D, Lehman AJ, Ensworth S, Kopec J, Esdaile JM, Liang MH. Determination of the minimal clinically important difference for seven fatigue measures in rheumatoid arthritis. J Clin Epidemiol 2008;61:705–13.

[44] Rendt-Nielsen L, Drewes AM, Svendsen L, Brennum J. Quantitative assessment of joint pain following treatment of rheumatoid arthritis with ibuprofen cream. Scand J Rheumatol 1994;23:334–7.

[45] Riemsma RP, Kirwan JR, Taal E, Rasker JJ. Patient education for adults with rheumatoid arthritis. Cochrane Database Syst Rev 2002;CD003688.

[46] Robinson V, Brosseau L, Casimiro L, Judd M, Shea B, Wells G, Tugwell P. Thermotherapy for treating rheumatoid arthritis. Cochrane Database Syst Rev 2002;CD002826.

[47] Roddy E, Zhang W, Doherty M. Aerobic walking or strengthening exercise for osteoarthritis of the knee? A systematic review. Ann Rheum Dis 2005;64:544–8.

[48] Roos EM, Lohmander LS. The knee injury and osteoarthritis outcome score (KOOS): from joint injury to osteoarthritis. Health Qual Life Outcomes 2003;1:64.

[49] Schaible HG, Ebersberger A, Von Banchet GS. Mechanisms of pain in arthritis. Ann NY Acad Sci 2002;966:343–54.

[50] Scott DL. Osteoarthritis and rheumatoid arthritis. In: McMahon SB, Koltzenburg M, editors. Wall and Melzack's textbook of pain. London: Elsevier; 2006. p. 653–67.

[51] Scott DL. Early rheumatoid arthritis. Br Med Bull 2007;81–82:97–114.

[52] Suarez-Almazor ME, Belseck E, Shea B, Wells G, Tugwell P. Methotrexate for rheumatoid arthritis. Cochrane Database Syst Rev 2000;CD000957.

[53] Suarez-Almazor ME, Belseck E, Shea B, Wells G, Tugwell P. Sulfasalazine for rheumatoid arthritis. Cochrane Database Syst Rev 2000;CD000958.

[54] Suarez-Almazor ME, Spooner C, Belseck E. Azathioprine for treating rheumatoid arthritis. Cochrane Database Syst Rev 2000;CD001461.

[55] Suarez-Almazor ME, Spooner C, Belseck E. Penicillamine for treating rheumatoid arthritis. Cochrane Database Syst Rev 2000;CD001460.

[56] Suarez-Almazor ME, Spooner CH, Belseck E, Shea B. Auranofin versus placebo in rheumatoid arthritis. Cochrane Database Syst Rev 2000;CD002048.

[57] Takken T, Van Der NJ, Helders PJ. Methotrexate for treating juvenile idiopathic arthritis. Cochrane Database Syst Rev 2001;CD003129.

[58] Towheed T, Shea B, Wells G, Hochberg M. Analgesia and non-aspirin, non-steroidal anti-inflammatory drugs for osteoarthritis of the hip. Cochrane Database Syst Rev 2000;CD000517.

[59] Towheed TE, Maxwell L, Judd MG, Catton M, Hochberg MC, Wells G. Acetaminophen for osteoarthritis. Cochrane Database Syst Rev 2006;CD004257.

[60] Wallen M, Gillies D. Intra-articular steroids and splints/rest for children with juvenile idiopathic arthritis and adults with rheumatoid arthritis. Cochrane Database Syst Rev 2006;CD002824.

[61] Wells G, Haguenauer D, Shea B, Suarez-Almazor ME, Welch VA, Tugwell P. Cyclosporine for rheumatoid arthritis. Cochrane Database Syst Rev 2000;CD001083.

[62] Wessel J. The effectiveness of hand exercises for persons with rheumatoid arthritis: a systematic review. J Hand Ther 2004;17:174–80.

[63] Wienecke T, Gotzsche PC. Paracetamol versus nonsteroidal anti-inflammatory drugs for rheumatoid arthritis. Cochrane Database Syst Rev 2004;CD003789.

[64] Zhang W, Moskowitz RW, Nuki G, Abramson S, Altman RD, Arden N, Bierma-Zeinstra S, Brandt KD, Croft P, Doherty M, et al. OARSI recommendations for the management of hip and knee osteoarthritis, part I: critical appraisal of existing treatment guidelines and systematic review of current research evidence. Osteoarthritis Cartilage 2007;15:981–1000.

Correspondence to: Prof. Kathleen A. Sluka, PT, PhD, Graduate Program in Physical Therapy and Rehabilitation Science, The University of Iowa, 1-252 Medical Education Building, Iowa City, IA 52242-1190, USA. Tel: 1-319-335-9791; fax: 1-319-335-9707; email: kathleen-sluka@uiowa.edu.

Case Studies

19

Kathleen A. Sluka and Carol Vance

Graduate Program in Physical Therapy and Rehabilitation Science,
The University of Iowa, Iowa City, Iowa, USA

The following 10 case studies describe pain in a selection of patients with a variety of diagnoses. Assessments are outlined, and normative values for tests are given where applicable. Each case is followed by a general description of the rationale for the patient having primarily a peripheral or central mechanism or a combination of peripheral and central components for the pain. The physical therapy treatment is then outlined, along with other treatments or referrals as appropriate. Finally, the clinical evidence to support the treatment plan is given, based on evidence presented in prior chapters. We refer the reader to these chapters for further information.

These case studies are intended to serve as a tool for learning and synthesizing the evidence presented within this book. The reader should first review the cases and define the signs and symptoms that support peripheral or central mechanisms underlying the pain (we outline this rationale under "General Considerations"). The reader should then develop an evidence-based treatment plan based on content presented in various chapters within the book. After developing the plan and reviewing the

Mechanisms and Management of Pain for the Physical Therapist
edited by Kathleen A. Sluka
IASP Press, Seattle, © 2009

evidence, the reader should then review the treatment plan put forth by the authors and the evidence that supports this plan.

Under "Pain Assessment," the McGill Pain Questionnaire (MPQ) was used to obtain a sensory (S), affective (A), evaluative (E), and total (T) pain rating index (PRI). The VAS refers to pain intensity score on a visual analogue scale. P1 and P2 refer to the first and second point of pain in the range of motion for the joint. Under "Quality of Life," the SF-36 scale (the quality-of-life subscale of the Medical Outcomes Study 36-item Short-Form Health Survey) is norm-based with 50 as average; scores below 50 are viewed as deficits in this area.

For each condition, the reader should be aware of other disciplines that should receive a referral to help improve care. The ideal treatment of any patient with chronic pain is clearly multidisciplinary. If a multidisciplinary pain treatment facility is not available for the patient, then the therapist should strive to facilitate multidisciplinary care through active communication and interaction with health care providers in the community (see Chapter 11).

Case 1

Subjective Assessment

This patient is a 42-year-old black male computer programmer who has a 4-month history of low back pain after having lifted a heavy suitcase out of his car. He states that the pain has not gone away as it did on other occasions when he had sprained his back. He decided to go to the doctor, who referred him to you for evaluation and treatment, stating that his X-ray showed some narrowing between some of the "back bones," and his MRI showed "bulging disks" in the lumbar spine. He reports that over the past few years he has had several bouts of low back pain that have lasted only a few days; otherwise, he is healthy and active and attends a fitness center three times per week. As the patient is talking, you observe that he frequently rubs his right calf, so you ask him if he has any other symptoms. He replies that his leg falls asleep a lot, but that "it is probably only poor circulation."

He states that for the past 4 weeks or so, his right leg "sort of falls asleep and aches," and he feels it more when he sits down or bends over. When you ask what decreases it, he says the problem is always there but is not so bad on awakening and on standing.

Case 1

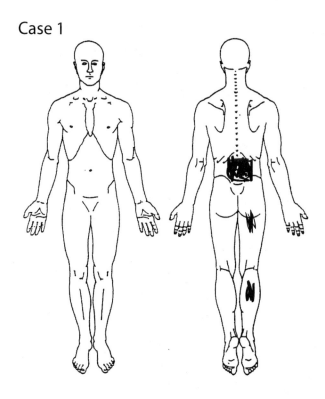

Pain Assessment

Words chosen on the MPQ: cramping, tingling, dull, annoying. PRI-S: 6/42; PRI-A: 0/14; PRI-E: 1/17; PRI-T: 7/78. VAS score: 6/10 for lower back pain and 3/10 for leg symptoms. P1 for lumbar flexion: 10°; P2 for lumbar flexion: 40°.

Objective Assessment

A gross postural scan shows that the patient's trunk has shifted to the left. He seems to be standing straight. There is guarding of the lumbar spine that creates a slight lumbar scoliosis to the left and a decreased lumbar lordosis. Trunk active range of motion (ROM): flexion, 40° (limited by pain); extension 10° (increases pain but is not limited by pain); side bending, left 30°; side bending, right 10°. Flexion and right side bending increase the patient's lower-extremity symptoms, so you ask him to remain standing in extension for a few seconds to see if it changes his numbness and pain. He says his leg feels better, but now his back is more uncomfortable.

As the patient tries to get into the supine position, you notice guarded transfers and grimacing, but once he is supine, he feels better. The patient then lies on his stomach and states that he cannot tolerate this position for very long because of back pain. You place a pillow under his abdomen for comfort and ask him how his legs and back feel now. Much to his surprise, the leg symptoms are considerably less (1/10), but his back continues to bother him.

Deep tendon reflexes for the lower extremity are normal. The patient reports diminished sensation to light tough on the posterolateral aspect of his right leg. His lower-extremity muscle strength is normal. Straight leg raise test, right: 30°, with increased low back and leg pain. Straight leg raise test, left: 70°; pain free except for mild pulling on the hamstring muscles.

Quality of Life

On the SF-36 quality-of-life survey, the patient received the following scores: Physical Function: 53; Role Physical: 35; Bodily Pain: 46; General Health: 58; Vitality: 61; Social Function: 45; Role Emotional: 45; Mental Health: 60. Summary: Physical Component: 44; Mental Component: 55.

Self-Efficacy

The patient filled out a self-efficacy questionnaire rating significant problems in work capability and in hobbies (0 = not at all confident; 6 = completely confident): I can enjoy things despite the pain (6/6). I can do most of the household chores despite the pain (4/6). I can socialize with my friends or family members as often as I used to despite the pain (3/6). I can cope with my pain in most situations (4/6). I can do some form of work despite the pain (3/6). I can still do many of the things I enjoy doing such as hobbies or leisure activities despite the pain (3/6). I can cope with my pain without medication (3/6). I can still accomplish most of my goals in life despite the pain (6/6). I can live a normal life-style despite the pain (5/6). I can gradually become active, despite the pain (5/6).

General Considerations

The patient appears to have pain that is driven primarily from a peripheral component. Signs that his pain centralizes with extension are a reduction in leg pain with standing in extension, lying supine, and prone positioning. He also has increased symptoms with flexion of the lumbar spine. He has altered posture, pain in his back, diminished sensation on his lower leg, and reduced ROM as a result of pain. He appears to have signs of radiculopathy because he has diminished sensation and accompanying pain in the posterolateral aspect of his leg, although his strength is normal. Although he appears to have a radiculopathy, imaging studies show signs of bulging disks and not herniated disks, suggesting minimal compression of the nerve from the bulging disks. Thus, this patient fits the paradigm for centralization-specific exercises (see Chapter 16). The pain is recurrent, and this bout has lasted for 4 months, and thus we must consider the involvement of central factors that may contribute to the pain. However, the self-efficacy questionnaire shows minimal deficits, with the greatest deficits in socialization, hobbies and leisure activities, and coping. Quality-of-life assessment shows minimal decreases in physical functioning.

Treatment

The pain is substantially lessened with extension, so the focus should be on a specific exercise program aimed at centralizing pain to the lower back (extension exercises). The patient continues to exercise at a fitness center three times per week, so you should discuss this program to ensure that it includes an aerobic conditioning program and proper weight-lifting techniques that do not strain the back.

If centralization-specific exercises do not improve symptoms and pain within the first week, pain control techniques should be added. These could include transcutaneous electrical nerve stimulation (TENS) or joint mobilization/manipulation. Using TENS or joint manipulation for pain reduction could produce effects in the central nervous system geared to reducing central sensitization in your patient.

Lastly, if centralization-specific exercises and the addition of pain-reducing treatments are still ineffective, a multidisciplinary approach should be considered; the addition of psychological treatment aimed at teaching coping skills could benefit this patient.

Evidence

Evidence from randomized controlled trials (RCTs) supports the use of a treatment-based classification system aimed at specific exercise programs for people with acute low back pain who show centralization of symptoms (see Chapter 16). For pain control, evidence from systematic reviews shows that TENS reduces pain for chronic musculoskeletal pain conditions (see Chapter 8), and evidence from clinical practice guidelines and systematic reviews indicates that joint manipulation reduces pain in both acute and chronic low back pain conditions (see Chapters 10, 16). Evidence from clinical practice guidelines and systematic reviews supports the use of cognitive-behavioral treatments for the management of chronic low back pain conditions (see Chapters 11, 13, and 16).

Case 2

Subjective Assessment

Mrs. H is an active 63-year-old, right-hand-dominant Hispanic woman who presents to you with a diagnosis of status post right Colles fracture sustained as a result of a fall in which she landed on her flexed wrist. She was immobilized in a cast for 6 weeks. The cast was removed 3 days ago. Mrs. H appears to understand and speak English, but her primary language is Spanish. She drives to her son's house daily to take care of her young grandchildren during working hours. She is widowed and lives independently, but she has a strong social support group from her church. Functional activity levels prior to the accident were normal. She complains of stiffness and pain, especially when she tries to move, and of inability to perform activities of daily living because she is so "right-handed." Her elbow and shoulder ache and feel stiff. She states that the cold outside makes the hand hurt much worse (the temperature outside is 20°F or minus 6.67°C), and she is unable to wear gloves because it increases her pain. As your examination commences, you realize that she is guarding her arm, which is maintained in a sling position even though there is no sling. Once she decides that she will let you evaluate the hand, you notice that the hand and wrist are swollen, paler, and cold to the touch compared to the left. The wrist appears somewhat malaligned. You are unable to test accessory joint mobility due to the patient's sensitivity to touch.

Case 2

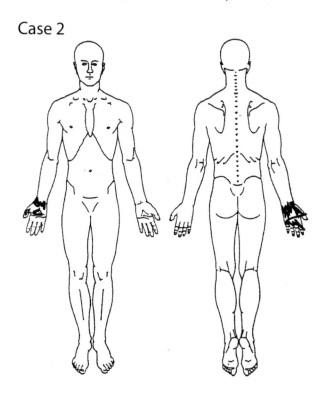

Pain Assessment

Words chosen on the MPQ: pulsing, pricking, stinging, sore, fearful, troublesome, cold. PRI-S: 6/42; PRI-A: 1/14; PRI-E: 2/5; PRI-T: 10/78. VAS: 5/10.

Objective Assessment

Active ROM: wrist extension: 10°; wrist flexion: 5°; ulnar deviation: 5°; radial deviation: 5°; supination: unable to obtain neutral; pronation: 30–60°; elbow: 20–100°. Strength: wrist extension: 3/5, within available ROM; wrist flexion: not tested; grip dynamometer: right 3 pounds (1.4 kg), left 40 pounds (18 kg).

Quality of Life

The patient filled out the SF-36 quality-of-life survey and received the following scores: Physical Function: 38; Role Physical: 28; Bodily Pain: 33; General Health: 44. Vitality: 40; Social Function: 35; Role Emotional: 55; Mental Health: 41. Summary: Physical Component: 29; Mental Component: 49.

General Considerations

This patient shows evidence of both peripheral and central components to her pain. The allodynia to cold and touch (inability to tolerate cold and gloves), decreased temperature of the hand, guarding, joint swelling, and stiffness suggest that she has complex regional pain syndrome (CRPS) as a result of a fracture followed by immobilization. CRPS is a centrally mediated pain condition. The fact that she has fractured her wrist, along with the reduction in ROM and strength related to the fracture, suggest peripheral changes in the joint structures. The malaligned wrist suggests that you may not be able to restore full ROM but will focus on regaining functional ROM.

Treatment

Initial treatment will be an active exercise program aimed at increasing ROM and strength of the wrist. Initial exercises will begin with active ROM exercises, progressing, as permitted, to light strengthening exercises for the wrist and hand. In addition, mirror therapy or desensitization therapy will be added to the treatment plan to improve symptoms of allodynia and reduce guarding of the limb.

For treatment of the pain and stiffness, thermal modalities (such as whirlpool, paraffin wax, or fluidotherapy) will be used prior to the active exercise program. The patient will be instructed in the use of warm water baths at home before performing her home program of active ROM exercises.

Once the allodynia is reduced or eliminated, you will assess for hypomobility of the wrist and hand. Treatment will then include joint mobilization to regain ROM, as indicated by the evaluation for hypomobility. Both dynamic and passive joint mobilizations will be performed.

It will be important to coordinate treatment with the physician to ensure that proper pharmacological treatments for CRPS are given at the same time as physical therapy.

Evidence

Evidence from RCTs indicates that active ROM exercises and mirror therapy are beneficial for reducing allodynia associated with CRPS (see Chapter 17). Further evidence suggests that an active exercise program will not only decrease pain but also improve function for people with joint stiffness and loss of motion after a fracture (see Chapter 7). Evidence from systematic reviews shows that exercise with heat therapy improves ROM and decreases pain in people with arthritis, who would have similar swelling, stiffness, and loss of motion (see Chapters 9, 18).

Case 3

Subjective Assessment

This patient is a 30-year-old, left-hand-dominant male dentist with complaints of left elbow pain of 1 year's duration that has gradually worsened. He states that there is no specific injury, but he notices the pain more after working a full day and after playing racquetball. However, the patient is not experiencing discomfort at rest. He decided to prescribe anti-inflammatory drugs for himself, but they have given him only mild relief. He saw an orthopedic surgeon, who injected the painful area with an anesthetic and a corticosteroid, but he continued to feel pain when performing work and sports. He has already been to see a physical therapist, who gave him ultrasound, ice, stretching exercises for the wrist, and an arm band.

The patient feels more pain as the day progresses. He wakes up at night only if he sleeps on his arm; in the morning he wakes up feeling relatively well, albeit somewhat stiff. He rates his pain during activities as 6/10 (verbal rating scale), describing it as a "toothache in his arm." He states that he has not experienced any numbness or tingling, but that his pain does occasionally radiate down into his knuckles, and he now fears that his work and patients may be at risk if this symptom continues. He demonstrates to you that merely upon extending his wrist he feels pain. The patient has no history of heart disease, diabetes, psychological illnesses, cancer, or arthritis. He reports no previous injury of the arm and reports his general health status as excellent.

Case 3

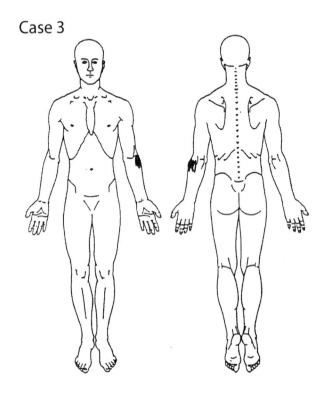

Pain Assessment

Words chosen on the MPQ: throbbing. shooting gnawing, heavy, tender, tiring, suffocating, frightful, grueling, troublesome, radiating, tight, agonizing. PRI-S: 16/42; PRI-A: 7/14; PRI-E: 2/5; PRI-T: 31/78. VAS at rest: 1/10; VAS with grip: 5/10.

Objective Assessment

A general inspection shows that the proximal posterior forearm is warmer to the touch than the non-involved side, and the tissue feels edematous ("boggy") in the same area. Girth measurements taken with a tape measure reveal no difference between right and left sides. Palpation of the extensor muscle group reveals a positive twitch response with increased localized pain. Light palpation of the head of the radius, the radiohumeral joint line, and the lateral epicondyle increases pain. Testing of accessory joint motion shows that radiohumeral and ulnohumeral joint distraction and radiohumeral anterior-posterior glides are not restricted but are positive for pain at grade III.

Active ROM: wrist flexion: 75°; wrist extension: 50°; pronation: within normal limits; supination: 80°. Passive ROM: wrist flexion: 85°; wrist extension: 65°; pronation: within normal limits; supination: 80°. Finger, elbow, shoulder, and cervical ROM: within normal limits. Strength: wrist extension: 4/5 with pain; wrist flexion: within normal limits. Grip dynamometer: left, 65 pounds (29 kg); right, 100 pounds (45 kg).

Quality of Life

The patient filled out the SF-36 quality-of-life survey and received the following scores: Physical Function: 47; Role Physical: 35; Bodily Pain: 42; General Health: 51; Vitality: 44; Social Function: 46; Role Emotional: 45; Mental Health: 46. Summary: Physical Component: 41; Mental Component: 47.

Self-Efficacy

The patient filled out a self-efficacy questionnaire rating significant problems in all domains (0 = not at all confident; 6 = completely confident): I can enjoy things despite the pain (3/6). I can do most of the household chores despite the pain (2/6). I can socialize with my friends or family members as often as I used to despite the pain (2/6). I can cope with my pain in most situations (3/6). I can do some form of work despite the pain (4/6). I can still do many of the things I enjoy doing such as hobbies or leisure activities despite the pain (3/6). I can cope with my pain without medication (4/6). I can still accomplish most of my goals in life despite the pain (5/6). I can live a normal lifestyle despite the pain (3/6). I can gradually become active, despite the pain (2/6).

General Considerations

This patient has lateral epicondylalgia, and a mixture of both peripheral and central mechanisms probably underlie his pain. Evidence for peripheral mechanisms includes localized pain, pain on palpation at the primary site of pain, and pain with movement. However, the year-long duration of the pain, the unrestricted but painful accessory joint movements, the fear of using the arm at work, and the minimal effects of nonsteroidal anti-inflammatory drugs (NSAIDs) and local injections all suggest a central component to his pain. His self-efficacy questionnaire and quality-of-life survey show significant deficits in all aspects, including coping skills and the ability to do chores, socialize, and work. The MPQ shows that the patient has chosen aspects related to all three dimensions of pain.

Treatment

Initial treatment will be aimed at educating the patient on ways in which he can use the arm during work and leisure activities without putting stress on the joint and soft tissues. During work you will have the patient wear a wrist cockup splint to maintain neutral wrist extension until the patient can maintain this position without the splint. The patient would benefit from an exercise program aimed at improving the strength of the upper extremities, with an emphasis on wrist extension and hand strength, to regain function of the arm. To reduce pain from lateral epicondylalgia in this patient, you will add local mobilizations of the elbow, as well as TENS, which will activate central inhibitory mechanisms aimed at reducing the central components of the pain. Since the pain is of long duration, and the patient has significant deficits in self-efficacy and quality of life, a multidisciplinary treatment program should be started. This program should include coordination of services with a physician and psychologist specializing in pain management.

Evidence

Evidence from systematic reviews suggests that mobilization of the elbow for people with lateral epicondylalgia (see Chapter 10) decreases pain and that TENS reduces pain associated with chronic musculoskeletal pain (Chapter 8). Evidence from a systematic review shows that strengthening exercises for lateral epicondylalgia reduce pain at rest and during activity [2]. Evidence from systematic reviews suggests that multidisciplinary treatments that involve physicians, nurses, physical therapists, and psychologists can improve pain and function in people with chronic pain (see

Chapter 11). There is also evidence that cognitive-behavioral treatment improves pain in a variety of chronic pain conditions (see Chapter 13).

Case 4

Subjective Assessment

This patient is a 50-year-old, left-hand-dominant, Asian female who presents with gradual onset of left shoulder pain that started approximately 6 months ago without apparent cause. She complains of a constant dull ache that radiates from her shoulder to the dorsal aspect of the forearm. The ache increases with motion and decreases with rest. She comes to you now because of increased difficulty reaching overhead and combing her hair. She works as a clerk and lately has needed help to retrieve file boxes located on top of the filing cabinets. She relates no prior history of left shoulder problems but states that she had bursitis of the right shoulder 10 years ago, which resolved with cortisone injections. Thinking that she

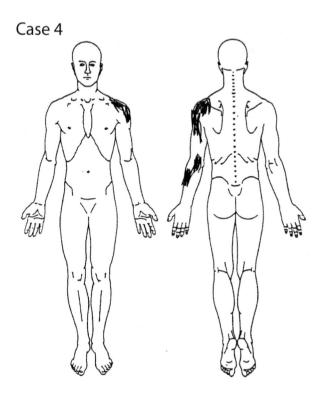

Case 4

had the same thing on the left side, she asked her doctor if he could inject it. Two shots over the last 3 months did not diminish her symptoms, nor has she attained significant relief with NSAIDs. Other medical history includes a hysterectomy 7 years ago and hypertension that is controlled with medication. She also takes calcium supplements at her physician's request. Otherwise, she is healthy and sedentary.

Pain Assessment

Words chosen on the MPQ: throbbing, gnawing, aching, fearful, miserable, nagging. PRI-S: 11/42; PRI-A: 3/14; PRI-E: 3/5; PRI-T: 18/78. VAS: resting 7/10; with arm elevation 9/10. Patient has significant guarding of the shoulder. P1 for external rotation of the shoulder = 5°; P2 for external rotation of the shoulder = 25°.

Objective Assessment

The patient's posture shows a mild kyphosis—rounded shoulders and a forward head. Scapular position reveals the medial angle of the left scapula to be one-half inch (~1.3 cm) higher than that of the right scapula. Scapulothoracic rhythm is asynchronous. Cervical ROM is complete, but with a feeling of tightness on the left during right side bending. Right shoulder ROM and strength are within normal limits.

Left shoulder: active ROM: flexion: 96°; abduction: 63°; adduction: within normal limits; external rotation: 25°; internal rotation: 70°. Passive ROM: flexion: 115°; extension: 35°; abduction: 110°; adduction: within normal limits; external rotation: 30°; internal rotation: 50°.

Accessory joint motion of the left glenohumeral joint: hypomobility in anterior and inferior directions. Manual muscle testing: 3+/5 on all shoulder girdle muscles, with the exception of external rotation, which is 3/5. All manual muscle test values are done within the available range. Palpation of shoulder region: diffuse tenderness of the upper trapezius, the medial border of the scapula, and the anterior and lateral shoulder.

Quality of Life

The patient filled out the SF-36 quality-of-life survey and received the following scores: Physical Function: 34; Role Physical: 28; Bodily Pain: 33; General

Health: 41; Vitality: 37; Social Function: 30; Role Emotional: 34; Mental Health: 39. Summary: Physical Component: 30; Mental Component: 39.

Self-Efficacy

The patient filled out a self-efficacy questionnaire, rating significant problems in all domains (0 = not at all confident; 6 = completely confident): I can enjoy things despite the pain (4/6). I can do most of the household chores despite the pain (2/6). I can socialize with my friends or family members as often as I used to despite the pain (3/6). I can cope with my pain in most situations (4/6). I can do some form of work despite the pain (4/6). I can still do many of the things I enjoy doing such as hobbies or leisure activities despite the pain (4/6). I can cope with my pain without medication (3/6). I can still accomplish most of my goals in life despite the pain (6/6). I can live a normal lifestyle despite the pain (2/6). I can gradually become active, despite the pain (3/6).

General Considerations

This patient's pain is primarily central in nature, but has resulted in tightening of the shoulder capsule in a capsular pattern. Signs of central mechanisms include insidious onset and pain lasting more than 6 months without relief from standard treatments aimed at reducing peripheral inflammation (NSAIDs and local injections). The patient has referred pain, i.e., pain radiating into the forearm, and this radiating pain increases with movement. She has significant impairments in all areas of the self-efficacy and quality-of-life questionnaires, and the MPQ shows aspects of all three dimensions of pain. Peripheral signs include loss of ROM, localized shoulder tenderness, and localized pain. The patient's pain significantly affects her function and ROM.

Treatment

The patient's pain is primarily central in nature, so treatments must be aimed at modulating central sensitization of the pain. Further, because the pain is chronic and has a significant impact on function and daily activities, the patient should be managed in a multidisciplinary system that includes coordination of services between a physician, psychologist, and physical therapist. The patient has significant pain (7/10 at rest and 9/10 with movement), and initial physical therapy treatments must be aimed at reducing pain scores. Thus, initial treatments will use TENS (alternating between low and high frequencies) to activate central inhibitory mechanisms. Use of the TENS unit during an exercise program and during work should allow the patient to increase function. Initial exercise treatments will start slowly, increasing active ROM through stretching. Once the pain has decreased to a moderate level, a more progressive exercise program will be instituted aimed at increasing the strength of the shoulder, along with a walking program to encourage normal arm use and to reduce guarding and activate central inhibitory mechanisms to reduce pain, as well as joint mobilizations of the shoulder to decrease any remaining hypomobility of the shoulder.

Evidence

Evidence from a meta-analysis shows that TENS reduces pain in chronic musculoskeletal conditions. Alternating between low- and high-frequency TENS will activate both μ-and δ-opioid receptors to improve pain reduction and reduce tolerance with repeated use (see Chapter 8). Aerobic exercise is effective for treatment of chronic pain conditions with a central component such as chronic low back pain and fibromyalgia (see Chapter 7). Increasing ROM with an active exercise program is expected to increase the available ROM and reduce the mechanical irritant and the activation of nociceptors in the shoulder. Joint mobilizations will similarly be used to increase the active ROM and reduce the mechanical activation of nociceptors in the shoulder (see Chapters 6, 10). Evidence from systematic reviews suggests that cognitive-behavioral therapy and multidisciplinary treatment are effective in reducing chronic pain and improving function (see Chapters 11, 13).

Case 5

Subjective Assessment

This patient is a 44-year-old black woman who states that she developed left lower-extremity pain about 3 months ago. She has no history of trauma or inappropriate lifting. Pain increases to a 10/10 at times, and it is felt all the way down to the foot, especially with prolonged sitting. The medical history is unremarkable. Examination reveals a slightly overweight female. Posture is normal, with the exception of a slight bilateral genu recurvatum and outward toe position (45°). Her trunk ROM is normal without reproduction or relief of pain, except for a tight feeling in the left posterior thigh during forward flexion. She works as an engineer, spending most of her time sitting and working at a computer.

Case 5

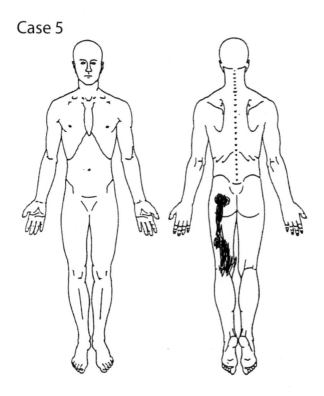

Pain Assessment

Words chosen on the MPQ: shooting, crushing, intense, radiating, agonizing. PRI-S: 8/42; PRI-A: 0/14; PRI-E: 4/5; PRI-T: 15/78. VAS at rest: 4/10.

Objective Assessment

Left straight-leg raise is positive for left leg pain at 60°; deep tendon reflexes and sensation to light touch are intact; Slump test and Gillet's test are negative. Manual muscle tests: 4+/5 for the left lower-extremity muscles, except for external hip rotation, which is 4/5 with slight pain; 5/5 for the right lower-extremity muscles, except for external hip rotation, which is 4/5. Palpation: there is tenderness on the left sacroiliac joint area and the left mid-buttock toward the greater trochanter. Pain in the leg is reproduced with pressure over the mid-buttock. With the hip in 90° flexion, stretching into hip internal rotation is painful during the stretch but results in slightly reduced pain after the stretching is finished.

Active ROM of the right or left hip: flexion: right 120°, left 110°; extension: right 15°, left 15°; abduction: right 45°, left 40°; adduction: right 40°, left 40°; internal rotation: right 35°, left 20°; external rotation: right 45°, left 45°.

Quality of Life

The patient filled out the SF-36 quality-of-life survey and received the following scores: Physical Function: 47; Role Physical: 42; Bodily Pain: 46; General Health: 60; Vitality: 66; Social Function: 46; Role Emotional: 55; Mental Health: 62. Summary: Physical Component: 42; Mental Component: 63.

Self-Efficacy

The patient filled out a self-efficacy questionnaire rating significant problems in all domains (0 = not at all confident; 6 = completely confident): I can enjoy things despite the pain (4/6). I can do most of the household chores despite the pain (5/6). I can socialize with my friends or family members as often as I used to despite the pain (4/6). I can cope with my pain in most situations (4/6). I can do some form of work despite the pain (6/6). I can still do many of the things I enjoy doing such as hobbies or leisure activities despite the pain (3/6). I can cope with my pain without medication (4/6). I can still accomplish most of my goals in life despite the pain (5/6). I can live a normal lifestyle despite the pain (4/6). I can gradually become active, despite the pain (4/6).

General Considerations

The patient's pain in this condition probably results primarily from peripheral mechanisms. The pain is reproduced with pressure on the buttock and is relieved by stretching, which suggests myofascial pain. She has reduced motion in internal rotation of the hip, as well as reduced strength and pain in external rotation of the hip. All other movements are within normal range. She has minimal limitations in self-efficacy, and her quality of life is good. Although she has symptoms of referred pain, these symptoms can be reproduced by pressing on the trigger point, suggesting that the referred pain is of myofascial origin.

Treatment

Treatment of this individual will be coordinated with a physician, who will give trigger point injections. Physical therapy will begin immediately after this injection, with active ROM and stretching in combination with ischemic pressure (trigger point massage) over the trigger point in the piriformis muscle. If this treatment approach is ineffective, the addition of electrotherapy, either interferential or TENS, should provide pain relief.

Evidence

Evidence from RCTs shows that trigger point injections are effective for treatment of myofascial pain syndrome (see Chapter 14). Further, an RCT shows that active ROM and stretching exercises, in combination with other therapies that provide ischemic pressure, reduce pain in people with myofascial pain syndrome (see Chapter 14). The same RCT shows that addition of electrotherapy to the active ROM and ischemic pressure combination further reduces the pain associated with myofascial pain syndrome (see Chapter 14).

Case 6

Subjective Assessment

This patient is a 45-year-old white woman who came into the office complaining of pain that has gradually worsened over the last year. It initially started in her shoulders, extending down her arms and into her hands. The pain also seems to travel up into her neck and cause "migraine" headaches. Later on, she felt pain in her lower back, her legs, and her feet. She now feels as if her whole body is in a state of constant pain. The pain came on gradually, without any pre-existing traumatic episode. She also complains of difficulty sleeping and says she has not slept an entire night in the last 6 months. She is also unable to work, garden, or do her normal walking because she is too tired. She complains of not having enough energy to even do the housework regularly. She says she has gained 30 pounds (13.6 kg) in the last year because she has been unable to do anything physical. She says she used to be a very active person and now cannot do anything because of the pain.

Case 6

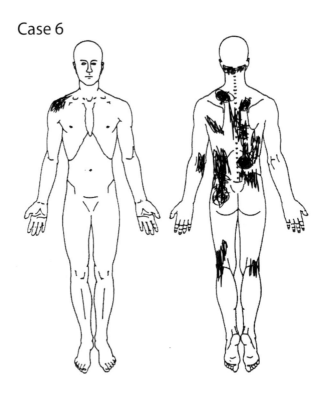

Pain Assessment

Words chosen on the MPQ: pounding, stabbing, crushing, wrenching, heavy, splitting, exhausting, suffocating, terrifying, vicious, wretched, unbearable, spreading, tight, dreadful. PRI-S: 27/42; PRI-A: 12/14; PRI-E: 5/5; PRI-T: 68/78. VAS: sensory-discriminative scale: 6/10; motivational-affective scale: 8/10.

Objective Assessment

Postural scan: rounded forward shoulders, forward head, increased lumbar lordosis and protuberant abdomen. Genu valgum, slight knee hyperextension, and pes planus. Palpation: multiple tender points located bilaterally at the occiput, C5–C7, trapezius, second rib, lateral epicondyle, gluteal region, and left medial knee. Trunk manual muscle testing: lower abdominals: 1/5; upper abdominals: 2/5; thoracic/lumbar extension: 3/5. Six-minute walk test: 100 yards (91.44 meters), but the patient stops after 3 minutes and refuses to complete the test due to increased pain and distress.

Quality of Life

The patient filled out the SF-36 quality-of-life survey and received the following scores: Physical Function: 28; Role Physical: 28; Bodily Pain: 33; General Health: 26; Vitality: 30; Social Function: 25; Role Emotional: 24; Mental Health: 30. Summary: Physical Component: 28; Mental Component: 28.

Self-Efficacy

The patient filled out a self-efficacy questionnaire, rating significant problems in all domains, including inability to enjoy social activities, perform household chores, go to work, and cope with the pain (0 = not at all confident; 6 = completely confident): I can enjoy things despite the pain (0.5/6). I can do most of the household chores despite the pain (1/6). I can socialize with my friends or family members as often as I used to despite the pain (1/6). I can cope with my pain in most situations (1/6). I can do some form of work despite the pain (0/6). I can still do many of the things I enjoy doing such as hobbies or leisure activities despite the pain (1/6). I can cope with my pain without medication (0/6). I can still accomplish most of my goals in life despite the pain (2/6). I can live a normal lifestyle despite the pain (0/6). I can gradually become active, despite the pain (0/6).

General Considerations

This patient appears to have pain that is driven primarily from a central origin, with a probable diagnosis of fibromyalgia. Signs of central mechanisms include the duration of the pain for more than 1 year, the widespread nature of the pain, difficulty sleeping, fatigue, multiple tender points, limited walking ability due to the pain, and high scores on the MPQ in all three dimensions of pain and overall score. Her self-efficacy questionnaire and quality-of-life survey suggest significant impairments in all aspects of her life, from physical functioning to mental health.

Treatment

Treatment of this patient must be multidisciplinary and would be best managed in a multidisciplinary pain center. Treatment will include coordination of services from pain management specialists in medicine, nursing, psychology, and physical therapy. The physical therapy treatment approach will be an active aerobic exercise program starting with only 2–3 minutes of walking 2–3 times per day because the patient was unable to complete the 6-minute walk test. The long-term goal will be to reach 20–30 minutes of daily walking in one session. The patient will be progressed slowly, with an emphasis on success, which may include increases as small as 1 minute per day. A strength training program will be added once the patient is actively participating in the aerobic exercise program and has made significant progress toward the goals. The strength training program will emphasize trunk muscles and proper postural support. If necessary, electrotherapy or massage can be added to help reduce the pain (1) once the patient is actively participating with the aerobic conditioning program or (2) prior to exercise to decrease pain and allow her to increase her exercise levels.

Evidence

A Cochrane systematic review and evidence-based clinical practice guidelines for fibromyalgia show strong evidence for a multidisciplinary treatment program and aerobic conditioning exercises to reduce pain and improve function (see Chapters 11, 12, 13, 14). Moderate evidence is found in the Cochrane review and evidence-based clinical practice guidelines for the use of strengthening exercises for people with fibromyalgia (see Chapters 7, 14). There is minimal evidence to support electrotherapy and massage therapy, and therefore these modalities are used only if the other treatments are not progressing or to enhance the patient's ability to exercise (see Chapter 14).

Case 7

Subjective Assessment

This patient is a 31-year-old white man who was playing basketball 2 weeks ago and "twisted" his right ankle, resulting in a Grade II sprain. He did not see a physician until 3 days ago. The physician put him in a removable ankle brace and sent him to physical therapy. He drives and delivers for a local beer distributor. He says he has difficulty driving and finds it difficult to unload the truck. He is currently on sick leave. He has no significant medical history.

Case 7

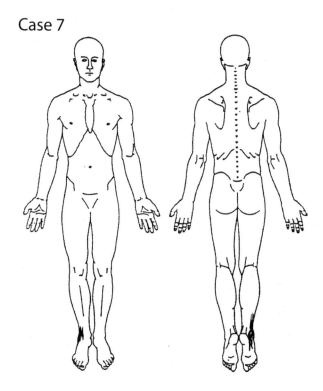

Objective Assessment

He has obvious swelling around the ankle joint, decreased active ROM (50% or greater decrease in plantar flexion, dorsiflexion, and internal and external rotation of the ankle). All ROM is limited as a result of pain. Passive ROM is similar and has an empty end feel (i.e., absence of end feel when the patient stops movement before sensing resistance). The patient complains of pain around the ankle that sometimes radiates into the calf and lower leg. Pain is rated at 4/10 at rest and at 8/10 when standing. There is increased pain with pressure on the lateral portion of the ankle (the anterior talofibular ligament and surrounding soft tissue).

General Considerations

This patient has an acute ankle sprain with inflammation of the joint and associated pain. There are likely to be increases in inflammatory cytokines, prostaglandins, and tumor necrosis factor, which are activating and sensitizing nociceptors. In addition, inflammatory neuropeptides, substance P, and calcitonin gene-related peptide are probably contributing to the inflammation by enhancing plasma extravasation and vasodilation, and by activating non-inflammatory cells to further enhance the release of inflammatory substances into the joint. The pain is probably a direct result of nociceptor sensitization. Signs of peripheral components are the acute injury, local pain, pain with pressure over the ankle, ROM that is limited as a result of pain, and swelling. The patient also has referred pain radiating into the calf and lower leg on occasion.

Treatment

Treatment of this patient will be aimed at reducing the peripheral inflammation and pain with local treatments, as well as increasing pain-free ROM. An active ROM program will maintain and increase movement in the ankle. The patient will be educated on home use of ice and elevation to decrease inflammation and reduce pain. Treatment with pharmacological agents for reduction in inflammation and pain will be managed by the physician and will probably include NSAIDs and weak opioids. The intermittent referred pain will most likely be resolved with removal of the peripheral irritants.

Evidence

Systematic reviews show limited evidence for ice in reducing inflammation and improving pain, and these effects are short-term (see Chapter 9). There is no evidence at present to suggest that active ROM exercises in acute pain will maintain ROM and improve function in the long term. However, general principles of physical therapy for acute injury are aimed at maintaining function and reducing the pain associated with the acute injury. If ice and ROM exercises do not produce a desirable reduction in pain and inflammation, then one can try electrotherapeutic modalities, such as TENS for pain or high-voltage electrotherapy to reduce inflammation and pain. Basic science evidence shows that TENS can reduce hyperalgesia associated with acute inflammation and that low-frequency TENS activates peripheral μ-opioid receptors (see Chapter 8), which are upregulated during inflammation (see Chapters 2 and 3). Basic science evidence also shows that cathodal high-voltage pulsed electrotherapy can reduce inflammation (see references in [1]).

Case 8

Subjective Assessment

This patient is a 45-year-old white woman who complains of low back pain that started one and a half years ago after an automobile accident. The pain is in the lower back, the left hip, and the back of the left thigh. The pain is worse with walking and better with sitting. However, if the patient sits too long, the pain again increases. She can sit for about 2 hours before she has to get up because of the pain. She says she is also tired all the time and is sore in the upper back and both legs. She reports pain and tenderness in the upper back and legs. She was initially able to work for the first year after the accident, but the pain has became progressively worse, and now she cannot work. She works as a secretary for a university department of anthropology and has been on an extended leave of absence for the last 3 months. She has had X-rays, an MRI scan, and nerve conduction tests, all of which are normal. She does not routinely exercise and did not do so before the accident (she says she did not have the time to do so, although she knows it is important). Previous treatments include exercises given by her family practitioner and medications consisting of muscle relaxants, naproxen, and acetaminophen (paracetamol) with codeine. She is now attending the multidisciplinary pain clinic at the university.

Pain Assessment

Words chosen on the MPQ: pounding, shooting, stabbing, cramping, cramping, tingling, aching, exhausting, frightful, cruel, intense, radiating,

Case 8

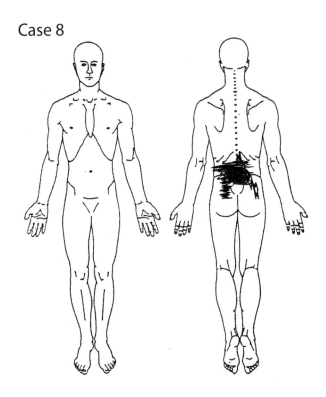

agonizing. PRI-S: 22/42; PRI-A: 7/14; PRI-E 4/5; PRI-T: 38/78. VAS for pain in the lower back: 5/10; for pain in the hip: 4/10: for pain in the leg: 2/10.

Objective Assessment

Posture: forward head, forward shoulders, flattened lordosis. Strength: upper abdominals: 3/5; lower abdominals: 2/5; back extensors: 2/5; hip extensors: 3/5. Straight-leg raise, left: positive for pain in the low back at 45°; hamstrings are tight. Straight-leg raise, right: positive for pain in the low back and leg at 60° degrees; hamstrings are tight. Palpation: there is tenderness over the lower back bilaterally with greater tenderness on the left side. The patient has mild muscle tightness over the left back. She also has tenderness over the hip area, and it hurts to shift her body weight and sit on the left hip.

Lumbar active ROM is reduced: forward flexion: 50%: extension: 0%, with pain; side bending, right: 20%; side bending, left: 50%, with pain;

rotation, right: 10%; rotation, left: 10%. Hip ROM is reduced: flexion: 100°; pain in back; internal rotation: 30°, with pain; external rotation: 30°, with pain; extension: 0° (unable to do).

Quality of Life

The patient filled out the SF-36 quality-of-life survey and received the following scores: Physical Function: 32; Role Physical: 35; Bodily Pain: 33; General Health: 37; Vitality: 35; Social Function: 35; Role Emotional: 45; Mental Health: 44. Summary: Physical Component: 28; Mental Component: 46.

Self-Efficacy

The patient filled out a self-efficacy questionnaire rating significant problems in work capability and in hobbies (0 = not at all confident; 6 = completely confident): I can enjoy things despite the pain (1/6). I can do most of the household chores despite the pain (0/6). I can socialize with my friends or family members as often as I used to despite the pain (3/6). I can cope with my pain in most situations (1/6). I can do some form of work despite the pain (1/6). I can still do many of the things I enjoy doing such as hobbies or leisure activities despite the pain (2/6). I can cope with my pain without medication (0/6). I can still accomplish most of my goals in life despite the pain (2/6). I can live a normal lifestyle despite the pain (3/6). I can gradually become active, despite the pain (0/6).

General Considerations

This person's pain is primarily maintained by central mechanisms. Signs of central involvement include referred pain into the hip, leg, and upper back; normal imaging and tests; the duration of the pain; inability to work; tenderness over the hip and upper back; and fatigue. She has significant deficits in self-efficacy, reduced quality of life in all domains, and high scores in all three dimensions of the MPQ. Peripheral signs are few, but they might include tenderness over the lower back, postural changes, and muscle tightness and weakness. However, this patient's peripheral components could be a direct result of long-term deconditioning, poor posture, and guarding as a result of the pain. It is likely that these peripheral components are secondary to the pain condition.

Treatment

This person is best treated with a multidisciplinary program that would include medicine, psychology, nursing, physical therapy, and potentially vocational rehabilitation. Goals for treatment will be to treat the strong central component to the pain, and to engage the subject as an active participant. As a member of the medical team, the physical therapist will coordinate all treatments with those of other disciplines through team meetings. Physical therapy treatments should begin with an active exercise program including spinal stabilization exercises and aerobic conditioning exercises. Education on posture, sleeping, and movement strategies to reduce pain should be added. If pain and function do not improve significantly with this treatment approach, joint mobilization, massage, or electrotherapy should be added. These additional strategies, which are passive treatments, will be added only when the patient has made a commitment to take part in an active exercise program.

Evidence

Data from systematic reviews and clinical practice guidelines show that spinal stabilization and aerobic conditioning exercises in a supervised setting are effective for decreasing pain and improving function in people with chronic low back pain (see Chapters 7, 16). There is also evidence from clinical practice guidelines and systematic reviews that joint manipulation is effective for chronic low back pain (see Chapters 10, 16), and from one meta-analysis that electrotherapy is effective for chronic musculoskeletal pain conditions (see Chapter 8). Further evidence from systematic reviews shows that multidisciplinary treatment is more effective than single-disciplinary standard care for the treatment of chronic low back pain to improve function and decrease pain (see Chapters 11, 16). Evidence-based guidelines suggest the use of certain pharmacological agents such as benzodiazepines, antidepressants, and tramadol, which have moderate to strong efficacy (see Chapter 16). Cognitive-behavioral treatments and patient education also have strong evidence to support their use in people with chronic low back pain (see Chapter 13).

Case 9

This patient is a 54-year-old married white woman with a part-time job as a greeter at a discount department store. She has been diagnosed with Grade II osteoarthritis of the right knee joint by a rheumatologist, with the initial diagnosis 4 years ago. She is currently taking tramadol, acetaminophen (paracetamol), and aspirin for the knee pain. Her height is 5′6″ (1.524 m), and her weight is 249 pounds (113.2 kg) (BMI = 40). She has high blood pressure and diabetes that is controlled with medications. Otherwise, she says she is generally healthy. Her pain is better when she wakes up in the morning, but it gets worse as the day progresses. Her current VAS pain rating at rest is 2/10, but she says it is as high as 7/10 when climbing stairs, which is a problem for her because she lives in a two-story house with a basement and has to climb stairs daily to do laundry and get to the bedroom.

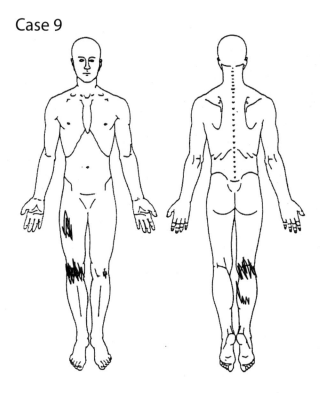

Case 9

Objective Assessment

Palpation of the knee reveals tenderness to pressure along the medial joint line of the right knee. Pressure pain thresholds of the knee (medial joint line): right: 145 kPa; left: 279 kPa. Active ROM of the right knee is 0° extension and 110° flexion and is limited by soft-tissue approximation. Her left knee joint has the same ROM.

The strength of the right knee is 3+/5 for knee extension and 4/5 for knee flexion. The strength of the left knee is 5/5 for both extension and flexion. Timed up-and-go test: 15 seconds to complete, with a pain rating of 9/10.

Functional Questionnaire

The WOMAC shows a function score of 1,465 (range 0–1,700), a pain score of 393 (0–500), and a stiffness score of 155 (0–200).

Quality of Life

The patient filled out the SF-36 quality-of-life survey and received the following scores: Physical Function: 45; Role Physical: 35; Bodily Pain: 42; General Health: 51; Vitality: 49; Social Function: 41; Role Emotional: 55; Mental Health: 57. Summary: Physical Component: 35; Mental Component: 57.

General Considerations

The subject has knee osteoarthritis with degenerative changes that are producing pain. The pain is clearly associated with peripheral changes, but the pain (9/10 during movement) is out of proportion to the degree of changes in the joint (grade II osteoarthritis). Thus, she probably also has significant central sensitization that will need to be addressed to obtain adequate treatment results. Treatment should be aimed at both peripheral and central mechanisms to relieve pain and improve function. The patient's function and quality of life in the physical domains are significantly compromised. The patient has difficulty working, doing household chores, and performing general self-care (bathing and dressing).

Treatment

The patient is currently being managed by an orthopedic surgeon for osteoarthritis. Her physical therapy intervention program will be aimed at (1) increasing the strength of the knees through an active strengthening program and (2) increasing function through a general aerobic exercise program that puts minimal stress on the knee joint, such as aquatic therapy or a stationary bicycle. Because the patient has significant pain with walking (during the timed up-and-go test), you will also add pain relief with high-frequency TENS and educate the patient on the use of heat and cold therapies at home for pain reduction. You will also include education on weight control and on avoiding excess stress on the joint during activities of daily living.

Evidence

There is strong evidence from systematic reviews that strengthening and/or aerobic conditioning exercises in people with knee joint osteoarthritis can decrease pain and improve function (see Chapters 7, 18). This evidence suggests that there are equal effects with strengthening, land-based or aquatic-based therapy, or with group therapy, and thus any type of exercise program should be considered and assessed for each individual patient. There is also good evidence from systematic reviews that high-frequency TENS reduces pain associated with osteoarthritis of the knee (see Chapters 8, 18). Although there is minimal evidence to support the use of heat and cold for arthritis, thermal modalities are recommended for palliative care in systematic reviews. Further, they have minimal side effects, can be applied by the patient at home, and probably have short-term effects (see Chapter 9).

Case 10

This patient is a 43-year-old white woman who has had neck pain for 5 months, with no other medical problems. She has not seen a physician or any other health professionals for her neck pain. She had prior experience with physical therapy for her knee that she found very helpful in the past, so she thought she would come first to the physical therapist. Pain started after she rotated her neck at work to one side and felt a sharp twinge on the left side. Her pain is now an ongoing aching pain on the left, with sharp pain when she moves her neck too fast. Her pain is worse at the end of the day. She gets occasional headaches that start in the back of the head and radiate to the front. She states that she has had these types of headaches for years, but they are more frequent now, occurring at least once a week. She also has aching in her left shoulder and upper arm on "bad days." She works as a technical writer, spending most of her time at a computer during the day. She continues to work but is unable to do activities at night. Lying down on her back makes the pain better. When asked, she denies nausea, dizziness, blurred vision, sweating, or changes in bowel or bladder habits.

Case 10

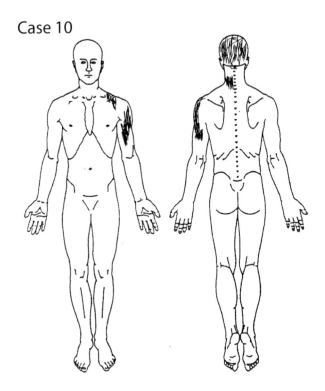

Pain Assessment

Words chosen on the MPQ: throbbing, sharp, cramping, aching, tender, troublesome, nagging. PRI-S: 13/42; PRI-A: 0/14; PRI-E: 1/5; PRI-T: 17/78.

Current neck pain on VAS: sensory-discriminative scale: 4/10; motivational-affective scale 2/10.

Objective Assessment

Active ROM: shoulder, neck, and lower back normal. Reflexes: normal, brisk and symmetrical; localized light touch: within normal limits at C1–T1 bilaterally; manual muscle testing of upper extremity: within normal limits bilaterally. Palpation: there is tenderness located from C3 to T1 bilaterally next to the spine. Tenderness is also located over the upper trapezius on the left, and the pain is referred to the base of the skull. Muscle spasms are felt with palpation of the left cervical spine from C4 to C7.

The patient has increased pain with cervical flexion. Cervical ROM: flexion: P1, 3" from chest; P2, full, to chest. Extension: P1, 30°; P2, 45° (full ROM). Rotation, right: P1, 10°; P2, 40° (patient stops due to stiffness). Rotation, left: P1, 70°; P2, 80°.

Quality of Life

The patient filled out the SF-36 quality-of-life survey and received the following scores: Physical Function: 49; Role Physical: 28; Bodily Pain: 46; General Health: 46; Vitality: 54; Social Function: 46; Role Emotional: 55; Mental Health: 50. Summary: Physical Component: 36; Mental Component: 56.

Self-Efficacy

The patient filled out a self-efficacy questionnaire and has minimal deficits (0 = not at all confident; 6 = completely confident): I can enjoy things despite the pain (6/6). I can do most of the household chores despite the pain (6/6). I can socialize with my friends or family members as often as I used to despite the pain (6/6). I can cope with my pain in most situations (5/6). I can do some form of work despite the pain (6/6). I can still do many of the things I enjoy doing such as hobbies or leisure activities despite the pain (5/6). I can cope with my pain without medication (5/6). I can still accomplish most of my goals in life despite the pain (6/6). I can live a normal lifestyle despite the pain (6/6). I can gradually become active, despite the pain (6/6).

General Considerations

This patient has signs of primarily central sensitization: long duration of pain, normal muscle strength, and referred pain to the head, arm, and shoulder. Her range of motion shows minimal decreases but is painful. Several factors suggest that the pain is not irritable and that treatment can be more aggressive: (1) a minimal difference between P1 and P2; (2) minimal limitations in ROM, and normal strength; (3) a minimal affective component to the pain (2/10 on VAS, 0 on the McGill affective scale); and (4) limitation in rotation on the right side as a result of stiffness, and not pain. She does have limited ROM in rotation to the right due to stiffness, suggesting soft-tissue tightness that may limit movement. Her tension-type headaches are long-standing and appear to be aggravated by the neck pain. Her quality of life is good, and she has high self-efficacy, so she should respond well to treatment.

Treatment

Given that the patient presented to you without seeing a physician, you must consider whether referral is appropriate. Her quality of life is relatively normal, her self-efficacy is high, she shows moderate pain on the sensory-discriminative dimension (MPQ and VAS), and there is minimal to no motivational-affective component to the pain, suggesting that this patient is coping effectively with the pain at this time. She does not appear irritable and has no "red flags" on evaluation (normal neurological examination and no constitutional symptoms). As such, the course of treatment should consist of (1) education on the disease process, posture, and work environment; (2) neck stretching and strengthening exercises; (3) massage over the cervical spine, particularly aimed at the muscle spasms; and (4) TENS for pain control during activities and work. If the patient does not make significant improvements, remains unchanged, or gets worse within 1–2 weeks, then referral to a physician for more extensive screening is appropriate.

Evidence

Evidence from systematic reviews supports the use of postural and strengthening exercises for neck pain, as well as for headache (see Chapters 15,

16). Evidence-based guidelines for low back and neck pain support the use of education (Chapter 16). A meta-analysis supports the use of TENS for chronic musculoskeletal pain (see Chapter 8), and there is evidence from systematic reviews and evidence-based guidelines for massage for neck and low back pain (see Chapters 10, 16). For headaches, RCTs support a combined treatment of postural education and exercises, along with massage (see Chapter 15).

References

[1] Vance CG, Radhakrishnan R, Skyba DA, Sluka KA. Transcutaneous electrical nerve stimulation at both high and low frequencies reduces primary hyperalgesia in rats with joint inflammation in a time-dependent manner. Phys Ther 2007;87:44–51.
[2] Vicenzino B, Paungmali A, Buratowski S, Wright A. Specific manipulative therapy treatment for chronic lateral epicondylalgia produces uniquely characteristic hypoalgesia. Man Ther 2001;6:205–12.

Correspondence to: Prof. Kathleen A. Sluka, PT, PhD, Graduate Program in Physical Therapy and Rehabilitation Science, The University of Iowa, 1-252 Medical Education Building, Iowa City, IA 52242-1190, USA. Tel: 1-319-335-9791; fax: 1-319-335-9707; email: Kathleen-sluka@uiowa.edu.

Arcadia University
Department of Physical Therapy
450 S. Easton Road
Glenside, PA 19038-3295

Index

Page numbers followed by f refer to figures, and by t to tables.

A

Aβ fibers, 19, 173
ACE (acetylcholinesterase) inhibitors, 179
Acetaminophen, 242
　for nociceptive pain, 247
　for osteoarthritis, 353
　for rheumatoid arthritis, 354
Acetylcholinesterase (ACE) inhibitors, 179
Acid-sensing ion channels, 27–28
Acupuncture, 210
Acute pain
　animal models, 31
　characteristics, 5–7
　conceptualization, 231
　pharmacotherapy for, 247
　TENS efficacy for, 182–183
Aδ fibers, 23, 173
Adenosine, 50
Adolescent Pediatric Pain Tool, 122
Aerobic exercise
　exercise-induced hypoalgesia and, 145
　ischemic pain and, 144
　pain management mechanisms, 136
Afferents
　Aβ fibers, 19, 173
　Aδ fibers, 23, 173
　cutaneous, TENS activation of, 173
　peripheral, classification of, 20t
　primary. See also Nociceptors
　　convergence of, 42f, 43
　　joint innervation by, 19
　　neuroanatomy, 19, 21, 21f
　　neurotransmitters, 26
　　small-diameter, 26
African Americans, 82, 83
Age factors in pain, 78t, 89
Allodynia
　in CRPS, 338
　definition, 5
　measurement, 125f, 126
　mechanisms, 64
　response to innocuous stimuli, 43

wide-dynamic-range neuron sensitiza-
　tion, 53
American Physical Therapy Association,
　13
Amitriptyline
　for fibromyalgia, 249, 290, 290t, 291
　for temporomandibular disorders, 311
AMPA/kainite (AMPA/KA) receptor
　complex, 49
Amygdala, 57
Animal models of pain, 31–34. See also
　specific types of pain, animal models
　TENS analgesia in, 174–175
Ankle sprain, case study, 383–385
Ankylosing spondylitis, 181, 349
Anterior cingulate cortex, 54
Anterior pretectal nucleus, 57
Anticonvulsants, 246
　for fibromyalgia, 290t, 291
　for neuropathic pain, 340
　for temporomandibular disorders, 311
Antidepressants, 311, 340. See also
　Tricyclic antidepressants
Anti-emetics, 181
Anti-inflammatory agents, 340. See also
　Nonsteroidal antiinflammatory drugs
　(NSAIDs)
Arthritis. See also Osteoarthritis; Rheuma-
　toid arthritis
　epidemiology, 349
　psychological management, 354–355
　TENS and joint function in, 178
Arthrocentesis, 311
Arthroscopic surgery, 311
Ascending pathways, 52–54
Asian Americans, 82
Astrocytes, 47
Aura, in migraine, 300
Autonomic nervous system, 176
Avoidance of activity, fear-related
　assessment, 84, 85–86, 110, 112t, 323
　and biopsychosocial pain model, 12

B

Back pain. *See* Low back pain
Beat frequency, 169f, 171
Behavior, nociceptive. *See* Pain behaviors
Behavior observation, 100
Behavior rating scales, 100
Behavior therapy, 263, 264t. *See also*
     Cognitive-behavioral therapy (CBT)
Benzodiazepine, 290t, 291
Beta-blockers, 303
Beta-endorphins
     exercise and release of, 60, 157–158
     in exercise-induced hypoalgesia,
       157–159, 162
Biofeedback
     for migraine, 269, 303
     for myofascial pain, 284
     objectives, 260
     for pain management, 268–269
     for tension-type headache, 269, 306
Biological factors, in hypoalgesia, 160
Biomedical model of pain, 11
Biopsychosocial model of pain, 11f, 11–12,
     160
     of chronic pain, 219, 222
     synergistic relationships in, 273
Blood flow, 176, 194
Blood pressure, 161
Bradykinin, 30
Brief Pain Inventory (BPI), 107, 108f
Buprenorphine, 243

C

C fibers
     in nociception, 19
     repetitive stimulation in wind-up, 62
     in visceral nociception, 23
Calcitonin gene-related peptide (CGRP),
     26, 50
Calcium channel blockers, 303
Cancer pain
     pharmacotherapy for, 243, 247
     TENS efficacy for, 181
Capsaicin
     in animal pain models, 31, 32
     for neuropathic pain, 340
Carbamazepine, 340
Carrageenan, 31, 32

Case studies
     overview, 361–362
     ankle sprain, acute, 383–385
     back pain
       with central sensitization, 385–388
       with radiculopathy, 362–366
     complex regional pain syndrome,
       366–369
     fibromyalgia, 379–382
     knee osteoarthritis, 389–391
     lateral epicondylalgia, 369–373
     myofascial pain of lower extremity,
       376–379
     neck pain, 391–395
     shoulder pain, 373–376
Catastrophizing, 84, 85, 234
Catechol-O-methyltransferase (COMT)
     gene, 87–88, 310
Caucasians, 82
Causalgia (CRPS-II), 10, 337
CBT. *See* Cognitive-behavioral therapy
     (CBT)
Central hyperexcitability, 237, 241
Central pain processing mechanisms,
     41–64, 42f
     ascending pathways, 52–54
     descending modulation, 54–61
     glial cells, 45, 47, 48f
     neurotransmitters, 47–52, 48f
     sex differences, 78–79
     spinal cord, 42–52
Central sensitization, 43, 62
Cervical manipulation and mobilization,
     211, 303
Cervical radiculopathy, 332
CGRP (calcitonin gene-related peptide),
     26, 50
Children's pain. *See* Pediatric pain
Cholecystokinin, 137
Chronic pain
     biopsychosocial approach to, 11–12,
       219, 222
     characteristics, 7
     intensity, 231
     multifactorial nature of, 217
     opioid therapy for, 243–244
     TENS efficacy for, 181–182
     treatment trends, 225
Chronic Pain Self-Efficacy Scale, 110, 111t

Chronic widespread pain, 32–33. *See also*
    Fibromyalgia
Cingulate cortex, anterior, 54
Clonazepam, 311
Codeine, 243
Cognitive impairment, 122–123
Cognitive restructuring, 266
Cognitive-behavioral therapy (CBT)
    for arthritis, 354–355
    for chronic pain, 234–235
    components, 265–267
    for CRPS, 343
    efficacy, 272
    for fibromyalgia, 291
    for migraine, 303
    for myofascial pain, 284
    for neuropathic pain, 341
    for temporomandibular disorders, 312
    for tension-type headache, 306
    theoretical perspectives, 265, 265t
Cognitive-evaluative dimension of pain, 4
Cold therapy, 193, 194. *See also* Thermo-
    therapy
Coloured Analogue Scale, 122
Commission on Accreditation of Rehabili-
    tation Facilities (CARF)
    on interdisciplinary pain rehabilitation
        programs, 222
    pain management standards, 218,
        220t–221t
Complete Freund's adjuvant, 31, 32
Complex regional pain syndrome (CRPS)
    case study, 366–369
    epidemiology and diagnosis, 337–338,
        339t
    exercise therapy, 342–344
    physical therapy, 342t, 342–345
    psychological management, 341
    sensory re-education, 344–345
    sympathectomy for, 341
Compliance, 155–156, 224
COMT gene, 87–88, 310
Conduction, 191
Contracts, treatment plan, 224
Convection, 191
Convergence-projection theory, 64
Corticospinal tract, 161
Corticosteroids
    for osteoarthritis, 353
    for rheumatoid arthritis, 354
    for temporomandibular disorders, 311

Counterirritants, 135
COX (cyclooxygenase) inhibitors, 242, 247
Cryotherapy, 193, 194. *See also* Thermo-
    therapy
Cutaneous nociceptors, 23
Cutaneous pain, 7–8, 31
Cyclobenzaprine, 290t, 291, 311
Cyclooxygenase (COX) inhibitors, 242, 247
Cytokines, proinflammatory, 30, 47

D

Deep-tissue massage, 206, 210
Deep-tissue pain, 7–8, 168
Degenerative disk disease, 186
Degenerative joint disease. *See* Osteoar-
    thritis
Delayed-onset muscle soreness, 149, 210
Deltorphin, 57
Depression, 234
Descending modulation of pain, 54–61
    inhibitory systems, 56–59
        joint mobilization and manipula-
            tion and, 208
        massage and activation of, 206
        TENS analgesia and, 174
    neurotransmitters in, 59–61
    pain facilitation, 56
Desensitization therapy, 344–345
Dextromethorphan, 50, 340
Dextropropoxyphene, 243
Diabetic neuropathy, 340
Diathermy, shortwave, 192–193, 195–196
Diazepam, 311
Diffuse noxious inhibitory controls
    (DNIC), 58–59, 83
Dimensions of pain, 4
Disabilities of the Arm, Shoulder and Hand
    (DASH), 115
Disability, definition, 14
Disablement model of pain, 13f, 13–14
Disease-modifying antirheumatic drugs
    (DMARDs), 354
DNIC (diffuse noxious inhibitory controls),
    58–59, 83
Dorsal horn neurons
    classification, 43
    neuroanatomy, 42f, 42–43
    nociceptor modulation, 9
    sensitization mechanisms, 45, 46f, 62

Dorsal root ganglion (DRG) neurons,
    339–340
Dorsolateral pontine tegmentum, 57
Drug therapy. *See* Pharmacotherapy
Dry needling, 284
Dual reuptake inhibitors. *See* Serotonin-
    norepinephrine reuptake inhibitors
    (SNRIs)
Duloxetine, 249
Dynorphins, 60
Dysfunctional pain, 237, 241, 248–249
Dysmenorrhea, primary, 183

E

Effleurage, 205
Electromagnetic therapy, 343
Electromyography, 305
Electrophysical treatment agents, 191–201.
    See also Interferential therapy
    (IFT); Transcutaneous electrical
    nerve stimulation (TENS)
    evidence base for, 200–201, 201t
    laser therapy, low-intensity, 8–10. *See
    also* Laser therapy
    thermotherapy. *See* Thermotherapy
    ultrasound. *See* Ultrasound therapy
Endomorphins, 60
Epicondylalgia, lateral
    case study, 369–373
    joint mobilization/manipulation, 208,
    212
    ultrasound therapy, 198
Epicondylitis, lateral, 200
Epidemiology of pain, 15–16. *See also
    specific types of pain*, epidemiology
Ethics, medical, 140
Ethnicity and race, 81–83
Evidence-based practice, 138–140, 139f
Exercise therapy. *See also* Aerobic exercise;
    Strength training
    for delayed-onset muscle soreness, 149
    electromagnetic therapy and, 343
    for fibromyalgia, 149, 152f, 154, 294
    joint stabilization, 205
    for low back pain, 149, 153, 154
    for myofascial pain, 286–287
    for neuropathic pain and CRPS,
    342–344
    non-aerobic, 147–148

for osteoarthritis, 152–153, 154,
    355–356
for rheumatoid arthritis, 357
stretching, 286–287
Exercise-induced hypoalgesia, 143–163
    overview, 143–144
    biopsychosocial model, 160
    compliance and, 155–156
    exercise type and, 153–154
    exogenous opioid cross-tolerance and,
    159
    in healthy subjects, 144–148
    intensity and duration in, 147, 147f,
    157–158, 162
    isometric contraction and, 144, 145,
    146f, 148, 162
    long-term benefits, 152–153
    low-intensity programs, 149, 153
    non-opioid mechanisms, 159–161, 163
    noxious stimulus location and, 145
    opioid mechanisms, 156–159, 162–163
    pain measurement in, 145
    sex differences in, 148
    strengthening exercises and, 147–148
    in subjects with pain, 149, 150t–151t,
    152–154, 162
Exposure therapy, cognitive-behavioral,
    260
Extended Personal Attributes Question-
    naire, 80
Extraversion, 83, 84
Eysenck Personality Questionnaire, 84

F

Faces Pain Scale, 121, 121f
Facial expression scales, 99–100
Fatigue, in exercise-induced hypoalgesia,
    148
Fear, pain-related, 84
    experimental pain and, 85–86, 86f
    treatment outcome and, 85, 234
Fear-Avoidance Beliefs Questionnaire
    (FABQ), 84, 85–86, 110, 112t, 323
Fear of movement, 234, 236
Fear of Pain Questionnaire (FPQ), 84
Fentanyl, 243
Fibromyalgia, 287–294
    case study, 379–382
    central hyperexcitability in, 241–242

epidemiology and diagnosis, 287–288
exercise therapy, 149, 152f, 154, 294
laser therapy, 200, 294
medical management, 290t, 290–291
operant conditioning, 263
as pain of unknown origin, 241
pathobiology, 288–289
pharmacotherapy, 249
physical therapy, 291, 294
psychological management, 291
tender points, 288, 289f
treatment compliance and, 155
Fibromyalgia Impact Questionnaire (FIQ),
115, 290, 292f–293f
Fitness training, vs. strength training, 153
Fluoromethane vapocoolant spray, 284
Formalin, 31
Frequency, in TENS therapy, 170
Functional assessment scales, 123–124
Functional disability, 185
Functional examination, 123–127
Functional limitation, definition, 13
Functional measures, 126–127
Functional Status Index, 123

G

Gabapentin, 246
    for fibromyalgia, 291
    for neuropathic pain, 340
    for temporomandibular disorders, 311
Gamma-aminobutyric acid (GABA),
    50–51, 176
Gate control theory, 9f, 9–10
    in exercise-induced hypoalgesia, 160
    physical therapy treatments and, 135
    in TENS analgesia, 171–172
GCH1 gene, 88
Gender and pain variability, 79–80. See
    also Sex differences
Gender Roles Expectations of Pain
    (GREP), 80
Generalization and maintenance, 266–267
Genes
    in pain perception, 87–88
    transcription in central sensitization,
        62
Genetics and heritability
    clinical pain, 88
    experimental pain, 88

fibromyalgia and, 290
pain variability and, 86–88
in temporomandibular disorders, 310
Glial cells, 45, 47, 48f
Glutamate
    as excitatory neurotransmitter, 27
    high-frequency TENS and release of,
        176
    in spinal cord nociceptive transmis-
        sion, 47, 48f, 49–50
Gout, 349
G-protein-coupled receptors, 51
Guided imagery, 268

H

Habenula, medial, 57
Headache. See also Migraine; Tension-type
        headache
    classification and prevalence, 299
    cluster headache, 304
    pain areas, 300f
Heat therapy, 192–193, 194–195. See also
    Thermotherapy
Heritability. See Genetics and heritability
High-threshold neurons, 43
Hispanics, 82
History, pain, 98, 233
Hot packs, 192
Hyaluronic acid, 353
Hydromorphone, 243
Hyperalgesia
    definition, 5
    measurement of, 125, 125f
    mechanical, 51
    NMDA antagonists preventing, 47
    opioid-induced, 245
    primary, 8, 62, 179
    secondary, 8, 56, 64
Hyperexcitability, central, 237, 241
Hypoalgesia, exercise-induced. See
    Exercise-induced hypoalgesia
Hypothalamus, 57

I

Ice treatments, 193, 194. See Thermo-
    therapy
Idiopathic pain, 241–242
IFT. See Interferential therapy (IFT)

Imagery, 268, 344
Immunosuppressive agents, 354
Impairment, definition, 13
Inflammation, 26–27
Insight-oriented psychotherapy, 261–262
Insular cortex, 54
Interdisciplinary pain management,
    217–228
  for chronic spinal pain, 332
  evidence for, 225–227
  history of, 217–218
  interdisciplinary care, definition, 219
  modality-specific clinics, 217
  multidisciplinary pain centers vs. pain
    clinics, 218–219
  pain practice providers, 219
  pain programs, outcome documenta-
    tion, 224–225
  patient assessment and treatment plan,
    222–224
  physical therapy in, 133, 135
  team unity in, 224
  treatment contracts with patients, 224
Interferential therapy (IFT)
  overview, 168, 168f
  analgesic mechanisms, 181
  clinical efficacy, 184–186
  for deep-tissue pain, 168
  inconsistent effects in experimental
    pain, 184–185
  parameters, 171
Interleukin-1 (IL-1) inhibitors, 353
Interleukins, in inflammation, 30
International Association for the Study of
    Pain (IASP), 3–4
International Classification of Diseases,
    10th revision (ICD-10), 14–15
International Classification of Functioning,
    Disability and Health (ICF), 14–15, 15t
Interview, structured, 99
Intracellular messengers, 51–52
Intracellular receptor proteins, 51
Ion channels, 27–28
Irritable bowel syndrome, 7
Ischemic pain, 144
Ischemic pressure, 284
Isometric contraction, 144, 145, 146f, 148,
    162

J

Joint Commission on Accreditation of
    Healthcare Organizations (JCAHO),
    96, 218, 220t–221t
Joint manipulation and mobilization
  in lateral epicondylalgia, 208, 212
  mechanisms, 207–208
  for osteoarthritis, 356
  peripheral, clinical evidence for, 212
  techniques, 205–206
Joint nociceptors, 23, 43
Joint pain, 32. See also Arthritis
Joint replacement, total, 353–354
Joint stabilization exercises, 205

K

Kaolin, 32
Ketamine, 50, 340
Kinesiophobia, 234, 236
Knee, osteoarthritis in. See Osteoarthritis
Knee Injury and Osteoarthritis Outcome
    Score, 352

L

Labor pain, 183
Laminae, 42–43
Laser therapy
  for fibromyalgia, 200, 294
  low-intensity, 198–200
    effectiveness, 199–200
    mechanisms, 199
  for temporomandibular disorders,
    312–313
  for osteoarthritis, 356
Leg pain, 317, 320
Leucine enkephalin, 60
Lidocaine, 250, 340
Loaded reach task, 126–127
Locus ceruleus/A7 cell groups, 57
Low back pain. See also Spinal pain
  acute, treatment-based classification,
    326–328, 327f
  catastrophizing and outcome, 85
  causes of, 318–319
  central hyperexcitability in, 241
  central sensitization in, case study,
    385–388

course of, 319–320, 320t
diagnosis and treatment guidelines,
    329–330
epidemiology, 319
exercise therapy, 149, 153, 154
fear-avoidance and, 85–86
laser therapy, 200
massage therapy, 210
multifactorial nature of, 318
operant conditioning, 263
operational definition, 317
physical therapy, 323–324, 325t
prognosis, 320
radiculopathy and, case study, 362–366
societal impact of, 320
TENS for, 178, 181
thermotherapy, 195
Low-threshold neurons, 43
Lumbar abnormalities, 318–319
Lumbar manipulation and mobilization,
    211–212

M

Manipulation and mobilization
    cervical, 211, 303
    effectiveness, 209t, 213
    of joints. *See* Joint manipulation and
        mobilization
    in lateral epicondylalgia, 208, 212
    lumbar, 211–212
    neural, 212
    soft-tissue, 210–211
    techniques, 205–206
Manual therapy
    clinical evidence for, 208–212, 209t
    for myofascial pain, 284
    techniques, 205–206
    for tension-type headache, 307
Massage
    clinical evidence for, 210–211
    deep-tissue, 206, 210
    for fibromyalgia, 294
    mechanisms, 206–207
    traditional, 205
McGill Pain Questionnaire (MPQ),
    104–106, 105f
    for adolescent pain assessment, 122
    for fibromyalgia, 289
    short form (SF-MPQ), 106f, 106–107

for temporomandibular disorders, 310
    TENS efficacy, 183
Mechanical hyperalgesia, 51
Mechanoreceptors, 19
Medial thalamic nucleus, 52, 53
Medical management of pain, 231–250.
    See also Pharmacotherapy
    clinical assessment in, 232–236
    fibromyalgia, 290t, 290–291
    migraine, 302–303
    myofascial pain, 283
    neuropathic pain, 340–341
    osteoarthritis, 353–354
    pain types and, 236–242
    patient referral, indications for, 236
    rheumatoid arthritis, 354
    spinal pain, 329–332
    temporomandibular disorders,
        310–311
    tension-type headache, 306
Meditation, 269–270
Memantine, 50, 340
Memory, 96–98, 97f
Menstrual cycle, 79
Meperidine, 243
Methadone, 243
Methionine, 60
Methotrexate, 354
Methylprednisolone, 331
Microglia, 47
Migraine
    biofeedback for, 269, 303
    diagnosis, 300, 301t
    epidemiology, 300
    ethnic/racial prevalence, 81
    medical management, 302–303
    pain assessment, 301–302
    pathobiology, 300–301
    physical therapy, 303
    psychological management, 303
Migraine Disability Assessment Scale
    (MIDAS), 301–302, 302t
Milnacipran, 249
Mindfulness meditation, 269–270
Mirror feedback therapy, 344
Morphine, 57, 179, 243
Motivational-affective dimension of pain,
    4, 53
Motor imagery, 344
Movement, fear of, 234, 236

MPQ. *See* McGill Pain Questionnaire (MPQ)
Multidimensional pain analysis, 103–104, 234–236, 235f, 289
Multidisciplinary care, definition, 219
Multidisciplinary pain centers, 218–219
Muscle nociceptors, 23, 43
Muscle pain, animal models, 32–33
Muscle relaxants, 311
Muscle soreness, delayed-onset, 149, 210
Muscle spindles, 19, 194
Musculoskeletal pain. *See also* Fibromyalgia; Myofascial pain
    massage for, 210
    prevalence, 279
    TENS efficacy for, 181
    thermotherapy, 195
    ultrasound therapy, 197–198
Myofascial pain, 279–287
    assessment, 283
    characteristics, 280t
    epidemiology and diagnosis, 279–282, 282t
    lower-extremity, case study, 376–379
    medical management, 283
    pain referral, 7, 280
    pathobiology, 282–283
    physical therapy, 284–287, 287t
    psychological management, 283–284
    temporomandibular disorders, 299, 309
    TENS efficacy for, 181, 285–286
    trigger points, 279–280, 281f, 282–283
    twitch response, 280, 282
    ultrasound therapy, 198
Myofascial therapy, 205
Myositis, animal models, 32

N

Naloxone, 137, 159
Naproxen, 311
Neck pain. *See also* Spinal pain
    acute, treatment-based classification, 328f, 328–329
    case study, 391–395
    causes of, 321
    clinical practice guidelines, 330–332
    epidemiology and course of, 321–322
    massage therapy, 210

operational definition, 318
    pharmacotherapy, 331–332
    physical therapy, 324
    prognosis, 322
    severity classification, 331t
    societal impact of, 320
    strength training vs. fitness training for, 153
Negative emotionality (neuroticism), 83–85
Neonatal Facial Coding System, 119t, 119–120
Neonatal Infant Pain Scale, 120, 120t
Neonatal pain assessment, 118–120
Nerve conduction, 194
Neural mobilization, 205, 206, 212
Neurogenic inflammation, 26
Neurogenic pain, 198
Neurokinin-1 (NK1) receptor, 50
Neurological impairment, 122–123
Neuromuscular electrical stimulation (NMES), 167, 285–286
Neuropathic pain
    animal models, 33, 175
    definition, 239–240
    epidemiology and diagnosis, 337, 338t
    grading system, 240
    medical management, 340–341
    pathology, 338–340
    pharmacotherapy, 250
    physical therapy, 342t, 342–345
    psychological management, 341
    referred pain vs., 237–239
    sympathetic nervous system in, 339–340
    TENS for, 175, 344
Neuropeptides, 26–28, 50
Neuroticism (negative emotionality), 83–85
Neurotransmitters, 59–61, 62
Neutral cells, 57
Newborns, pain assessment in, 118–120
NMES (neuromuscular electrical stimulation), 167, 285–286
N-methyl-D-aspartate (NMDA) receptor antagonists, 47, 340
Nocebo effect, 137–138
Nociception. *See* Pain processing
Nociceptive pain, 237–239
    pharmacotherapy, 247–248

Nociceptors
    definitions, 22
    dorsal horn modulation, 9
    joint and muscle, 23, 43
    polymodal, 23
    specificity theory and, 8
    types of, 19, 20t, 23–24
Non-aerobic exercise, 147–148
Nonsteroidal anti-inflammatory drugs
        (NSAIDs)
    enhancing effectiveness of TENS, 179
    ineffectiveness for fibromyalgia, 290t,
        291
    for nociceptive pain, 247
    for osteoarthritis, 353
    for pain relief, 242
    as prostaglandin inhibitors, 30
    for rheumatoid arthritis, 354
    for temporomandibular disorders, 311
    for tension-type headache, 306
Norepinephrine, 57, 61
Nucleus raphe magnus, 56
Nucleus reticularis gigantocellularis pars
        alpha, 56
Nucleus reticularis paragigantocellularis
        lateralis, 56
Numerical rating, 102, 103f

O

Observation of behavior, 100
OFF cells, 57, 58f
ON cells, 57, 58f
Operant conditioning, 262–264, 263t
Opioid receptors
    in descending inhibition of pain, 57
    distribution of, 243
    types of, 60
Opioids
    analgesic vs. affective effects, 244
    for chronic nonmalignant pain,
        243–244, 248
    contraindications, 244
    exercise and cross-tolerance to,
        158–159
    hyperalgesia caused by, 245
    ineffectiveness for fibromyalgia, 290t,
        291
    for pain management, 243–245, 250
    tolerance and TENS, 179–180, 180f

    tolerance vs. dependence, 244–245
    weak vs. strong, 243
Opioids, endogenous
    in descending modulation of pain,
        59–60
    in exercise-induced hypoalgesia,
        156–159, 161
    in inflammation, 27
    physical therapy activation of, 135
    sex differences in analgesia, 157, 159f
    in TENS analgesia, 172, 175–176, 177
OPRM1 gene, 87, 88
Osteoarthritis
    cognitive-behavioral therapy, 354–355
    diagnostic criteria, 349–350, 350t
    epidemiology, 349
    exercise therapy, 152–153, 154,
        355–356
    ice packs, 195
    joint replacement, 353–354
    knee
        case study, 389–391
        IFT efficacy, 185
        joint mobilization, 208
        laser therapy, 199
        TENS efficacy, 181
    medical management, 353–354
    pain assessment, 352–353
    pathology, 352
    peripheral joint mobilization/manipu-
        lation, 212
    physical therapy, 355–356, 356t
    referred pain in, 7
    treatment compliance, 155
    ultrasound therapy, 198
Oswestry Disability Questionnaire, 115,
        116
Oswestry Disability Scale, 123
Output type, TENS therapy, 170
Oxycodone, 243
Oxytocin, 206

P

PAG. See Periaqueductal gray (PAG)
Pain. See also Pain terms below
    acute. See Acute pain
    age factors in, 78t, 89
    cancer. See Cancer pain
    chronic. See Chronic pain

conceptualization of, 231
cutaneous, 7–8, 31
deep-tissue, 7–8, 168
definitions and terminology, 4–5, 6t, 74
dimensions of, 4
drug therapy. *See* Pharmacotherapy
dysfunctional, 237, 241, 248–249
epidemiology, 15–16
exercise and. *See* Exercise-induced
    hypoalgesia
as fifth vital sign, 3, 95
idiopathic, 241–242
ischemic, 144
in labor, 183
medical management. *See* Medical
    management of pain
models of, 11–15
multidimensionality of, 10, 231–232
musculoskeletal. *See* Musculoskeletal
    pain
myofascial. *See* Myofascial pain
neuropathic. *See* Neuropathic pain
nociceptive, 237–230
pediatric. *See* Pediatric pain
postoperative. *See* Postoperative pain
psychogenic, 242
referred. *See* Referred pain
sensory-discriminative aspect, 4, 52,
    81–82
spinal. *See* Low back pain; Neck pain;
    Spinal pain
theories of, 8–10
types of, 62, 63t, 236–242
of unknown origin, 241–242, 248–249
variability. *See* Variability of pain
visceral, 7, 33
widespread, chronic, 32–33. *See also*
    Fibromyalgia
Pain adjective descriptors, 99
Pain assessment, 95–128. *See also* Pain
    measurement
in adults, 102–119
in arthritis, 352–353
in children and adolescents, 121–122
clinical assessment, 232–236
definition, 96
in fibromyalgia, 289–290
goals, 95–96
history of pain, 98, 233
memory and, 96–98, 97f

in migraine, 301–302
multidimensional pain analysis,
    103–104, 234–236, 235f
in myofascial pain, 283
in neurological or cognitive impair-
    ment, 122–123
in newborns, 118–120
physical and functional examination,
    123–127, 233–234
questionnaires, 104–118
recommendations, 96
techniques, 98–101
in temporomandibular disorders, 310
in tension-type headache, 306
Pain behaviors
in biopsychosocial model of pain, 12
in pain assessment, 100–101
reinforcement of, 262–263, 263t
Pain Catastrophizing Scale, 84
Pain centers, multidisciplinary, 218–219
Pain clinics, multidisciplinary, 219
Pain measurement
body diagrams, 103, 103f, 233
in children, self-report techniques,
    99–100
definition, 96
in exercise-induced hypoalgesia, 145
functional measures, 126–127
multidimensional measures, 103–104,
    234–236, 235f
pain rating scales, 102, 103f
physiological parameters, 101
techniques, 98–101
Pain practice providers, 219
Pain processing
ascending pathways, 52–54
in biopsychosocial model, 11
central mechanisms, 41–64, 42f
definitions, 22t
descending modulation, 54–61
peripheral pathways, 19–34
spinal cord and, 42–52
Pain rating scales, 102, 103f
Pain receptors. *See* Nociceptors
Pain Self-Efficacy Questionnaire, 107, 109f,
    110
Parabrachial region, 57
Paracetamol. *See* Acetaminophen
Pathology, definition, 13
Patient compliance, 155–156, 224

Patient education
 in cognitive-behavioral therapy, 266
 for fibromyalgia, 291
 for rheumatoid arthritis, 356–357
Patient referral to pain specialist, 236
Pattern theory, 8
Pediatric pain
 assessment in children and adolescents, 121–122
 assessment in newborns, 118–120
 behavioral assessment, 101
 facial expression scales, 99–100
Pediatric Pain Questionnaire, 122
Percutaneous electrical nerve stimulation
 (PENS), 167, 181
Periaqueductal gray (PAG)
 in descending modulation of pain, 54,
  55, 55f, 56, 58f
 in TENS analgesia, 174
Peripheral sensitization, 24–26, 25f
 mediators of, 28, 29f, 30
 primary hyperalgesia and, 62
Personality traits, 83–84
Pethidine, 243
Petrissage, 205
Phantom limb pain, 8, 10, 344
Pharmacotherapy, 242–250
 acetaminophen, 242
 anticonvulsants, 246
 COX inhibitors, 242
 for dysfunctional pain, 247–248
 for fibromyalgia, 290t, 290–291
 for neuropathic pain, 250, 340–341
 for nociceptive pain, 247–248
 NSAIDs, 242
 opioids, 243–245
 for osteoarthritis, 353
 for pain of unknown origin, 247–248
 practical aspects of, 246–247
 for rheumatoid arthritis, 354
 serotonin-norepinephrine reuptake
  inhibitors, 245–246
Physical examination, 123–127, 233–234
Physical therapy
 alliances with other pain care providers, 227–228
 for back and neck pain, 323–324, 325t
 disablement model of pain and, 13f,
  13–14
 ethics in, 140

evidence-based practice, 138–140
 for fibromyalgia, 291, 294
 guidelines, 134, 134f
 interdisciplinary pain management,
  133, 135
 mechanisms of action, 135–138, 136f
 for migraine, 303
 for myofascial pain, 284–287, 287t
 for neuropathic pain and CRPS, 342t,
  342–345
 for osteoarthritis, 355–356, 356t
 pain evaluation, 137
 pain models and practice of, 16–17
 patient referral, indications for, 236
 placebo effect, 137
 practice of, 133–141
 principles of, 133–135
 for rheumatoid arthritis, 356–358, 357t
 for temporomandibular disorders,
  308t, 311, 312–313
 for tension-type headache, 306–308,
  308t
 therapeutic goals, 134
Physiological parameters, in pain measurement, 101
PKA (protein kinase A), 51
PKC (protein kinase C), 51–52
Placebo effect, 137
Polymodal nociceptors, 23
Pontine tegmentum
 dorsolateral, 57
 lateral, 54, 55, 55f
Pool therapy, 294
Positive and Negative Affect Schedule, 84
Postherpetic neuralgia, 198, 340
Postoperative pain
 animal models, 33–34
 ethnic/racial prevalence of, 81
 TENS for, 178, 183
Prefrontal cortex, 57
Pregabalin, 246, 249, 291
Pressure pain threshold, 183
Presynaptic inhibition, 10
Pretectal nucleus, anterior, 57
Proglumide, 137
Propranolol, 303
Prostaglandins, 30
Protein kinase A (PKA), 51
Protein kinase C (PKC), 51–52
Psychoanalytic treatment, 261

Psychodynamic perspective, 261–262
Psychodynamic therapy, 261
Psychogenic pain, 242
Psychological factors
    chronic pain, 234
    clinical pain, 84–85
    definitions, 83
    exercise-induced hypoalgesia, 160
    experimental pain, 85–86, 86f
    pain variability, 83–86
    traits vs. states, 83
Psychological interventions, 257–273.
        See also Biofeedback; Cognitive-
        behavioral therapy (CBT)
    for arthritis, 354–355
    characteristics, 259t
    for chronic pain, 257–258, 258t
    efficacy of, 271–272
    guided imagery, 268
    hypnosis, 270–271
    meditation, 269–270
    for myofascial pain, 283–284
    for neuropathic pain, 341–342
    objectives, 260
    operant conditioning, 262–264, 263t
    psychodynamic, 261–262
    psychological perspectives affecting,
        260t
    psychosocial treatments vs., 259–261
    relaxation, 267–268
Pulse amplitude and duration, in TENS,
    170
Pulsed electromagnetic energy, 193

Q

Quality-of-life surveys, 110–111, 113t–
    115t, 116, 117t–119t
Questionnaires, self-report, 99

R

Race and ethnicity, 81–83
Radiculopathy
    in back pain, 362–366
    cervical, 332
    MRI scan, 330
Randomized controlled trials, 139
Range of motion (ROM), 124
Receptive fields, 43–44, 44f

Red nucleus, 57
Referral of patients, 236
Referred pain
    convergence-projection theory, 64
    cutaneous vs. deep-tissue pain, 7–8
    definition, 5, 237
    distribution, 238f, 238–239, 239f
    myofascial, 7, 280
    neuropathic pain vs., 237–239
    primary afferent convergence, 43
    sex differences, 78–79
Reflex sympathetic dystrophy (CRPS-I),
    337
Reinforcement, 262–263, 263t
Relaxation, 267–268
    for fibromyalgia, 291
    for migraine, 303
    for myofascial pain, 284
    for tension-type headache, 306
Repetitive strain injury, animal model, 32
Resistance training. See Strength training
Reticulospinal tract, 57
Rheumatoid and Arthritis Outcome Score,
    353
Rheumatoid arthritis
    anti-TNF therapy, 30
    cognitive-behavioral therapy, 354–355
    corticosteroids for TMD in, 311
    diagnostic criteria, 351, 351t
    epidemiology, 349
    laser therapy, 199–200
    medical management, 354
    pain assessment, 352–353
    pathology, 352
    physical therapy, 356–358, 357t
    TENS efficacy, 181
    thermotherapy, 195
    ultrasound therapy, 198
Roland-Morris Disability Scale, 123
ROM (range of motion), 124
Rostral ventromedial medulla (RVM)
    in descending modulation of pain, 54,
        55, 55f, 56, 58f
    in TENS analgesia, 174
Rubrospinal tract, 57

S

Sciatic nerve ligation, 33
Second-messenger pathways, 51

Selective serotonin reuptake inhibitors (SSRIs)
for fibromyalgia, 290t, 291
lacking analgesic effects, 246
for neuropathic pain, 340
for pain inhibition, 61
prolonging effects of low-frequency TENS, 179
Self-care, for temporomandibular disorders, 311–312
Self-efficacy questionnaires, 107, 109f, 110, 111t
Self-mobilization exercises, 205
Self-rating scales, 99
Self-report measures, 99–100
Sensation, 8
Sensitization, 24. See also Peripheral sensitization
Sensory receptors and pathways, 19–24
activation, 22
cutaneous, 19
in nociception, definitions, 22t
peripheral afferent classification, 20t
Sensory re-education, 344–345
Sensory-discriminative dimension of pain, 4, 52, 81–82
Serotonin
in descending inhibition of pain, 60–61
in migraine, 301, 303
in nociception, 28, 30
Serotonin-norepinephrine reuptake inhibitors (SNRIs), 245–246
for fibromyalgia, 249, 290t, 291
for neuropathic pain, 250
for pain inhibition, 61
Sex differences
age and pain prevalence, 78t
clinical pain, 76
in exercise-induced hypoalgesia, 148, 157, 159f
experimental pain, 78–79
gender roles and pain perception, 79–80
pain prevalence, 77t
pain variability, 76–79
Short Form 36 Quality of Life Questionnaire (SF-36), 110–111, 113t–115t, 178
Shortwave diathermy, 192–193, 195–196
Shoulder pain
case study, 373–376

laser therapy for, 200
poststroke, TENS efficacy for, 181
Sickness Impact Profile, 123–124, 307
Silent nociceptors, 23–24
Skills acquisition and consolidation, 266
SNL (spinal nerve ligation), 33
SNRIs. See Serotonin-norepinephrine reuptake inhibitors (SNRIs)
Social support, 160
Sodium channels, 28
Soft-tissue mobilization, 205
Somatosensory cortex, 54, 57, 58–59
Spared nerve injury, 33
Specificity theory of pain, 8
Spinal cord, 42–52
ascending pathways, 52–54
laminae, 42–43
neurotransmitters, 47–52, 48f
nociceptive input to, 43
stimulation for neuropathic pain and CRPS, 341
Spinal interneurons, 42–43
Spinal manipulation
clinical evidence for, 211–212
mechanisms, 207
for migraine, 303
patient expectation and effectiveness, 138
for tension-type headache, 307
Spinal nerve ligation (SNL), 33
Spinal pain, 317–332. See also Low back pain; Neck pain
acute, treatment-based classification, 325–326, 326f
chronic, interdisciplinary management, 332
general presentation, 318–322
medical management, 329–332
physical therapy, 322–324, 325t
terminology, 317–318
Spinomesencephalic tract, 53
Spinoreticular tract, 53
Spinothalamic tract, 52–53
Splints, for temporomandibular disorders, 311
SSRIs. See Selective serotonin reuptake inhibitors (SSRIs)
Steroids. See Corticosteroids
Strength assessment, 124

Strength training
    benefits of, 235–236
    exercise-induced hypoalgesia and,
        147–148
    for fibromyalgia, 294
    fitness training vs., for neck pain, 153
    opioid activation and, 158
    for osteoarthritis, 355–356
Stress management, 306
Stress-induced analgesia, 161
Stretching exercises, 286–287
Structured interview, 99
Substance P, 26, 50, 176
Substantia gelatinosa neurons, 9
Suffering, 12
Sumatriptan, 303
Supraspinal pathways, 137
Sweep frequency, 171
Sympathectomy, 341
Sympathetic nervous system, 339–340
Synovitis, inflammatory, 351
Systemic lupus erythematosus, 349

T

T cells, 9
Temporal summation, 62, 64
    gender roles and, 80
    sex differences in, 78
    spinal manipulation and decrease in,
        207
Temporomandibular disorders (TMD)
    categories, 299, 309
    central hyperexcitability in, 241
    COMT polymorphisms in, 310
    epidemiology and diagnosis, 308–309
    ethnic/racial prevalence, 81
    laser therapy, 200
    medical management, 310–311
    pain areas, 313f
    pain assessment, 310
    pathobiology, 309–310
    physical therapy, 308t, 311, 312–313
    psychological management and self-
        care, 311–312
    tension-type headaches with, 299
Tender points, 288, 289f
TENS. See Transcutaneous electrical nerve
    stimulation (TENS)

Tension-type headache
    biofeedback for, 269, 306
    diagnosis, 304–305, 305t
    epidemiology, 304
    manual therapy, 210
    medical management, 306
    pain assessment, 306
    pathobiology, 305
    psychological management, 306
    in temporomandibular disorders, 299
Thalamic nucleus, medial, 52, 53
Thalamus, 54, 57
Thermotherapy
    cryotherapy, 193, 194
    effectiveness, 195–196
    evidence base for, 201t
    heat therapy, 192–193, 194–195
    for osteoarthritis, 355
    pain relief mechanisms, 194–195
    processes for, 191–192
    for rheumatoid arthritis, 357–358
    for temporomandibular disorders, 312
Timed up and go test, 126
TMD. See Temporomandibular disorders
    (TMD)
TNF-α (tumor necrosis factor-α), 30
Topical agents, 250, 340, 354
Total joint replacement, 353–354
Tramadol, 243, 249, 250, 353
Transcendental meditation, 269–270
Transcription factors, 51
Transcutaneous electrical nerve stimula-
        tion (TENS), 167–186
    afferent fiber activation, 173
    analgesia theories and, 171–173
    in animal models, 174–175
    clinical applications, 178–179
    clinical efficacy, 181–184, 182t
    devices for, 168f
    electrode placement and analgesic
        response, 173–174
    gate control theory and, 10
    high-frequency, 175–177
    history of, 167–168
    low-frequency, 177–178
    mechanisms of action, 136, 172t,
        172–173
    medications and outcome, 178–179
    modes of, 171
    for myofascial pain, 285–286

neuronal pathways activated by, 174
for neuropathic pain, 344
opioid mediation of, 175–176, 177
opioid tolerance and, 179–180, 180f
for osteoarthritis, 355, 356
parameters of, 170–171
for rheumatoid arthritis, 357
targeting supraspinal control sites, 10
for temporomandibular disorders, 312
for tension-type headache, 307
terminology, 167, 170
Transmission cells, 9
Trapezius myalgia, 241
Treatment compliance, 155–156, 224
Treatment outcomes
chronic pain programs, 226
documentation of, 224–225
interdisciplinary pain programs, 225–226
pain rehabilitation programs, 225
physical therapy in interdisciplinary programs, 226–227
psychological predictors for, 234
Tricyclic antidepressants, 246
for fibromyalgia, 249, 290, 290t, 291
for migraine, 303
for neuropathic pain, 250, 340
for pain inhibition, 61
for tension-type headache, 306
Trigger points
injections, 283
manual therapy, 205, 284
in myofascial pain, 279–280, 281f, 282–283
Triptans, 301, 303
TRPV1 gene, 87, 88
Tumor necrosis factor-α (TNF-α), 30
Twins, pain variability in, 86–87
Twitch response, 280, 282

U

Ultrasound therapy, 196–198
effectiveness of, 197–198
ineffectiveness for osteoarthritis, 356
for myofascial pain, 284–285
for rheumatoid arthritis, 357

V

Vanilloid receptor-1 (TRPV1), 28, 88
Variability of pain, 73–89
age factors, 89
complexity in, 89
ethnicity and race, 81–83
factors influencing, 74–75, 75f
gender roles and, 79–80
genetics and heritability, 86–88
intensity ratings, 74f
overview, 73–75
psychological factors, 83–86
sex differences, 76–79
Ventroposterior lateral nucleus (VPL), 52–53
Verbal rating scales, 102, 103f
Vertebral fractures, 186
Visceral nociceptors, 23
Visceral pain, 7, 33
Visual analogue scales (VAS), 99, 102, 103f, 122, 183

W

Walking tests, 126
Western Ontario and McMaster Universities Osteoarthritis Index (WOMAC), 115, 352
Whiplash injuries
central hyperexcitability in, 241
methylprednisolone for, 331
referred pain in, 238, 239f
Whirlpool baths, 191
Wide-dynamic-range (WDR) neurons, 43, 53
Widespread pain, chronic, 32–33. See also Fibromyalgia
Wind-up, 62
Wong-Baker Faces Pain Scale, 121, 121f
World Health Organization Quality of Life Assessment (WHOQOL), 111, 115, 116t–118t
Wound healing, TENS for, 181
Wrist pain, case study, 366–369

ADD THESE BOOKS TO YOUR COLLECTION!

FROM IASP PRESS®

Functional Pain Syndromes: Presentation and Pathophysiology

Editors: Emeran A. Mayer, M. Catherine Bushnell
This book explores the connection of functional pain syndromes with anxiety, depression, chronic fatigue syndrome, and post-traumatic stress disorder. The authors address possible common pathophysiologies and review a range of treatment options, from antidepressants to cognitive-behavioral therapy.
2009 ■ Softbound ■ 578 pages

Fundamentals of Musculoskeletal Pain

Editors: Thomas Graven-Nielsen, Lars Arendt-Nielsen, Siegfried Mense
Musculoskeletal pain is a major medical and economic problem that encompasses a broad range of conditions, including fibromyalgia, work-related myalgia, low back pain, and arthritis. This book integrates research findings from the field of musculoskeletal pain into a comprehensive publication that explores translational aspects relevant to clinical pain.
2008 ■ Hardcover ■ 496 pages

Immune and Glial Regulation of Pain

Editors: Joyce A. DeLeo, Linda S. Sorkin, Linda R. Watkins
This authoritative volume describes immune and glial factors within the peripheral and central nervous systems that relate to chronic pain states.
2007 ■ Hardcover with CD-ROM ■ 443 pages

Sleep and Pain

Editors: Gilles Lavigne, Barry Sessle, Manon Choinière, Peter Soja
This book focuses on the interaction between sleep disorders and chronic pain syndromes, bridging the information gap between the sleep and pain communities.
2007 ■ Hardcover ■ 474 pages

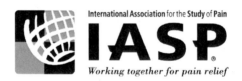

International Association for the Study of Pain

IASP®

Working together for pain relief

Visit the IASP Bookstore: www.iasp-pain.org/Bookstore
Email: books@iasp-pain.org   Tel: +1.206.283.0311   Fax: +1.206.283.9403